THE
WILD DIET

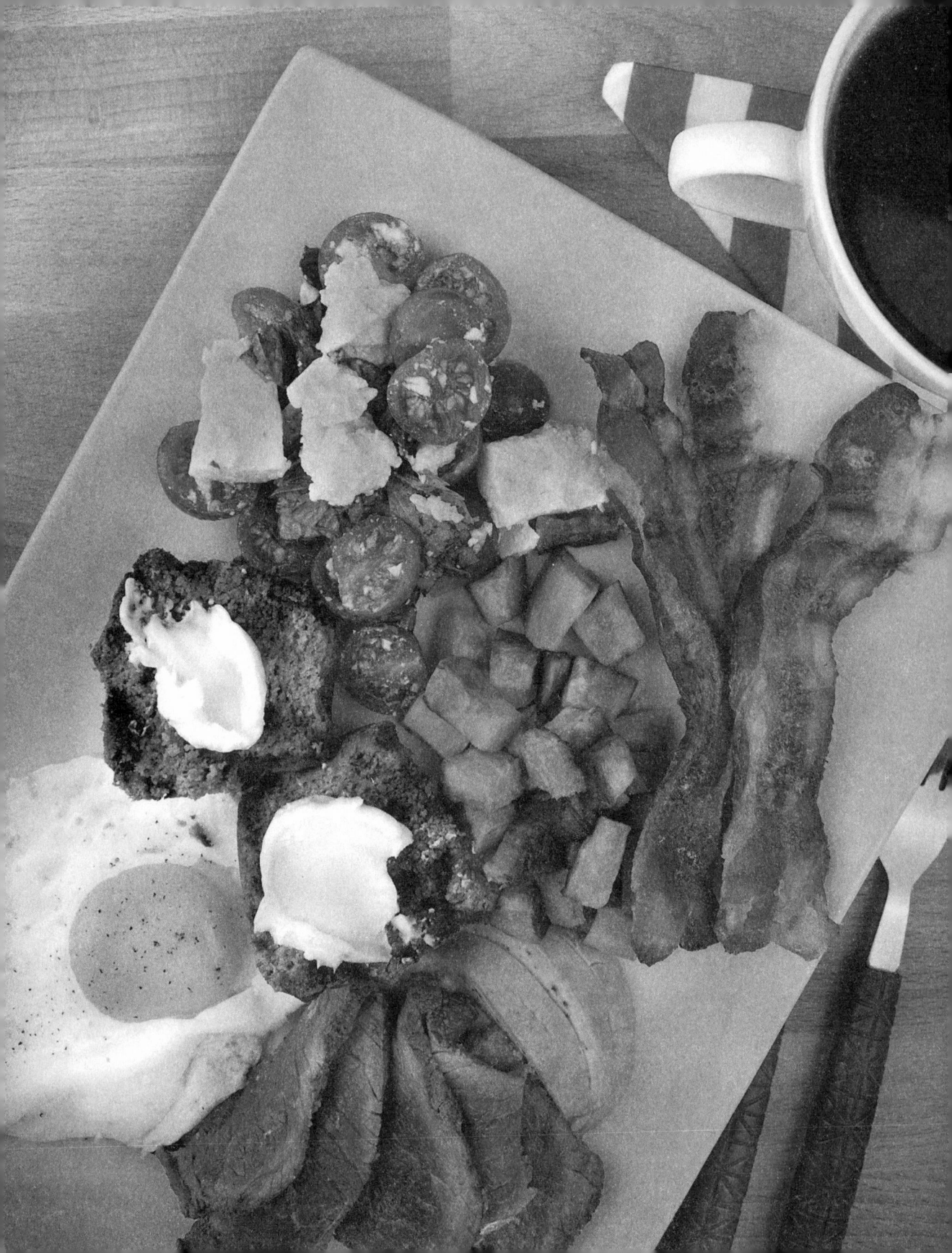

THE
WILD DIET

Get Back to Your Roots, Burn Fat, and Drop Up to 20 Pounds in 40 Days

ABEL JAMES

AVERY · A MEMBER OF PENGUIN GROUP (USA) · NEW YORK

AVERY

Avery, an imprint of
Penguin Random House LLC
375 Hudson Street
New York, New York 10014

Photographs © 2015 by Melinda Bryce

Excerpt on pages 347–349: Originally published in the December 1965 *Ladies' Home Journal* ® magazine

Library of Congress Cataloging-in-Publication Data

James, Abel.
The wild diet : get back to your roots, burn fat, and drop up to 20 pounds in 40 days/Abel James.
p.   cm.
ISBN 978-1-58333-573-4
1. High-protein diet—Recipes.   2. Reducing diets—Recipes.
3. Prehistoric peoples—Nutrition.   4. Cooking (Wild foods).   I. Title
RM237.65.J36   2015   2014047008
641.5'638—dc23

Printed in the United States of America
1   3   5   7   9   10   8   6   4   2

BOOK DESIGN BY MEIGHAN CAVANAUGH

Most Avery books are available at special quantity discounts for bulk purchase for sales promotions, premiums, fundraising, and educational needs. Special books or book excerpts also can be created to fit specific needs. For details, write SpecialMarkets@penguinrandomhouse.com.

DEDICATION AND A TOAST

———————

This book is dedicated to my grandparents
Marion and Horace Bascom.

From Our Family to Yours: Nan's Favorite Toast

"Here's to thee and thy folks

from me and my folks.

Sure there never was folks

since folks was folks,

ever loved any folks

half as much as me and my folks

love thee and thy folks!"

Wild |wīld| *adjective (of an animal or plant)*
Living or growing in the natural environment; not domesticated or cultivated. Passionate, vehement, unrestrained. Untamed.

"Wild with excitement."

Di·et |dī-it| *noun*
The kinds of food that a person, animal, or community habitually eats.

"The native human diet."

AUTHOR'S NOTE

Earlier this year, my wife, Alyson, and I dined at a farm-to-table restaurant in Florida with twenty leaders in the health movement, a motley crew of bestselling authors, nutritionists, Olympians, cooks, and physicians. After a long week, we were ready for a feast.

Our waiter scribbled furiously as Alyson, my cute-as-a-button, 105-pound wife, and I ordered:

- Bacon deviled eggs
- Two roasted marrow bones with local herbs and spices
- Two hearty farm-fresh salads with aged meat, nuts, and avocado
- Charcuterie board with a trio of duck, lamb, and pork pâtés; raw artisanal cheese; and a side of homemade sauerkraut
- Sautéed sweetbreads
- Wild sea bass with mushroom butter sauce
- Grass-fed sirloin steak with heirloom vegetables (medium-rare, of course)

As others watched in awe, we polished off the lot, including more than our fair share of wine and champagne. One of the health experts said with a gasp, "How on earth do you two eat so much and stay so lean?"

This book is the answer to that question.

I hope you enjoy it.

In health and happiness,
Abel James Bascom
August 23, 2014

CONTENTS

AUTHOR'S NOTE   *ix*

INTRODUCTION: BAND GONE WILD   *1*

PART I

How "Healthy" Food Made Us Fat and Sick   *9*

PART II

The Wild Body   *41*

PART III

Wild Movement   *73*

PART IV

The Wild Diet   *89*

PART V

Wild Cooking, Meals, and Recipes *129*

PART VI

The Wild Diet Challenge *283*

PART VII

The Wild Diet Survival Guide *297*

PARTING WORDS *347*

NOTES *353*

INDEX *359*

INTRODUCTION:
BAND GONE WILD

As we hop aboard Tim McGraw's tour bus idling outside a Quality Inn in Austin, Texas, I suddenly realize that being healthy is cool again.

Instead of smoking ashtrays, passed-out groupies, and stale beer, the smell of strong coffee wafts through the country superstar's Zen-like tour bus. A veritable cornucopia of fresh produce, organic seaweed snacks, and an imposing 5-pound sack of Brazil nuts fill the mini-kitchen. Despite filming the *Today* show in New York City twenty-four hours earlier, these road warriors are bright-eyed and bushy-tailed. Denny, enjoying an unprecedented twenty-year reign as Tim's guitarist and musical director, introduces us to the rest of the band.

Fresh off his feature on the cover of *Men's Health* after losing 40 pounds, forty-seven-year-old Tim McGraw is a specimen of health. He credits his pumped-up biceps and six-pack abs to his band's new routine of clean eating and intense outdoor workouts on the road. His tour bus even pulls a trailer dedicated to unconventional exercise gear—hauling heavy chains, sledgehammers, and sandbags across the country.

"Whoa, the Fat-Burning Man. . . . It's so surreal you're here!" Deano, the fiddle player, muses, somehow expressing precisely how I feel at that moment. I'm not sure exactly when it happened, but more people seem to know me as "Fat-Burning Man," the tongue-in-cheek title of my hit health show, than as the road-weary musician I've been for most of my life. I'd taken time away from music to focus on inspiring others to live better by eating real food and breaking a good sweat. As far as I was concerned, I was just a regular guy babbling into a microphone on my computer and doing my best to make my show valuable to whoever happened to be tuning in. It wasn't until I received my favorite thank-you note ever from a musician named Denny that I realized people were actually *listening*. Better yet, these newfound health nuts were actually getting results that blew my mind.

A loyal listener of *Fat-Burning Man*, Denny has been following the Wild Diet for more than a year. Enjoying hearty meals that include plenty of butter, bacon, and eggs, he's dropped 46 pounds. Impressed by Denny's transformation, several bandmates came along for the ride.

"Billy, our keyboard player, only decided to try the Wild Diet because he's allowed to eat coffee cake." Denny grins. "It really isn't that complicated—you just listen to your body and eat when you're hungry. It's great. I'm full of energy and feel fifteen years younger."

"My kids love eating this way," adds Deano. "They're totally into organ meats and headcheese. Their friends think eating brains is cool."

After Deano convinces us to taste his latest culinary fascination, emu oil (it's not bad, actually), we take Denny back to our place to play a few tunes. On the way, we grab two cups of fresh-roasted "fatty coffee" (see page 249) with butterfat and pure cocoa, our first "meal" of the day. To fuel an epic jam session, we polish off a few pints of green smoothie, sample asparagus and bacon quiche, and indulge in homemade blueberry muffins, pumpkin scones, and Alyson's newest cheesecake recipe (Peanut Butter Chocolate "Cheesecake" with Hazelnut Crust—try it yourself on page 250) with our afternoon tea. A few hours later, our luxurious dinner includes bacon-wrapped sea scallops, wild Atlantic salmon, creamed spinach with toasted prosciutto, and a wee bit of wine. This ain't no ordinary diet.

Sound incredible? Well, the truth is that I haven't always had the body of an underwear model while feasting like a rock star. Before people knew me as my fat-burning alter ego whose abs are plastered all over the Internet, I was the chubby kid with chipmunk cheeks.

I've always loved food. As a toddler in the eighties, I discovered that the spiral cord on our kitchen phone didn't quite reach the candy cupboard. So every time the phone rang, I sprinted to the candy and drooled like Pavlov's dog. As soon as Mom picked up the phone, now safely out of reach, I'd stuff my face with as much chocolate, candy, and cookies as humanly possible.

One night, still dressed in my suspenders and bow tie after playing clarinet at the local diner for pocket money, my dad took me aside for an important talk.

"Abel, your body is about to go through some changes," he explained with a gentle smile. "With our genes, you can grow up to be overweight . . . or strong and athletic. It all depends on how you eat and exercise in the next few years as you grow into a teenager."

An athletic strapping stonemason for most of his life, Dad had packed on nearly 30 pounds after he was forced into a desk job when the economy tanked. I listened closely and took heed. I didn't want to be overweight, and for the first time in my life I realized I had a choice. And then I was off.

I learned in one of Dad's magazines that "fat makes you fat and clogs your arteries." So I declared that I would switch to fat-free milk, shun red meat, and I even started to carry around extra napkins to sponge the grease off pizza in order to avoid excess cholesterol. I was eight years old.

I took up every sport I could. A little too excited after watching *Rocky* for the first time, I choked down a full glass of raw eggs before my morning workout and chased chickens around the backyard. I cranked the brittle gears of my yard-sale Huffy to the summit of the legendary Piper Hill and trained like a Ninja Turtle to get my purple belt in karate. By seventh grade, my baby fat and chipmunk cheeks grew into a chiseled frame with a strong jaw to match. The girls even started calling me "Mr. Buff," my first stupid nickname.

I'd done it—the chubby kid who played clarinet at Christmas parties had transformed into a handsome, athletic teen. But getting fat doesn't happen all at once. Sometimes it sneaks up on you.

After speeding through Dartmouth College, studying brain science, music, and technology, it was time to pay off a few nasty student loans and chase the American Dream. Turning down offers from Wall Street and the CIA, I took a job as a strategy consultant for Fortune 500s in Washington, D.C., moonlighting as a computer programmer. I quickly learned that spending nearly all of my waking hours under fluorescent lights takes its toll. But there was work to be done, loans to be paid, and no time for hikes in the woods.

My fancy new office had a "Healthy Snacks" program to help us get through the long hours consulting with the bigwigs. I was pleased to find that many of the snacks lined up perfectly with the fat-free, low-calorie diet praised by the media and health magazines. I nibbled on fat-free whole-grain crackers, nonfat yogurt, and zero-calorie Jell-O, and I sipped cholesterol-free soy milk; cloudy, experimental diet soda; and other oddities provided by our Fortune 500 clients in the food and beverage industry.

When I sat down with my new physician for my first checkup as an adult, he avoided eye contact at first, shuffling papers on his desk. His brow suddenly furrowed as he looked up at me with a wide-eyed grin.

"You have *great* insurance!" he blurted.

From that point on, I peed in a cup and had my blood drawn every time I set foot in the doctor's office, which was often. My results didn't look good. I had high blood pressure, high cholesterol, elevated triglycerides, thyroid problems, insomnia, and many other disorders and diseases of civilization that we're somehow conditioned to "expect" as our youth evades us.

"You have the body of a middle-aged man," the doctor admitted grimly. "With your blood pressure and family history, you might be looking at heart disease, thyroid disorder, and even diabetes if you don't cut out dietary fat and do more cardio starting right now."

Doc put me on a new painkiller for a running injury, a prescription-strength antiperspirant, several sleep meds, and even an antidepressant that he promised would "help me sleep."

Gritting my teeth, I followed the doc's advice. I popped the pills, counted every last calorie, grew accustomed to constant hunger, nibbled on low-fat food that tasted like cardboard, and jogged five times a week.

I proudly became a vegetarian, swapped real butter for zero-cholesterol vegetable oil spread, and replaced farm-fresh eggs with 100% whole wheat bagels with nonfat cream cheese and zero-calorie jam from the supermarket. Without fresh veggies from our family's garden, I stocked up on bananas, 100% orange juice (with pulp, obviously), and reduced-sodium canned vegetable juice from the Safeway down the street.

But every time I went to see my doctor, I was fatter and sicker than ever . . . and people started to notice. Subtlety was never my boss's strong suit. One day, he just laid it right out there.

"Whoa, Abel, you've put on a few pounds! What *happened* to you? Too many sweets, eh?" Nope—I was dieting harder than ever.

I took a good, hard look in the mirror and I didn't like what I saw.

Instead of a strong, vital twenty-four-year-old, I had the flab of an unhealthy man twice my age. The impossibly low-fat diet recommended by doctors, diet books, magazines, and the media didn't appear to be working. Fed up, I diverted my energy to healing myself. I scoured medical textbooks, underground bodybuilding manuals, and the nooks and crannies of the Internet to find the perfect protocol to drop my excess fat and regain my vitality.

I quickly discovered that everything I thought I knew about diet was wrong.

When I started my new "diet," I did the opposite of what most well-meaning nutritionists might tell you. I chowed down on the most delicious and rich foods of my life—real butter, scrambled eggs, fresh veggies, rich meats, coconut, aged cheese, steak, and chocolate. I flushed my pharmaceuticals and called my mom, an author and herbalist, once a week to reincorporate adaptogenic herbs, teas, and tonics back into my daily habits.

HERE'S WHAT HAPPENED . . .

The mounting health problems that I'd been told were just part of getting older—high blood pressure, heartburn, low energy, thyroid issues, insomnia, dry skin, acne, kidney stones, the spare tire, and much more—quickly improved. My sugar cravings, nagging hunger, and mood swings gently faded with each passing week. I began to feel a glowing energy and clarity that reminded me of what it was like to be a young buck in his prime. My double chin quickly receded, and my belly fat followed close behind.

When I stepped on the scale, I was shocked. I had lost 20 pounds of flab in forty days. This fat loss revealed a muscular body and washboard abs that could be slapped right on the cover of a fitness magazine. More important, I had more energy and gusto than I'd felt in my entire life.

But as much as I enjoyed taking my new abs for a spin, I was angry. Why had I been trying so hard to stay on an expensive diet that was making me fat and sick for all those years? Everybody deserves to feel this way.

So I wrote a fat-loss manual and printed twenty copies at Kinko's to send to friends and family. After ten weeks, my dad, cousins, friends, coworkers, and bandmates each dropped around 20 pounds. Even my dental hygienist eventually lost more than 60 pounds by going Wild, just through what I could mumble during my cleanings every six months.

REAL FOOD, REAL RESULTS

After transforming my own body, I launched my health show, *Fat-Burning Man*, to educate and inspire others to be happy and healthy by optimizing their bodies with real food, a good sweat, and cutting-edge science and technology. I had a goal to change a million lives with real food and Wild movement, and word quickly spread. Within the first year, we hit that goal, and even beat out Jillian Michaels, head trainer on *The Biggest Loser*, for Apple's number-one-rated podcast in health. Eventually, the series hit number one in more than eight countries around the world and won three awards in independent media, including Best Health and Fitness Podcast at the Podcast Awards.

If you like this book, you'll enjoy the *Fat-Burning Man* show. I cover almost every subject in this book—from digestion to dead lifts—with detailed, topical interviews with top experts. You can listen in and watch the entire series for free at FatBurning Man.com.

In *The Wild Diet*, you'll find that we are not meant to starve ourselves or count calories. We're wired to eat and live well without getting fat. That's what we've been doing effortlessly for thousands of years, in fact, before we started following the wrong advice.

If you think that you're stuck with the genes you inherited and there's nothing you can do about it, read closely. *The Wild Diet* paints a different picture, one in which we have the power to influence our genetic expression by taking control of the environment around us. As a testament to the healing power of fresh food and a good sweat, I've seen my family, friends, fans, and clients lose many hundreds of pounds, reverse degenerative disease, recover from cancer, extend their life-spans, and win Olympic gold medals using the principles you're about to learn.

I made a conscious choice to write this book in layman's terms with minimal cryptic scientific jargon. Rest assured—*The Wild Diet* is based on proven scientific principles and a growing body of peer-reviewed and independent research. But instead of hurling studies and their equal-and-opposite counterparts back and forth, this book gets straight to the point and shows you what works so you can look and feel better than you ever thought possible. If you'd like to do your own homework, please explore the notes section.

Fair warning: Much of what you read in this book may be "controversial" and stand in direct opposition to current conventional wisdom and popular beliefs. While the principles in this program may seem radical today, I believe that they will be the "breakthroughs" of the future. I am confident that if you read this book with an open mind, the knowledge on the following pages will have the power to change your life.

Ready?

Great. Let's get started.

PART I

How "Healthy"
Food Made Us
Fat and Sick

WHY WE ALL GAINED 30 POUNDS

The average forty-year-old man in 1960 tipped the scale at 166 pounds. Weighing in at 196 pounds, the average man today is 30 pounds heavier.

What happened?

Like many of us, you've probably put on a few pounds over the past few years. And I bet you've tried to do something about it. Maybe you even went on a crash diet, forcing yourself to count every last calorie and buy expensive packaged dinners and a Shake Weight. Fighting through incessant cravings with shocking self-control, you probably even shed a few pounds. But as soon as you stopped depriving yourself, the fat came right back, didn't it? Most diets seem to imply that you can be lean, but only if you're hungry and miserable.

I'm here to tell you that it doesn't have to be like that.

When the Internet gurus tell you to subsist on cabbage soup, eat thirty bananas a day, or pop caffeine pills to melt off belly fat, don't listen. There's a better way to re-claim your youth and vitality. So get ready—I'm going to gently ask you to set aside nearly everything you've been told about diet, nutrition, and health. Many of the strate-gies and principles of *The Wild Diet* fly in the face of popular beliefs, fad crash diets, and advice from the droning, half-alive "experts" you see on daytime television.

You don't need me to tell you that our collective health seems doomed. Diabetes, cancer, and heart disease, rare until the turn of the twentieth century, are now predicted to affect almost everyone in the developed world at some point in their lifetime. Health care costs are increasingly crippling our economy, and eight-year-old children are weighing in at 300 pounds. One in three U.S. children born in 2000 will become diabetic in their lifetimes; nearly half of minorities are predicted to develop the disease; and the next generation of children is the first in centuries expected to have shorter life-spans than their parents. This is staggering . . . and also completely preventable.

If you're reading this, then conventional wisdom about nutrition and fitness has probably failed you. Confounded by special interests, misinformation from powerful industry lobbyists, and sleazy health and fitness gurus, the lion's share of conventional wisdom about diet and health is wrong, and those who trumpet its claims are misinformed, misguided, or simply misleading you. *The Wild Diet* will teach you to liberate yourself from the gimmickry, half-baked dogma, and empty promises of the diet and fitness industry.

As host of *Fat-Burning Man*, Apple's number-one-rated show, I've interviewed hundreds of the top experts across the world in weight loss, athletic training, physiology, brain science, and even indigenous tribespeople to figure out why America got fat. I quickly realized that losing fat and building muscle isn't a mystery. I've whittled this approach to health down to a few simple, easy-to-follow principles . . . some of which will surely surprise you.

What many seek to accomplish with extreme fad diets and the stapling of stomachs, we will achieve by restoring your mental and physical balance. Instead of fighting against it, we will work *with* your body to improve your health. Despite what you hear from the screaming maws of overcaffeinated weight-loss trainers on reality shows, you'll soon discover that taking pleasure in nourishing your body is essential to your success. You really can be happy and healthy at the same time.

THE SECRET TO FAT LOSS IN ONE SENTENCE

We don't need more diets, more books, or more information. We need trusted, step-by-step strategies from people who know what they're talking about. If you're familiar with my work, you already know that I've never claimed to be an expert or a guru. I'm just a regular guy who has spent the last decade obsessing about nutrition and fitness so you don't have to. And if you're not in the mood to read another diet book front to back, I'll give you the secret to fat loss in one sentence right now:

Stay away from sugar and processed grains, especially in the morning.

Disappointed? Let me give you some good news before you throw this book across the room.

If you've given up some of your favorite foods—like gooey cheese, chocolate, grilled steak, bacon, butter, full-fat cream, eggs, wine, cheesecake, ice cream, or anything else delicious—for the sake of "health," you're about to have a really good time eating this way. If you've exercised for hours a day, gritting your teeth and sweating pure misery, I'm going to teach you how to burn more fat with just minutes of exercise a week. Sound impossible? Take it from the Fat-Burning Man: Burning fat can be a lot of fun.

WHY DIET BOOKS DISAGREE WITH EACH OTHER

When I met with fancypants editors in Manhattan who were interested in publishing *The Wild Diet*, most said something like this: "So, Abel, your program makes a lot of sense. And your fans and followers clearly get great results. But what's *new* about your diet?"

Wrong question.

Take a second and type "diet" into Google. How many results did you get? I'm going to take a wild guess and say 14 bazillion.

Heard of the raw vegan diet? Dieters were arguing about it before we invented the automobile. How about low-carb? Check out "Banting," which became a fat-loss craze in England during the late 1800s. Last year, one of my blog posts went viral after I announced that I'd received a cease-and-desist letter from a fellow Paleo author. He threatened to sue me unless I removed the words "Paleo Diet" from my work because he had trademarked the term to sell supplements. But even the caveman diet has been around since the 1970s—or for the entire duration of human existence, depending on how you look at it.

And if all the fad diets weren't enough, most "scientific discoveries" touted by the media are ridiculous.

SCIENTIFIC DISCOVERY: EGGS ARE GOOD FOR YOU AGAIN!

MAN LOSES 20 POUNDS BY CUTTING OUT HIS STOMACH!

BREAKING NEWS: MUFFIN TOPS ARE ACTUALLY MADE OF MUFFINS!

Here's the truth—there is no such thing as a "new" diet. Anyone who tells you different is trying to sell you something. The philosophy of the Wild Diet is to honor the natural rhythms of your body and get food as close to its source as possible. Know that this is an ancient way of eating, not a new one. This isn't a diet book, but a book about how to reclaim your health by following the laws of nature (with a few delicious recipes to boot) for people who don't like diet books.

Some of what you read in this book will seem like no-brainer common sense. Good. We don't need more conflicting information and fads—it's time to get back to fundamentals. Not too long ago, "dieting" and losing weight weren't even considerations, since most people remained lean throughout their lifetimes. Our body isn't an adversary that we must "diet" and "exercise" into submission, but a remarkable biological system that adapts to the way we eat, train, and live.

WHY PROCESSED FOOD IS A
WASTE OF YOUR MONEY

Modern food manufacturers have overwhelmed grocery store shelves with foodstuff that is nutrient-poor, rotten, spoiled, dead, old, and tainted with antibiotics, synthetic hormones, and petroleum-based flavors. They saved a buck on cheap ingredients and didn't tell us they ruined our food in the process. Instead of nourishing our bodies with the fresh bounty of small family farms and gardens, we have been conditioned to subsist on marked-up, overhyped industrial-strength Frankenfoods from Fortune 500 corporations.

Since the rise of convenience food following the Second World War, Big Food has cut corners, capitalized on cheap oil, and embraced backward government policy to doctor our food beyond belief. While we continued to eat foods that go by the same names as those made at home by our parents and grandparents, the ingredients quietly shifted: The honey and natural sugars in our sweets, sauces, and sodas became genetically engineered corn syrup; the hand-churned grass-fed butter on our kitchen table became corn oil; wheat was bred into a plant that would be utterly unrecognizable to our ancestors; and the spices that flavored our favorite dishes were pushed out by artificial chemicals from test tubes.

Assembly-line production may work well for the automotive industry, but its ruthless efficiency and profit-based bent don't serve us well when our health is concerned. Factory food may be convenient and "cheap," but it's killing us.

For the titans of industry who run Big Food, the pursuit of short-term profits has trumped good judgment and clouded ethics. After years of tweaking from legions of white-coated technicians and geneticists, the fundamental nature of our food has changed. The land of milk and honey became the land of soy milk and agave nectar. Today, many of the foods we eat "in the pursuit of health" are intentionally designed to encourage overeating.

Have you ever tried a dinky "100-calorie pack" of crackers, cookies, or chips? When you get to the end of the bag (in, if you're like me, about five seconds flat), you want another one, right? But how many times have you eaten a big, juicy apple (usually about 100 calories, by the way) and said to yourself, "Golly, I really want *another apple* right now"? Doesn't happen. Your brain knows when you eat real food. Processed food makes you crave more, so you *buy* more. Real food fills you up.

But the whole point of eating is to get full, isn't it? This is the first time in the history of man that we're tricked into thinking that we want less *food* in our food. We are surrounded by food, but we're nutritionally starving. Nutrient-poor processed foods distort your appetite and cause you to consume more calories than you need. This perpetuates a vicious cycle of stuffing your face but never feeling totally satisfied or nourished.

When you're hungry, your body doesn't necessarily want food; it craves *nutrition*. If you try to quell your hunger with empty calories or doctored food, your brain and body will never really feel totally satisfied. The key is to feed yourself nutrient-dense foods that satiate your hunger. As I'm sure you've noticed, today's concrete jungle of freeze-dried franchises and chain supermarkets can make life a challenge for any aspiring health nut.

In America, our standards for food are shockingly low. This section of the book may surprise or disgust you, but bear with me—you'll see that poor-quality food is easy to avoid once you know what to look for. But first, buckle up—it's about to get bumpy. What I learned as a consultant inside the diet and health industry made my stomach turn.

The Worst Thing Since Sliced Bread

Something happened to our wheat. Although it claims the same name, the hybridized dwarf wheat we eat today does not resemble the whole grain our parents once ate. For thousands of years, we used hardy ancient varieties of wheat like emmer, einkorn, and khorosan to make bread, pasta, and baked foods. However, the mutant, genetically altered grain that makes up 99 percent of the wheat we eat today has been "dwarfed"—it stops growing at just one-third of the height of the massive amber waves of grain our ancestors sang about.

The blunted stems, high yield, and ease of transport of "dwarf" wheat makes it cheap to produce, but it's also less nutritious and difficult to digest. Since agribusiness began genetically altering wheat in 1960, concentrations of zinc, copper, iron, and magnesium in the grain plummeted (19 to 28 percent lower in the years 1968 to 2005, compared to 1845 to 1967). Big Food has bred a wolf into a Chihuahua, but that's just the beginning of the madness.

It's a wonder to comprehend how expansive field grains are manipulated by man and machine into a 100% wheat bagel or hamburger bun. The truth isn't pretty. Let's travel with "dwarf" wheat on its journey from field to sack.

- After machines remove large contaminants like sticks and rocks, wheat endures high-temperature steam conditioning, which prevents the berries from naturally fermenting. Once the chaff is removed, the endosperm, the least nutritious and starchiest part of the wheat, is separated and ground into a fine powder.

- Chlorine, bromates, and azodicarbonamide are chemicals that are banned in Europe but are used widely in America to improve appearance, remove odors, and standardize texture. Bleaching and oxidizing agents (such as benzoyl peroxide, calcium peroxide, nitrogen dioxide, chlorine, or azodicarbonamide) are added to the flour made from the ground endosperm. Since the most nutritious part of the grain has already been removed during processing, the government mandates that food refiners must "enrich" their flour with synthetic vitamins, which can be difficult to absorb.

- The bleached wheat flour sits in containers for one to two months before being packed into sacks or large tanks to be shipped off to consumers or used to make processed food. Since the wheat hasn't been fermented, soaked, or sprouted to remove toxic antinutrients, this flour contains substances that can damage the gut, causing weight gain, autoimmune disorders, and disease.

TINY LITTLE VEGETABLES

We didn't always blast our modern wheat with heat and chemicals. Once upon a time, our grandparents knew well that grains needed to ferment, soak, and sprout before they were nutritious enough to eat.

Sprouting and fermenting grains essentially turns them into tiny, ready-to-eat vegetables that are more easily digested. Sprouting grains increases the amino acid lysine, reduces antinutrients like phytic acid and lectins, disables enzyme inhibitors, and releases enzymes to increase the absorbability of nutrients. Essentially, when you prepare grains (or any other food) the way that nature intended—through fermenting, soaking, sprouting, followed by low-and-slow cooking—you maximize the nutrient density of your food.

So what happens when we turn this modern flour into "heart-healthy, low-fat, whole-grain" bread? Here is a breakdown of store-bought bread with a label that screams in big, flashy typeface, "ALL NATURAL INGREDIENTS" and "NO ARTIFICIAL PRESERVATIVES ADDED":

Enriched bleached wheat flour (bleached wheat flour, malted barley, niacin, reduced iron, thiamine mononitrate, riboflavin), water, high-fructose corn syrup, yeast, wheat bran, vital wheat gluten, butter. Contains 2% or less of each of the following: rye meal, corn flour, molasses, rolled whole wheat, salt, dough conditioners (ammonium sulfate, sodium stearoyl lactylate), brown sugar, honey, vinegar, oatmeal, soy flour, mono- and diglycerides, partially hydrogenated soybean oil.

Here's what you should know about these ingredients:

- Enriched bleached wheat flour is refined white flour. "Enriched" is a confusing term—it sounds healthy, but it's not. The bran and the germ portion of the whole wheat have been refined out, leaving you with the least nutritious and most fattening portion of the wheat. To compensate for refining out approximately twenty nutrients, manufacturers add back four synthetic nutrients: niacin (vitamin B_3), reduced iron, thiamine mononitrate (synthetic vitamin B_1), and riboflavin (vitamin B_2). These meager synthetic nutrient additives are not digested or absorbed by your body as readily as whole food sources. Oh, and did you notice they bleached it, too? Awesome, thanks.
- High-fructose corn syrup is one of the most perniciously fattening substances on the planet. This genetically modified, sickly sweet syrup is associated with skyrocketing blood sugar, obesity, type 2 diabetes, B-vitamin deficiency, hyperactivity, tooth decay, and indigestion, among many other maladies.
- Dough conditioners can cause mineral deficiencies, and many processed breads include the same chemical that gives yoga mats their texture. I lived in an apartment above a Subway in college, and after smelling the noxious fumes of whatever substance was baking downstairs every morning, I can tell you that it's not bread. Subway was recently exposed by a blogger for using the same chemical used to

form little bubbles in yoga mats to give their breads a similar bubbly texture. A report from my friends at the Environmental Working Group found that the compound, azodicarbonamide, is used in close to five hundred food products, from Pillsbury Dinner Rolls to Little Debbie products to Wonder Bread.

- Ammonium sulfate may cause mouth ulcers, nausea, and kidney and liver problems.
- Sodium stearoyl lactylate may be corn, milk, peanut, or soy based, and may cause high blood pressure, kidney disturbances, and water retention.
- Brown sugar is frequently refined white sugar with molasses or artificial chemicals for coloring added. Sugar is sugar—stay away.
- Mono- and diglycerides are known to cause allergic reactions.
- Partially hydrogenated soybean oil is associated with obesity, heart disease, breast and colon cancers, atherosclerosis, elevated cholesterol, and reduced sperm count.

To your body, many of these substances are novel and unrecognizable as food. Before you buy anything in a package, take a look at the ingredients on the back and make sure that it's made with real food. Ask yourself: Where did these ingredients come from—a farm or a lab? As Joan Gussow quipped, "I trust cows more than chemists."

Pesticides in Our Corn

Here's a rhetorical question: Why is the same company that manufactured Agent Orange, a highly toxic herbicide responsible for poisoning millions since its use in the Vietnam War, making our corn?

Incredibly, scientists at this company, Monsanto, have discovered a way to genetically splice a *toxic pesticide* into the very DNA of corn itself. This genetically modified grain is known as "Bt [*Bacillus thuringiensis*] corn," and it already accounts for 65 percent of all corn grown in the United States. That means that when you eat this corn, or any product that contains corn-derived ingredients (such as high-fructose corn syrup, corn oil, or maltodextrin), you're swallowing a toxic pesticide.

Monsanto insists that Bt corn is perfectly safe for humans. Here's why that bothers me: Our bodies are less a single "human" organism than a high-level ecosystem comprising many different cells, bacteria, and organelles. In fact, you may be surprised to learn that nearly nine out of ten of the cells in and on your body right now are not technically "human," but belong to tiny bacteria that we've only just begun to study (you'll learn more about them on page 53).

Now, the toxic Bt pesticide that is engineered into the majority of corn grown in America is designed to rupture the stomach of any unfortunate bug that swallows it, causing death. We know that nine out of ten cells in our bodies are made of little bugs, necessary for our health. But wait a minute. . . . Isn't the Bt toxin designed to kill little bugs by making their stomachs explode?

And mind you, none of this genetic modification is done for the sake of your health and well-being, but for the profits of the same company that invented Agent Orange. Monsanto isn't exactly known for the safety of their products. How could we possibly trust them with our food?

In the United States, Big Food doesn't even have to tell you which foods contain this genetically altered corn on the label or whether it was used to feed the animals you're eating. No wonder Europe won't import our food. Even China, the country known for feeding poultry feces to its farmed fish, banned our meat and much of our processed food. We can do better.

I don't know about you, but I thought corn was perfectly fine before chemical companies started turning vegetables into toxic weapons. Growing up, my brothers and I would always fight over the first sign of sweet, crunchy sugar corn when harvest season came. You can't buy that in a package.

I would never tell you to deprive yourself of real, fresh corn straight off the stalk—but I will recommend you go organic. Organic certification lets you know that your corn is free of intentional GMOs (and toxic weapons) and grown without petroleum-based chemical fertilizer.

HOW TO AVOID GENETICALLY MODIFIED FOODS

The genetic engineering of foods is a contentious topic. Perhaps one day we'll actually develop GMO foods that are beneficial for our health, but we're not there yet. The truth is that foods today aren't genetically modified for the sake of your health, but to cut costs and increase profits for Big Food. While GMOs are banned in many other countries due to concerns about their safety for human consumption, the United States doesn't even require food manufacturers to disclose whether their products *contain* GMO ingredients. However, a growing number of consumer-conscious food manufacturers—usually organic—now display the "Non-GMO Verified" seal on their products. Avoid the products below and on the following page and seek organic and non-GMO verified options when you can.

Common Products That Contain GMOs

KELLOGG'S: Rice Krispies • Corn Flakes • Frosted Flakes • Special K • Apple Jacks • All-Bran • Corn Pops • Crispix • Froot Loops • Frosted Mini-Wheats • Raisin Bran • Pop-Tarts • Eggo Waffles • MorningStar Farms Vegan Veggie Burgers • MorningStar Farms Chik'n Nuggets • MorningStar Farms Veggie Sausage • Keebler Chips Deluxe • Famous Amos Cookies • Carr's Table Water Crackers

KRAFT/NABISCO: Chips Ahoy! Cookies • Capri Sun • Boca Burgers • Cheez Whiz • Cool Whip • Corn Nuts • Crystal Light • Country Time • Honey Maid Graham Crackers • Jell-O • Kool-Aid • Kraft Singles • Lunchables • Maxwell House Coffee • Miracle Whip • Fig Newtons • Oreos • Oscar Mayer • Philadelphia Cream Cheese • Planters Nuts • Polly-O • Ritz Crackers • SnackWell's • Teddy Grahams • Triscuits • Velveeta • Wheat Thins

FRITO-LAY: Lay's Potato Chips • Doritos • Tostitos • Cheetos • Fritos • Sun Chips • Cracker Jack • Rold Gold Pretzels • Ruffles • Munchies • Stacy's Pita Chips • Smartfood Popcorn

QUAKER OATS: Quaker Oats Oatmeal • Life Cereal • Oat Bran • Quick Oats • Instant Oatmeal • Natural Granola • Chewy Granola Bars • Rice Cakes • Grits • Wheat Germ

NESTLÉ: Nesquik • Butterfinger • Crunch Bars • Kit Kat • Nescafé • Buitoni • Lean Cuisine • Hot Pockets • Stouffer's • Coffee-Mate • Carnation • Juicy Juice • Nestea • Dreyer's • Häagen-Dazs • Nestlé Ice Cream

CAMPBELL'S SOUP: Condensed Soups • Chunky Soup • Select Harvest • Healthy Request • Pace • Pepperidge Farm • Prego • Swanson • V8

COMMON GMO INGREDIENTS

1. **Soy:** soy flour, lecithin, soy protein isolates and concentrates (protein shakes). May contain GMO soy derivatives: vitamin E supplements, tofu, cereals, veggie burgers, soy sausages, tamari, soy sauce, chips, ice cream, frozen yogurt, infant formula, sauces, protein powder, margarine, soy cheese, crackers, breads, cookies, chocolates, candy, fried foods, shampoo, bubble bath, cosmetics, enriched flours and pastas.
2. **Corn:** corn flour, cornstarch, corn oil, corn sweeteners, syrups. Products that may contain GMO corn derivatives: vitamin C supplements, corn chips, candy, ice cream, infant formula, salad dressings, tomato sauces, bread, cookies, cereals, baking powder, alcohol, vanilla, margarine, soy sauce, soda, fried foods, powdered sugar, enriched flours and pastas.
3. **Cotton:** oil, fabrics. Products that may contain GMO cotton derivatives: clothes, linens, chips, peanut butter, crackers, cookies.
4. **Canola oil.** Products that may contain GMO canola: processed foods, chips,

crackers, cereal, snack bars, frozen foods, canned soups, candy, bread, hummus, oil blends.

5. **Sugar beets:** sugar. Products that may contain GMO sugar beets: any product that doesn't specify "cane sugar" but just "sugar" on ingredients, cookies, cakes, ice cream, donuts, baking mixes, candy, juice, yogurt.

6. **Alfalfa:** used to fatten livestock. Products that may contain GMO alfalfa: all types of conventionally raised meat, pork, poultry, eggs, and dairy.

7. **Aspartame:** artificial sweetener. Products that may contain aspartame: diet soft drinks, diet foods, yogurt, gum.

8. **Dairy:** rBGH growth hormone. Products that may contain GMO rBGH: all conventionally raised dairy products: milk, cheese, butter, yogurt, ice cream, and whey.

According to the Non-GMO Project, the highest-risk genetically modified crops include:

Sugar beets (approx. 95% of U.S. crop in 2010)

Soy (approx. 94% of U.S. crop in 2011)

Canola (approx. 90% of U.S. crop)

Cotton (approx. 90% of U.S. crop in 2011)

Corn (approx. 88% of U.S. crop in 2011)

Alfalfa (first planting 2011)

Zucchini and yellow summer squash (approx. 25,000 acres)

Papaya (most of Hawaiian crop; approx. 988 acres)

Avoid Processed Grains

We've known that carbs make us fat for hundreds of years, but the fat-free craze drowned out our common sense. Any food that contains finely ground flour—whether from wheat, rice, or other grains—will stimulate an undesirable jump in blood sugar. The more finely ground the flour and glycemic the carb source, the more quickly your blood sugar will rise. We enjoy wild, black, brown, or red rice or sprouted ancient grains in the evening a few nights a week. But when fat loss is the goal, cutting back on grains is a time-tested trick to drop weight fast.

The proof is in the pudding. You can ask any rancher in Texas:

How do you fatten a cow?
Feed it grains.

How do you fatten a human?
Feed it grains.

Humor me for a moment. What is your favorite part of a hamburger? The meat, the bacon, the gooey cheese, grilled onion, tomato, and seasonings, right? And how about pizza? Most people don't even eat the crust unless it's stuffed with cheese. These days, bread, dough, and other starches are often little more than vehicles for their toppings. Flour isn't delicious in and of itself. Flour relies on added flavor, usually in the form of salt, sugar, or fat, to make most products palatable. Have you ever swallowed a spoonful of white flour? Ick.

DID DON DRAPER INVENT BETTY CROCKER?

While researching the history of food processing for this book, I discovered that the affable "Betty Crocker" was never in fact a real person but a personality carefully engineered by a marketing team. In 1921, the new star of food marketing, Betty Crocker, was invented by the advertising department at Washburn Crosby (which later became General Mills) as part of a calculated campaign to drive American women to the company's expanding catalogue of convenience foods. For nearly a century, on television, radio, and magazine advertisements, Betty has promoted processed grain-based products with catchy slogans like "grand time savers" to appeal to busy moms. Responsible for moving millions of products made from cheap, shelf-stable ingredients and sold for stiff markups, Betty Crocker is one of the most profitable commercial characters of the twentieth century.

Do you need to cut out bread, pasta, grains, and other starches forever? No way! I'd never deprive anyone of a few treats during holidays and special occasions. But that's just it: They're treats, not dietary staples. Indulgences, not health foods. If you do choose to eat grains, enjoy them in moderate quantities (ideally on exercise days) and go for whole grains like brown rice, buckwheat, or quinoa to limit digestive stress from high-glycemic domesticated modern grains. Sandwiches and pasta dishes are often convenient but grain-heavy, so look at the recipe section for hearty fat-burning meals that will help you reach your goals.

With few exceptions, including an occasional bite or two of fresh-baked bread as a special treat, I prefer life without wheat, GMO corn, and other modern grains. Once you drop them, it's like health starts to happen automatically.

The Sordid Story of Soy

For decades, we've endured marketing spin about how soy is a health food. But, like many other processed foods, soy isn't ubiquitous because it's healthy—it's being pushed because it's profitable. In reality, processed soy is no health food.

The soybean was an unpopular crop until food manufacturers intent on creating cheap vegetable oils successfully persuaded the government to subsidize it. After processing the soybean to oil, the manufacturers were left with an industrial waste product—isolated soy protein. In order to boost profits, food manufacturers took the waste soy protein isolate and effectively created a market for it.

Now a veritable cash cow, soy is present in roughly seven out of ten foods on grocery store shelves in the form of soy lecithin, soybean oil, vegetable oil, texturized vegetable protein, soy flour, soy protein isolate, and more. Since nearly all the soy produced in the United States and Canada is genetically modified and contaminated with pesticides, it's best to avoid any food with soy products or by-products in the ingredients. Be careful—soy can be found in everything from protein shakes and bars to veggie burgers and imitation cheese. Go for real cheese instead. And if you don't dodge soy for the sake of your health, do it for taste. Compare a soy burger with vegan cheese product to a grass-fed burger with a sharp aged cheddar, and you'll see what I mean.

Processed soy acts as a goitrogen that disrupts your body's absorption of iodine and reduces thyroid function. Your thyroid regulates your metabolism, so when it falters, you gain weight and encounter a slew of other negative effects. Soy is also packed with antinutrients including phytates, enzyme inhibitors that block mineral absorption in the digestive tract. Soy contains a variety of toxic chemicals that cannot be fully metabolized by the body unless it undergoes extensive fermentation, which doesn't happen when soy shows up in processed food products. If you choose to eat soy, go organic and stick to its uses in traditional fermented foods such as miso, tempeh, or natural soy sauce (tamari).

The False Promise of Processed Oil

Packed with trans fats, pesticides, and chemical solvents, industrial seed and vegetable oils have been making us fat and diseased for decades. Deep down, we all know that real old-fashioned butter gives us something that fake butter just can't—no matter how hard Big Food tries to convince us otherwise. (Yes, we *can* believe the off-white, tasteless, odorless whipped vegetable spread hocked by Fabio is not butter.) Because the natural fats we crave, like real butter from cows raised on pastures, aren't just more delicious, they're also much better for us than the fats we see on commercials.

While real butter is still made by simply churning milk, much like your grandmother may have, modern vegetable oil processing looks more like a meth lab than Grandma's kitchen.

Genetically modified canola oil, for example, is obtained through a combination of high-temperature mechanical pressing and solvent extraction. Traces of the solvent (usually the petroleum-derived hexane) remain in the oil even after extensive processing. Canola oil is subjected to caustic refining, bleaching, and degumming—all of which involve high temperatures and/or chemicals of questionable safety. And since canola oil easily becomes rancid and foul-smelling when exposed to oxygen and high temperatures, it must be deodorized.

Before canola reaches the supermarket shelves, the deodorization process removes a large portion of the beneficial omega-3 fatty acids and turns them into trans fats, which are linked to heart disease and cancer. Since these trans fats occur in trace amounts, food manufacturers are not required to disclose them on their labels.

By the way, did you know that the word *canola* was invented by food marketers, too? The real name of the canola plant is rapeseed, which marketers assumed wouldn't sell well for obvious reasons. Instead, Big Food renamed rapeseed oil "canola," an amalgam of "oil" and "Canada," where the seed was popularized and continues to be grown today.

WHAT THE NUTRITION FACTS DON'T TELL YOU

Watch out for deceptive marketing statements like these on product labels:

- Fat-Free!
- Reduced Fat!
- Sugar-Free!
- No Added Sugar!
- Diet!

What these phrases often mean in practical terms:

- Fat-free, but packed with sugar and chemicals to compensate for the lack of flavor.
- Reduced fat, but increased carbohydrates and stratospheric glycemic index.
- Sugar-free. Artificial everything else.
- No added sugar . . . because the insane amount of "naturally occurring" sugars are enough to give you type 2 diabetes.

- "Diet" food, because it is literally watered down to "reduce" calories. Oh, and it causes brain tumors in lab rats.

Be careful of statements like these as well:

- All Natural Ingredients!
- 100% Natural!
- No Preservatives!
- No Artificial Preservatives!
- No Artificial Ingredients!

Statements like these mean next to nothing. Snake venom is 100 percent natural, too, but I wouldn't spread it on my toast.

Whenever a food claims to be good for you because it *doesn't* have something in it, be wary. For decades, "sugar-free" has translated to "known carcinogens that kind of resemble sugar"; "fat-free" to "tastes like cardboard"; and "natural flavors" to "may or may not contain the anal secretions of beavers" (see page 32). Remember, you want your food to be nutrient-dense, which means no junk calories (or "calorie-free" chemicals).

The healthiest foods are often the simplest ones, so aim for the fewest ingredients possible. For example, if you're picking out almond butter, look for almonds and perhaps salt on the label, but put down the jar if it has added sugars, processed oils, emulsifiers, preservatives, or anything else. These additives make products cheaper and last longer on the shelf, but they will also make you fat and sick.

WHY COUNTING CALORIES IS
A WASTE OF YOUR TIME

FDA loopholes allow food manufacturers to manipulate the nutrition facts by omitting chemicals, additives, trans fats, and other substances from their labels. Nutrition facts are often doctored to make it appear that you're eating fewer calories than you actually are. Not only is it impossible to gauge your exact meal-to-meal calorie and macronutrient requirements, but trying to will drive you crazy.

If you're trying to lose weight by counting calories, you might want to reconsider. Does how much you eat have an impact on your weight? Sort of—fat loss doesn't depend on *how many* calories you eat, but on *which* calories you eat and *when*. Not only that, but because food manufacturers can manipulate the calorie counts listed on labels, most people drastically underestimate the number of calories they consume.

Even if the calorie counts on packaged food were accurate, the idea that your body "burns off" calories equally regardless of food source oversimplifies the matter. If you listen to Big Food, they'll tell you that drinking 100 calories of soda is the metabolic equivalent of eating a can of tuna fish. I don't buy it. Our bodies aren't like the incinerators they use in labs, burning calories one at a time—our bodies are incredibly complicated, intelligent, and self-regulating systems that want to be healthy. When you eat real food and trust your senses, you'll never have to count a calorie again.

BEWARE OF FOOD THAT DOESN'T SPOIL

If a food product can last on the shelves for extended periods of time, take a good look at its ingredients. Have you heard about the fourteen-year-old hamburger from McDonald's that still hasn't gone bad? Or the ice cream sandwich from Walmart that never melts, even on a hot day? If Mother Nature (and Father Time) won't even touch it, how confident are you that your body will recognize a bar of processed chemicals as food?

Real food gives your body the signals it needs to know that you just ate, while processed food encourages overeating, food intolerance, and eventually most of the diseases of the modern world. If your food doesn't go bad, or if ants refuse to eat it, drop that corn dog.

The Negative Effects of Industrial Food Processing

- As much as 90 percent of phytonutrients, which radically improve health and fight disease, are destroyed.
- The physical properties of foods are chemically altered in a manner that renders them dangerous. For example, homogenization and high-temperature pasteurization alter the fat molecules in milk, giving them properties that contribute to inflammation and heart disease.
- Minerals and natural cofactors are stripped from the food. Synthetic vitamins are often added into the flour to compensate, but synthetics are often not adequately digested since they lack the natural substances present in real food to increase bioavailability.
- Calories are concentrated in unnatural ways. For example, corn is processed into high-fructose corn syrup, which contains concentrated sugar devoid of fiber—a combination impossible to find in nature.

THE APPETITE ENHANCER
HIDDEN IN MORE THAN 700 FOODS

Many of us know that monosodium glutamate (MSG) is used as a chemical additive in most processed and fast foods. But do you know why?

MSG is a chemical used frequently by Big Food to *stimulate your appetite* and fool your brain into making low-quality food taste better than it actually does. But not only does MSG make you hungry, it also makes subjects predictably *gain fat* in the lab: Scientists frequently inject lab rats with MSG to literally *induce* obesity. Be careful—free glutamate, the damaging substance in MSG, can be hidden in almost anything, including sauces, condiments, jerky, chips, candy, chewing gum, and drinks.

Aside from appearing as monosodium glutamate, or MSG, this hunger-inducing substance often hides within the following more marketing-friendly ingredients:

- Autolyzed plant protein
- Autolyzed yeast
- Calcium caseinate
- Gelatin
- Glutamate
- Glutamic acid
- Hydrolyzed plant protein (HPP)
- Hydrolyzed vegetable protein (HVP)
- Monopotassium glutamate
- Senomyx (wheat extract labeled as "artificial flavor")
- Sodium caseinate
- Spices
- Textured protein
- Vegetable protein extract
- Yeast extract

No wonder we're all hungry. Avoid all packaged food with MSG or any of these ingredients on the label. When eating out, order your sauce and dressing on the side, as most are contaminated with MSG and other appetite-enhancing chemical additives.

DON'T BE DUPED BY "NATURAL" FLAVORS

The chemical flavoring industry is worth billions of dollars, practicing its furtive magic just off the New Jersey Turnpike. Although most consumers don't know much about the chemical flavoring business or its wily ways, chemicals are largely responsible for giving processed foods the smells and tastes that hijack your senses and create the illusion of real food. For example, you can sniff test tubes in the lab that smell exactly like your favorite burger, fries, or shake. Creepy.

Distinctions between artificial and natural flavors are relatively meaningless, based more on how the flavor has been manufactured than on the chemicals it actually contains. If you see "natural flavor" or "artificial flavor" on a label, you're holding a chemical soup.

For example, a typical artificial flavoring like the one in a McDonald's strawberry milk shake may contain some or all of the following ingredients:

amyl acetate, amyl butyrate, amyl valerate, anethol, anisyl formate, benzyl acetate, benzyl isobutyrate, butyric acid, cinnamyl isobutyrate, cinnamyl valerate, cognac essential oil, diacetyl, dipropyl ketone, ethyl acetate, ethyl amyl ketone, ethyl butyrate, ethyl cinnamate, ethyl heptanoate, ethyl heptylate, ethyl lactate, ethyl methylphenylglycidate, ethyl nitrate, ethyl propionate, ethyl valerate, heliotropin, hydroxyphenyl-2-butanone (10% solution in alcohol), a-ionone, isobutyl anthranilate, isobutyl butyrate, lemon essential oil, maltol, 4-methylacetophenone, methyl anthranilate, methyl benzoate, methyl cinnamate, methyl heptine carbonate, methyl naphthyl ketone, methyl salicylate, mint essential oil, neroli essential oil, nerolin, neryl isobutyrate, orris butter, phenethyl alcohol, rose, rum ether, g-undecalactone, vanillin, and solvent.

And that's just the short list; there are upwards of one thousand food-flavoring chemicals that can help your strawberry shake taste like a strawberry or your grape drink taste somewhat grape-like. I'd rather have a strawberry, thanks.

Think you're better off eating foods with "natural flavor"? Chew on this: Secretions from the anal glands of beavers produce a bitter, smelly, orange-brown substance known as castoreum that is used extensively in raspberry and vanilla flavoring. It's legally labeled as "natural flavoring."

This is what happens when you trust food manufacturers, my friends. I hope you like beaver butt.

Honestly, I'm not as worried about the natural flavors made from crushed beetles or the rear ends of rodents; I'm much more concerned about the chemicals that trick your brain into thinking processed food actually tastes like anything good. Unlike real food, since chemicals can be owned as property, these newfangled substances are sped through production and often remain untested for human safety.

In some cases, natural flavors—like citrus—are actually made from the thing they are trying to approximate, but usually they're made in the lab. With few exceptions, I avoid all artificial flavors and most natural flavors, especially vanilla and raspberry. Flavors should come from plants, not smoking cauldrons in labs off the New Jersey Turnpike.

IF YOU'RE ADDICTED TO FOOD, IT'S NOT YOUR FAULT

If you've ever been caught knuckle-deep in a bag of Fritos, you're not alone. Processed food is engineered to hijack your brain to tell you that you're hungry when you're not.

If you take a bite of something and immediately crave more, drop it. That craving is indication that the pleasure centers of your brain have been hijacked. This is what most processed foods are designed to do, since craving more makes you eat and purchase more of the product, which means higher profits for Big Food. Obviously, there's a conflict of interest between your health and their boardroom meetings, and I think you know to which side the executives with $400 haircuts lean. In my time as a consultant, I worked with several of the biggest food manufacturers in the world, and I can tell you that many of the executives don't even feed their own products to their children. I asked one executive why, and he huffed, "Because they're all chemicals!"

WHY WE'RE ADDICTED TO SUGAR

Can't kick your sugar habit? You're not alone. We're wired to love sugar, and Big Food knows it. Big Food uses cheap, concentrated sugar (or, more often, high-fructose corn syrup) in almost everything because sweetness makes even bad food taste reasonably good. The sugar in our food adds up quickly, leaving many of us overweight and addicted. Today, just by including processed and restaurant foods in our diets, we're being exposed to more sugar in a year than our ancestors would have seen in their entire lifetimes.

One hundred years ago, we consumed 4 pounds of sugar a year. Fifty years ago, we bumped it up to 12 pounds per year. Today, the U.S. Department of Agriculture reports that the average American consumes more than *152 pounds of sugar a year*. While we once ate minimally processed sugars like honey, molasses, and cane sugar, the vast majority of our sugar today comes in the form of processed high-fructose corn syrup and genetically engineered sugar beets.

Sugar is one of the most addictive substances on the planet. The sweet tooth is a vicious cycle that starts with eating sugar and ends (or doesn't end) with craving more sugar. But here's my promise: If you start whittling down the amount of sweet stuff you consume, your cravings will slowly but surely disappear. If you can get the sugar monkey off your back, you may never have to worry about your weight again. The less you cave, the less you crave.

As a rule, I do my best to avoid any packaged food with more than 3 to 5 grams of sugar per serving (or per bottle, if it's a drink). Be careful—Big Food knows that sugar on the label stops consumers from buying, so often the serving size you see on the label is much smaller than what any normal human being would eat or drink in one sitting. This is designed to make it seem like the food is less bad for you than it actually is. Look carefully at the number of servings in the package or bottle and keep the total sugar below 5 grams.

Hidden sugars are everywhere, especially in beverages and packaged, processed foods. Be vigilant. It doesn't matter what name it goes by—glucose, crystalline fructose, cane sugar, agave nectar—it's all sugar, and it will all cause you to store fat instead of burn it. Also, remember that anything ending in "-ose" is typically a form of sugar, as in high-fruct*ose* corn syrup, malt*ose*, dextr*ose*, and sucral*ose*, to name a few. And if you see something sweet with low or no sugar, make sure to look at the label to ensure that Big Food didn't add in any artificial sweeteners (aka "nasty chemicals") to compensate.

Don't worry—you won't have to go without sweet things when you go Wild. Alyson and I eat a treat or two most nights, and many of our favorite homemade desserts are included in this book. Try them yourself on pages 250 to 269.

HOW TO IDENTIFY HIDDEN SUGAR IN YOUR FOOD

Food manufacturers often hide sugar under more marketing-friendly terms such as "cane sugar," "crystalline fructose," or "brown rice syrup," but it's all the same once it crosses your lips. Spotting refined sugar in packaged food can be a harrowing task—you have to be a real ingredient sleuth to decipher the sugar code, but knowing some of the most common names for hidden sugar is a good place to start.

- Sucrose
- Brown rice syrup
- Barley malt
- Fructose
- Glucose
- Dextrose
- Galactose
- Lactose
- Maltose
- Maltodextrin
- Invert sugar
- Raw sugar
- Turbinado sugar
- Brown sugar

- Confectioners' sugar
- Granulated sugar
- Corn syrup
- High-fructose corn syrup
- Crystalline
- Cane syrup
- Mannitol
- Sorbitol
- White grape juice concentrate
- Date sugar
- Dextran

- Dextrose
- Diastase
- Diastatic malt
- Ethyl maltol
- Fruit juice concentrate
- Glucose
- Glucose solids
- Grape sugar
- Malt syrup
- Refiner's syrup
- Sorghum syrup

If you're eating out and you taste a sauce, dressing, or dish that seems sweet, it's likely packed with sugar or an artificial sweetener. Be careful—ignorance isn't bliss when nutrition is concerned. If something tastes too sweet, it's usually not worth finishing.

LIQUID SUGAR: SODA, SPORTS DRINKS, AND FRUIT JUICE

For many, the consumption of liquid calories is the single factor that means the difference between burning fat and storing it on a daily basis. Surprisingly, it's not just soda that destroys diets. Sports drinks, sweetened teas, and fruit juice can be just as catastrophic to your progress.

Packaged juice is a lot less natural than it appears. Although it's labeled as "fresh-squeezed 100% orange juice," for example, large juice manufacturers like Tropicana and Minute Maid store their juice inside giant vats for months on end, often in the belly of shipping tankers. Processing removes oxygen from the juice to aid in preservation, but the flavor goes with it. To compensate for the lack of flavor in their juice, Big Food contracts artificial chemical companies to synthesize fragrances to make your orange juice appear to smell and taste like real oranges. The same chemical fragrances that make perfume, laundry detergent, and household cleaners smell like citrus.

As Alfred E. Neuman, the buck-toothed, red-haired star of *MAD Magazine*, mused, "We are living in a world today where lemonade is made from artificial flavors and furniture polish is made from real lemons."

Not only does the industrial juicing process destroy flavor and most nutrients and antioxidants from the juice, but processing also strips the fruit of its natural fiber. When you eat fruit and vegetables whole, the natural fiber slows the absorption of fructose and other natural sugars into the bloodstream and prevents spikes in blood sugar. Remove the fiber and you have a fattening beverage indeed. The processed fruit juice you find in the supermarket has been shown to increase the risk of diabetes, and a high intake of fruit juice has been linked to childhood obesity.

If you really like fruit juice, have a few sips, but don't try to fill up on it or drink it for the sake of health—that's just fancy juice bars' way of overcharging you for a sugar bomb. Go for a whole piece of fruit or a green smoothie instead (see page 112).

Why Artificial Sweeteners Don't Count as Calories

One of the best strategies for cultivating vibrant health throughout your life is to know where your food comes from. But have you ever wondered about what an artificial sweetener actually is? Aspartame (NutraSweet) was discovered in the 1980s after the new substance was accidentally licked off the finger of a scientist who was trying to synthesize a new antiulcer drug. Sucralose (Splenda) is no better—it was discovered by two lab students while experimenting with a new type of *chlorinated pesticide*. Oops . . . I mean, yum!

Before you're enchanted by the suspiciously low calorie or carb count on the nutrition label of a packaged food, keep in mind that the only reason zero-calorie artificial sweeteners don't count as calories or carbs is because they're not technically food— they're chemicals. But don't be deceived—these substances have side effects (remember Olestra, which caused "anal leakage" in thousands of unsuspecting dieters?). While Big Food invents proprietary artificial sweeteners to make a quick buck, remember that many artificial sweeteners marketed to us, like saccharin, are eventually exposed as what they really are: carcinogenic chemical compounds that have no business being called food.

So How Do We Satisfy Our Sweet Tooth?

When you eat something sweet, do your best to make sure some amount of nutrients come along with it. Fresh fruit is a nutrient-dense and convenient treat, whether eaten whole, dried, or blended with other ingredients to sweeten baked goods (as we do in some of our dessert recipes). Minimally processed plant-based sweeteners like pure maple syrup and raw coconut nectar (if you can, get it raw and local—my parents have their own bees) contain trace minerals, making them good options for sweetening baked goods, beverages, and treats. Other flavorful sweeteners we use in moderation are coconut palm sugar, brown cane sugar, and blackstrap molasses.

Our favorite low-carb sweetener is the dried leaf of the stevia plant. Organic extracts of stevia can also work well in a pinch, but avoid processed "stevia" sweeteners. For example, Truvia, which is "made from stevia" and purports to be an "all-natural sweetener," goes through forty-two steps of processing to make it four hundred times sweeter than sugar. Sounds like a processed food to me. Instead, order the dried, crushed stevia leaf online or grow it yourself.

HOW BEBAC AND MOKOLO DROPPED 170 POUNDS

After a twenty-one-year-old male gorilla named Brooks died of heart failure in 2005 at the Cleveland Metroparks Zoo, biologists decided to investigate why their gorillas suffer from the same afflictions as humans in much of the developed world.

Although obesity is almost unheard of in wild animals, many creatures get fat and sick as soon as they're caged. From a young age, zoo gorillas show evidence of high blood pressure, high cholesterol and triglyceride levels, fibrosis of the heart, and obesity. In captivity, more than one-third of gorillas die of heart disease, much like modern humans.

Interestingly, before poor Brooks's heart stopped, his diet included bucketfuls of vitamin-rich biscuits that were specially formulated by nutritionists to meet the precise dietary needs of gorillas. Apparently, nutritionists have some work to do.

To see if they would have better luck with a more "natural" diet, the biologists decided to feed two surviving gorillas, Mokolo and Bebac, foods closer to what they would find in the wild. From that day forth, zookeepers wheeled out 10 pounds of fibrous vegetables including dandelion greens, romaine lettuce, endive, alfalfa, green beans, flaxseeds, and a multivitamin hidden in half a mashed banana for good measure.

Although Mokolo and Bebac consume about twice as many calories on their "wild" diet, the two gorillas dropped nearly 65 pounds each in the first year and now weighing in the range of their wild counterparts. But it's not just gorillas that benefit from going wild.

Many pet owners find that the weight, health, and vitality of their furry friends improves when fed their native, raw diet. We feed our Labrador, Bailey, raw meaty bones, scraps, and off-cuts of meat as often as we can, and she has more mojo than we know what to do with. See page 316 for tips on how to feed your pets Wild.

"BUT IF PROCESSED FOOD WERE SO DANGEROUS, SOMEONE WOULD HAVE TOLD ME!"

I'm telling you. We all want to believe that omnipresent regulatory agencies with their legions of scientists protect us from the profiteers in Big Food, or at least that chemical companies and food manufacturers act responsibly in the interest of public health.

Big Food execs work in an environment where profits and shareholders come first, not your health. After suffering through more boardroom meetings than I'd care to remember in my time as a consultant, I know for a fact that most processed food manufacturers won't go out of their way to tell you anything that might hurt their bottom line. They want you to buy their food, not be suspicious of it. But our sense of security is misplaced.

Big Food is expected to police itself, which it does just about as well as Wall Street. Unfortunately, regulators and advocacy groups—even if they do have your best interests at heart—are years behind Big Food, which can churn out newfangled chemicals and invent foodstuffs with incredible efficiency and speed to make a quick buck.

A century ago, four out of ten of us were farming. Today, farmers number four in *one hundred* and most work on large-scale petro-chemical-fueled monocrops like GMO corn, canola, and soy—a landscape that would have been utterly unrecognizable as a farm to previous generations that believed a good harvest came from working *with* the land, not against it.

This information is not meant to inspire paranoia or conspiracy theories. The people who run Big Food aren't evil, just shortsighted and often irresponsible with our health. As long as you limit your exposure, it's quite likely that the effects of all of these fake foods and foreign substances will be minimal. Do the best you can.

Remember: Your body is a biochemical marvel. It can squeeze every last bit of nutrition out of any substance remotely resembling food. Your body can literally turn Twinkies into fingernails. With mystical powers like that, is it really so hard to believe this simple, straightforward idea: that you can burn fat if you eat the foods our bodies are adapted to eat, and break a sweat from time to time? There is hope!

The takeaway? Real food—natural plants and animals that we have been consuming safely for thousands of generations—is always a safer choice than processed food. The closer you can get a food to its source, the better. Read the ingredients, take the extra step to find farm-fresh food, and meet the people who get dirt under their fingernails to make sure you have a hearty meal on your dinner table. Taking the extra effort to understand where your food comes from may be uncomfortable when you realize that some of it isn't as healthy as you once might have believed, but it's one of the most rewarding things you can ever do for your health and well-being.

PART II

The Wild Body

> **Life in all its fullness is Mother Nature obeyed.**
>
> —*Weston A. Price*

WHAT WONDERFUL GENES YOU HAVE

Most of us are "getting old" too soon and settling for far less energy and vitality than we deserve. Through instinct, animals stay lean and vital in the wild despite eating as they please when food is available. With a little bit of practice, you can do the same. In this part, you'll learn how to tweak your lifestyle and habits to make your Wild genes thrive.

We once thought that we were shackled to "bad genes"—the ones that steal our youth, cripple our bodies, and bum us out every time the doctors talk about them. But research is clear—lifestyle factors like how you eat, where you live, and how you move are each inputs of information your body analyzes to turn certain genes on and off. Any look at a "before and after" fat-loss picture reveals that the "after" often looks like a different person, with well-formed muscles, tight and clear skin, and improved posture. Your genes know how to thrive, too, and you can drive your body to adapt to remarkable health with careful tweaking to your lifestyle.

Epi-genetics is a cutting-edge science that demonstrates that the air you breathe, food you eat, way you move, and even the thoughts you entertain can reprogram your genes for better or worse. You are endowed with a genetic program 3.5 billion years in the making that knows how to build a healthy body. The code is there. But in the modern world, the ancient biological systems once designed to help us thrive can work against us.

The turbocharged, polluted, high-tech world we live in is a far cry from what our Stone Age genetics were expecting, and we're suffering as a result. We didn't always settle for a diagnosis of diabetes, cancer, or heart disease before our time. These diseases of the industrial world are not rooted in genetic inevitabilities but self-inflicted conditions that are a direct result of how we eat and the way we live. "Domesticated" bodies are overfed yet undernourished, sedentary but stressed, and confronted with an environment that is increasingly polluting our air, water, earth, and food.

Once upon a time, all humans were "wild" and nomadic hunter-gatherers. Before the industrial revolution, cities, and agriculture, everything was wild, native, and organic. This is how your body was, and is still, designed to live. But instead of fleeing terrifying beasts that want to eat us for lunch, now we need to use all the willpower and energy we can muster to dodge food all day.

Our bodies haven't adapted to the intentionally addictive products of Big Food and the environment of drive-thru convenience that comes along with it. Molten chocolate cakes don't exist in nature, nor do Slurpees or deep-fried ice cream; the sheer amount of sugar in these gut bombs would have been nearly impossible for our ancestors to obtain in the natural world. For instance, you'd need to down 3 pounds of carrots for the sugar equivalent of one bottle of Coke. Modern food products play to—and take advantage of—our instinct to binge on sweets designed to fatten us up in preparation for the meager times ahead.

The main philosophy of *The Wild Diet* is that the closer we can get to the environment our genes expect—the world of our ancestors—the more our bodies will thrive. Animals that eat their native diet in their natural habitat enjoy lives free of the diseases of modern civilization. But for better or worse, we don't live in the same world as our ancestors. The utopian wilderness our genes expect doesn't exist where most of us live but can still be found in camping trips and outdoor adventures. Thankfully, while industrial progress has left us with an increasingly unnatural world, it has also provided tools to fight back. In comes modern technology.

HOW TO LIVE WILD IN A WORLD OF TECH: A CASE STUDY

These days, most of us can't go out to forage for berries on the prairie or butcher our own wild boar. So to help explain how you can apply the back-to-roots principles of living Wild, I figure I might as well tell you precisely what's happening right now.

As I type this sentence, I'm soaking up the afternoon sun that peeks in through the live oak tree outside my window. My watch tells me that I slept like a rock last night. It's also tracking my movement, temperature, perspiration, heart rate, and sleep—uploading everything wirelessly from my wrist to the Cloud. This allows me to see how changes in my behavior, mind-set, and activity affect my biology. I'm barefoot, haven't eaten a meal in nearly twenty-four hours (don't worry, I feel terrific), and I'm wearing prescription lenses that block blue light to help regulate my circadian rhythm and reduce iStrain from my iMac. . . .*

Whenever I get stuck, I take a break to unplug and clear my head by avoiding visual, auditory, and other sensory distractions. In fact, I composed a few passages of this book while "floating" in a sensory deprivation tank, but I wrote most of it outside or in view of the window in daylight hours while fasting. By delaying my large meals until later in the day, I channel my energy to productive work throughout the day and save my feasting (and food coma) for the evening hours.

I do my best work in the woods, taking breaks for a hike with the dog, conquering a mountain on the bike, or howling old bluegrass songs where there's no one around to hear me. While I may edit and hone my work on machines, I do the vast majority of thinking when I'm on adventures in the wilderness, never without my notebook and a good pen.

*In case you were wondering how much of a nerd I am, I'm glad to have saved you the trouble. There's even a fitness tracker on my dog.

Later in this part, you will learn how to upgrade your health, productivity, and performance using what I call *holistic* biohacking. If you think of Western medicine as getting a patient from "sick" to normal, think of Holistic Biohacking as bringing your body from "normal" to "super-normal" by optimizing your lifestyle for health and performance. But first, let's talk about sex.

Like pretty snowflakes, we are all biochemically unique. Depending on your sex, genetics, body type, age, activity level, hormones, brain, rhythm, gut bacteria, enzymes, metabolism, and many other factors, the exact same diet will have different results for you than for your significant other, next-door neighbor, sibling, or even your identical twin.

You probably have an annoying friend or family member who never seems to gain a pound despite eating whatever they want, whenever they want. Good for them. But before you get envious, know that the genetic freaks with perpetual six-packs and see-through skin are also the first to starve in a famine. Variability in a population increases the likelihood of survival of the species as a whole. And that's good news for everyone.

HE SHED, SHE SHED: HOW MEN AND WOMEN BURN FAT DIFFERENTLY

Body Composition

Women are genetically designed to have a lower percentage of muscle and more body fat than men, principally to support the biological processes of pregnancy and childbirth. Because women naturally have less muscle than men, they typically have lower basal metabolic rates. This means that men, with a higher percentage of muscle, require more calories than women of comparable weight. Additionally, men are taller on average than women and require more daily calories to maintain their size.

Hormones

Women are naturally predisposed to store and retain more fat due to higher levels of estrogen, a hormone that works to keep the fat on the female body in preparation for pregnancy. Men, on the other hand, have twenty to thirty times more testosterone than the average woman, which often leads to lower body fat and increased muscle mass. This disparity in testosterone, the male sex hormone, is largely responsible for differences between men and women in total body fat percentage, fat distribution, and muscle mass. There are athletic trade-offs as well—men tend to be more muscular and women more flexible due to differences in genetics, hormones, and bone structure.

Fat Storage

Women typically store fat in their thighs, hips, and limbs, known as "peripheral" fat, and beneath the skin, which is called "subcutaneous" fat. Men tend to store more body fat in the upper body and within the body cavity, which is called "visceral" or intra-abdominal fat. Although all body fat is chemically similar, where it's stored on the body makes a significant difference in how hazardous it is to your health. While the female body tends to store the less-damaging peripheral fat underneath the skin, men tend to store damaging visceral fat that accumulates beneath muscles and surrounds organs. This often takes the form of the dreaded "beer belly."

Beer bellies aren't just unsightly, they're downright dangerous. The visceral fat that wraps around organs and forms beer bellies drastically increases the risk of diabetes, hypertension, sleep apnea, impotence, cancer, heart attack, and stroke. In fact, regardless of overall weight, men with waists exceeding 40 inches have double the death rate of those with normal waist circumference. Fortunately, hiding beneath every set of love handles and every beer belly there is a six-pack. We're going to find yours.

Muscle Gains

Many women hesitate to incorporate weight training into their weekly routines because they believe it will lead to brutish, hulk-like muscles. Unless you're taking growth hormones, testosterone, or steroids, that won't happen to you. The female body does not naturally have sufficient levels of hormones to achieve anything close to "bodybuilder" size. Trust me—you have nothing to worry about. My petite wife, Alyson, impresses onlookers at the gym with heavy dead lifts, squats, and swings and has never been slimmer or stronger.

Protein Consumption

Men generally carry higher muscle mass and lower body fat than women, so they tend to need more protein to maintain their size. That said, most people do not eat enough protein for optimal health; this is especially true for women. Meat is not a "man's" food. To support the biological processes of ovulation, menstruation, and pregnancy, some nutrients that are only found in animal foods are arguably even more critical for women's health. If you prefer not to eat meat, do your best to get protein from nuts, seeds, legumes, leafy greens, and whole grains. See "The Wild Diet for Vegetarians and Vegans" on page 312 for more.

Rate of Fat Loss

You may have noticed that while women often cut calories and exercise constantly with sluggish results, some men are mysteriously able to shed pounds seemingly without effort. This is not an illusion: Due to differences in hormones, metabolism, and body composition, males do tend to lose fat a bit more quickly while female bodies fight to hold on to it. Most of these sex differences stem from the fact that female hormones readily store extra fat to prepare a woman's body for the significant energy demands of ovulation, pregnancy, lactation, and childbirth.

If you're petite, you may lose weight more slowly than those who are larger. As such, pay attention to improvements in body composition rather than strict weight loss by the numbers. But there are some advantages to being smaller—even a small amount of weight loss will be quite evident on a small frame.

For both men and women, it is important not to measure success by looking at the scale but by how you look in the mirror, the way you feel in clothes, and/or by body fat percentage. Muscle weighs more than fat, water weight fluctuates according to a variety of factors, and weighing yourself constantly will drive you bananas. I've gained and lost 5 to 10 pounds in the same day on many occasions, none of which have anything to do with my love handles. Forget the scale and measure your progress by how you look and feel instead. Watching the scale won't help you lose fat more quickly, but watching what you eat will.

FAT-LOSS TIPS

For Women

INDULGENCE IS IMPORTANT, BUT SO IS MODERATION

What foods truly bring you pleasure? What foods could you eat less of? What foods do you eat to pointless excess? The pleasure comes in the first few bites of food—anything more is unnecessary and upsets the balance of your body. It is far more important and satisfying to eat small amounts of many tasty foods than enormous portions of one or two. You can really enjoy a little bit of anything as a treat.

LEARN THE ART OF BALANCE

Balancing your meals is an art learned with practice. If you have an extra glass of wine, then skip the cheese. If you have a rich lunch, have a light dinner. "Overdoing it" should always be followed by an active effort to restore balance. If it's easier, think of your nutrition in weeks, not days. Eating a vegetable or a protein every meal is a good guideline, but it's unnecessarily prescriptive. If you find that you don't have enough access to vegetables one day and eat several extra servings of protein, that's fine. On the next day, prioritize fibrous fruits and green veggies to maintain balance.

EMBRACE THE RULE OF QUALITY OVER QUANTITY

Most Americans are accustomed to eating very low-quality food. When you replace junk substitutes with the real thing, you immediately realize that less is more. Savoring one single piece of real chocolate is far more satisfying than eating a dozen Hershey's bars (which, oddly, contain more GMO corn than real chocolate [cocoa]). Go for the good stuff—you deserve it.

FASTING MAY BE MORE EFFECTIVE FOR MEN THAN WOMEN

In the next section, we'll cover my cyclical approach to eating, which I call "fasting and feasting." While the hormonal environment in the male body is relatively consistent, the fluctuating hormones in a woman's body are easily disrupted. While fasting works well for some women, fasting too much can stress the adrenals and cause your hormones to rebel. Adrenal burnout comes quickly when you combine hormetic stressors like exercise and fasting, especially if you're not sleeping well or you're emotionally drained. Listen to your body—if you find that going without a meal works well for you, know that there are many benefits to doing so. If not, plan ahead and make sure you have a steady source of healthy food that's always ready for when hunger strikes—like nuts, veggies, fruit, and the always-convenient leftovers.

For Men

TESTOSTERONE—GET SOME

If you're experiencing symptoms such as decreased sex drive, erectile dysfunction, memory problems, or depressed mood, low testosterone may be to blame. Testosterone plays a critical role in sexual and reproductive function, muscle mass, hair growth, bone density, and more. But a man's production of testosterone begins to decline around age thirty and continues to do so as he ages.

As a man gets older, he tends to lose muscle mass and gain fat, largely due to a natural reduction in the body's production of testosterone and growth hormone. Since fatty tissue doesn't require the same amount of energy to maintain lean muscle, he gains weight over time even if his diet remains consistent. While women put weight on their breasts, hips, and limbs, men store fat around the gut, where it circulates through the liver, causing metabolic problems like diabetes. This extra fat puts you at risk of cancer, heart attack, hypertension, and sleep apnea and can also affect your sex life.

What if one nut could increase your metabolism, raise your testosterone, and boost your sex drive? Say hello to your new friend, the Brazil nut. High in healthy fat, protein, and trace minerals, Brazil nuts are one of the highest dietary sources of selenium, an essential trace mineral and potent antioxidant. Selenium boosts testosterone levels in men and improves sperm production and motility. Brazil nuts are also rich in the amino acid arginine, which increases levels of blood to the genitals. That's right—in the supermarket, nature's Viagra is found in the "nut" section.

TROUBLE IN THE BEDROOM?

If you've ever had trouble getting your mojo workin', you're not alone. A recent study found that about 49 percent of men ages forty to seventy-nine with high blood pressure had erectile dysfunction. Another study, published in the *Journal of Urology*, found that 68 percent of men with high blood pressure had some degree of erectile dysfunction. For 45 percent of the men, it was considered severe.

While the ephemeral diagnoses of high blood pressure can be easy to ignore or deny, impotence gets a man's attention. Did you know that impotence isn't just a problem with your erectile capabilities but actually one of the most obvious symptoms of high blood pressure, elevated triglycerides, and the initial stages of heart disease?

High blood pressure prevents the arteries that carry blood into the penis from fully dilating, while the smooth muscle in the penis loses its ability to relax. As a result, the body fails to send enough blood into the penis to make it erect. For that reason and many others, you don't want high blood pressure.

Can't I Just Pop a Pill for That?

If you watch the commercials during football games—you know the ones, with the good-looking silver-haired man in his Mustang and a hot trophy wife sitting shotgun—you'd think that taking drugs for sexual dysfunction is fashionable. But many prescription drugs work against each other, fixing one problem but breaking something else. For example, commonly prescribed medications that treat high blood pressure—like diuretics and beta-blockers—actually *cause* erectile dysfunction, and statins can decrease production of testosterone.

If you want to improve your performance in the bedroom, get your diet in line and engage in high-intensity interval training and/or strength training. By balancing insulin and boosting growth hormone, fasting can also help normalize blood pressure. Spare yourself the embarrassing trip to the doctor and an expensive prescription by eating Wild and committing to high-intensity workouts to bulk up and lean down as quickly as possible.

BE A REAL MAN AND COMMIT

The male body seems to get away with more overeating, laziness, and misbehavior than the female body. I've seen men achieve the impossible—losing 20 pounds in a week, dropping down to a skeletal 3 percent body fat in less than a month eating mostly fat, and fast for weeks without losing muscle or strength. As long as they eat clean and exercise consistently, most men tend to have an easier time losing fat and building muscle than women. The problem is, women tend to pay more attention to their bodies, so their level of commitment tends to be higher.

I know it's not "cool" for a man to care about his "diet," but if you can't do it for yourself, do it for your family and friends who care about you and want to keep you around for a long time. The better your health now, the more years in your life and life in your years. When you commit to eating right and staying in shape, you'll have more time with the people you love.

"But my friends will make fun of me for being on a diet!"

Maybe, but they'll also start coming to you for fitness advice when you're the only one in the group with a six-pack.

YOUR MICROBIOME: THE HUMAN ECOSYSTEM

Humans are more of an "ecosystem" than a single organism. Believe it or not, the human digestive tract is home to a dizzying quantity of tiny gut bugs (bacteria) that outnumber human cells ten to one. These bacteria are storehouses for an enormous amount of genetic information—genes that are switched on and off depending on the health of your microbiome, how you exercise, your diet, stress, how much sugar you eat, and much more.

The quantity and quality of your gut flora play an essential role in how you digest your food and how well you are able to obtain nutrients from it. Gut bacteria predigest your food, provide immune protection, and even release neurotransmitters that affect your behavior and mood (some refer to the gut as your "second brain"). Let's meet the two main categories of bacteria, the good guys and the bad guys:

- Probiotic (good) bacteria aid digestion, release nutrients, and protect the digestive system against dangerous pathogens. Fiber and raw fermented food feed good bacteria. Traditional methods of food fermentation yield positive probiotic bacteria that are readily introduced into your digestive tract. Our favorite fermented foods that you might find fizzing on our counter include kimchi, sauerkraut, yogurt, kefir, and kombucha.
- Pathogenic (bad) bacteria invade the body, steal nutrients, and release toxins into the bloodstream. Sugar feeds the bad bacteria, or "sugar bugs," the bad guys. Fasting and eating low carb starves "sugar bugs" of their main fuel source, and eating probiotic-rich foods and vegetable fiber helps to heal your gut and expel pathogenic bacteria.

The old saying "you are what you eat" is true, but it's incomplete. Your body can't access the energy in food the second it crosses your lips—you must digest and metabolize the food first. You have to disassemble your food before it's "reassembled" as part of your body or eliminated as waste. You aren't what you eat, you're what you *absorb* and assimilate. Since the gut and liver alter nutrients before they enter the bloodstream, the nutritional content of the food (what it says on the label) is fundamentally different from the nutrients and energy that are absorbed by your cells.

The types of bacteria living in and on your body also dictate whether you store fat or burn it as fuel. Lab studies have shown that the wrong species of bacteria in mice can make them gain fat no matter what they eat. We're just beginning to understand how these bacteria affect our own biology, but suffice it to say that I do my best to be good to my gut.

Just like you eat and excrete nutrients, bacteria do, too. While the bad bugs (pathogenic bacteria) excrete toxins and other substances that can disrupt metabolic processes, good bugs (probiotics) release vitamins and nutrients into your bloodstream. Bad bugs thrive on sugar, and good bugs thrive on fiber. Make sure you feed the right ones.

ANTIBIOTICS, CANONS, AND MOSQUITOS

With many of us popping antibiotics like candy, it's important to note that taking an antibiotic kills off not just the bad bacteria but the good bacteria in your gut as well. When you think about the literal meaning of anti-biotics (anti-life), that starts to make sense. Take antibiotics with caution, and make sure you use them only when absolutely necessary. If you do take an antibiotic, eat extra fermented, probiotic foods and round it out with a soil-based probiotic supplement to get your gut back on track. While prescriptions can clearly be useful and, at times, lifesaving tools, pills are also very easy to abuse.

The average American age forty-five and older is on four different prescription medications, a number I'd argue is far too high. Not only are synthetic drugs expensive, but they also cause side effects, steal nutrients, and interact unpredictably within the body. When I started using food as a tool to heal, I noticed that the symptoms I used drugs to treat—high blood pressure, insomnia, nagging colds and viruses, joint pain, allergies, and more—resolved themselves without pill-popping. I noticed another benefit of going wild—the several hundred dollars a month once spent on prescriptions were delightfully redirected to artisanal cheese, pâté, aged prosciutto, and the occasional bold Cabernet.

Be Good to Your Gut

In these days of fake food and broken guts, food intolerances and sensitivities are incredibly common. Many people do not realize that their unknown, undiagnosed food allergies and intolerances—primarily to processed grains, legumes, and dairy—are responsible for their weight gain, inefficient digestion, bloating, skin problems, allergies, and other health issues. Despite individual variance in food sensitivity and allergy, nearly everyone can benefit from eating more fresh, nutrient-dense fruits and vegetables.

Processed foods damage the gut, while most real, whole foods help to heal it. The Wild Diet helps heal "leaky gut" and other afflictions by encouraging consumption of plant and fruit fiber (which determines the amount and type of bacteria that thrive in your system), adding regular fermented food to your diet, and creating an environment that allows probiotic bacteria to thrive. Sugar bugs, be gone!

We almost always have something fizzing, bubbling, or growing on the counter— kombucha, sourdough, sauerkraut, sprouting seeds, and more. My friend and fellow author Tucker Max taught me this trick: If you want to improve the probiotic punch of store-bought kombucha, twist the cap and let it sit on the counter for a few days. The good bacteria in the bottle will go straight to work digesting the residual sugars, which will leave you with an authentic low-sugar fermented drink without the weeks of attention it usually takes to make kombucha from scratch.

The Cyclical Rhythm of Fasting and Feasting

The concept of time doesn't play a factor in most diets. But failing to address *when* we eat misses a critical dimension, one that could be the difference between vibrant health and unshakable sickness.

Against the relentless onslaught of advertising that taunts our deep-seated, primal urge to eat as often as we can, willpower isn't enough. Every thirty seconds, most of us are interrupted by a boisterous distraction that demands our gustatory attention:

"Quarter-Pound Hamburger for 99 cents!"

"Pizza! Pizza!"

"Hungry? Grab a Snickers."

Unlike our ancestors, who spent all day chasing a beast and all evening enjoying it, the smells, sights, and sizzles of food nag at us 24/7. In a world where everyone is eating all the time, it's difficult to know when we should actually eat.

As it turns out, three square meals a day—breakfast, lunch, and dinner—is arbitrary, more a cultural artifact than a biological necessity. The modern man isn't just eating *more* than he ever has but—critically—*more often* than he ever has. Eating from dawn to dusk gives our bodies a steady stream of glucose, damaging in excess. Without a break from the taxing requirements of digestion, most of our population is faced with insulin resistance, weight gain, and disease.

"Fasting and Feasting" is what I call a rhythm of meal timing that maximizes the hormonal benefits of under- and overeating. While skipping just the occasional meal can be beneficial, cycling periods of fasting (usually in the morning) and feasting (usually at night) can aid detoxification, encourage fat burning, and improve immune function. Fasting and feasting isn't meant to be a dogmatic—it's simply the concept that your body thrives by following a cyclical approach to eating and digestion.

By one definition, fasting means "to abstain from all food." But it also means "to eat sparingly, or of certain types of foods." For the most part, I'm talking about the latter, less draconian definition. In the same way that our muscles and bodies recover from plenty of rest, wouldn't it hold that our digestive system would benefit from an occasional break from food?

Fasting Is Good for You

If you could put the mental, physical, and spiritual benefits of fasting in a pill, you would make billions. The many benefits of fasting include:

- Promoting human growth hormone production, which helps your body burn fat, build muscle, and slow the aging process
- Normalizing insulin sensitivity, which prevents chronic disease like diabetes, heart disease, and even cancer
- Normalizing ghrelin levels, also known as "the hunger hormone"
- Decreasing triglyceride levels
- Reducing inflammation and reducing free radical damage

While most nutritionists argue that we eat too much, I argue that we simply eat too *often*. By undereating most of the day and filling up at night, most people also find that they eat significantly less food (and save money) once they start fasting.

Let's dig a little deeper.

Calorie Restriction and Cyclical Undereating

Since the 1930s, animal studies have been telling us that restricting calories improves health and longevity. Until recently, we believed that it was necessary to "starve yourself" to reap the benefits. But you can actually trim your waistline, improve your biomarkers of health, and increase your longevity without the pain, suffering, and hunger that comes along with restriction. Fasting works, too, but since it's difficult for Big Food to profit from people going without their food, most of the benefits of skipping meals don't make it into common wisdom.

There's a monumental difference between "common" and "normal," however. Today, more than 67 percent of us in the United States are overweight or obese. Being overweight is common. But it's not normal. Fasting, on the other hand, is historically quite normal but isn't common in a world abundant with drive-thrus, meal-replacement shakes, and "eating 6+ times a day is healthy" dogmatism. For millions of people across the world, regular fasting is commonplace and has been part of spiritual practice for thousands of years. But before that, fasting was simply a way of life.

With no storable grains, and few other foods that stayed fresh for very long, most of our ancestors experienced both feast and famine on a regular basis. When game was scarce, seasons changed, or the pickings were slim, hunter-gatherers did without. To reap the full rewards of the Wild lifestyle, you might consider going without occasionally, too.

Antiaging Effects of Fasting

We've known for many years that eating less increases life-span in humans and animals, but "starving yourself" doesn't appear to be gaining much traction. Thousands of studies have shown that when animals are placed on a calorie-restricted diet, they invariably outlive their frequently fed counterparts. The longest-living and most disease-free cultures on the planet eat significantly less than the average American.

If you're over the age of thirty, and especially if you lead a sedentary lifestyle, you've likely entered a phase known as somatopause, or age-related growth hormone deficiency. Natural production of growth hormone declines beginning in our twenties, leading to a reduction in lean body mass and bone mineral density and an increase in body fat—especially abdominal fat. As growth hormone declines over time, you begin to look and feel older.

Here's the good news: Fasting sets in motion a hormonal chain of events that not only burns fat but also protects hard-earned muscle. After approximately sixteen to twenty-four hours in a fasted state, our bodies release a massive surge of growth hormone. One study showed that while fasting for twenty-four hours, human growth hormone increased an average of 1,300 percent in women and nearly 2,000 percent in men. But be careful: Depending on your unique situation, many find that you do begin to lose muscle with fasts that are longer than twenty-four hours. Listen to your body and eat when you're hungry.

Another activity that can lead to a dramatic increase in growth hormone is high-intensity interval exercise like the 7-Minute Wild Interval Workout (see pages 81 to 83). Combining fasting with high-intensity exercise can provide synergistic effects to boost growth hormone. In adulthood, the presence of growth hormone leads to a healthier body composition. Growth hormone:

- Keeps your body lean
- Increases synthesis of new protein tissues to promote muscle recovery and repair

- Decreases fat accumulation
- Strengthens bones
- Protects your organs from the decline that occurs with age
- Promotes healthy hair and nail growth
- Improves circulation
- Gives a more favorable cholesterol profile
- Decreases signs and symptoms of aging

Did I mention that fasting is free and you can start right now?

Breakfast: The Most Dangerous Meal of the Day

Would you eat donuts for a "healthy" breakfast? Believe it or not, most products marketed as heart-healthy "breakfast foods"—cereal, granola, oatmeal, bagels, yogurt, and muffins—pack more sugar than a deep-fried, sugar-coated Krispy Kreme donut. Some cereals are even packed with more processed sodium than a bag of potato chips.

Cereal is a shining example of a product that Big Food intentionally mislabels to make it appear "healthier" than it actually is. In an analysis of 1,556 popular cereals, researchers at the Environmental Working Group found that "97 percent of the most common class of cold cereals have labels that underestimate the amount of cereal people actually eat." Since the serving sizes on cereal labels are unrealistically small, many Americans unintentionally eat more than one "serving" in a single bowl.

Many popular cereals are packed with more sugar than a scoop of ice cream, a jelly donut, or a slice of chocolate cake. Honey Smacks contains more than 50 percent sugar, and Apple Jacks, Froot Loops, and Corn Pops all contain 12 grams of sugar and almost zero fiber in the paltry serving listed on the side of the box. For perspective, a glazed donut from Dunkin' Donuts contains 12 grams of sugar. Surprised?

When you look at the ingredients in cereal and donuts, you really don't see much of a difference. Donuts are made from processed flour, sugar, and industrial oil. Cereal is made from processed flour, sugar, and . . . industrial oil.

Here's why that's a problem: Nobody eats a donut for breakfast and thinks they're doing themselves a favor. But how many people eat cereal for breakfast (or dinner) and assume that it is good for them? Cereal and bagels got me through college, but I didn't know I was eating dessert for breakfast.

People who start their days with carb-y, high-glycemic foods like cereal, muffins, bagels, and fruit juice ignite a vicious cycle of hunger and snacking. The flood of insulin in the hours following breakfast leads to low energy, brain fog, and nagging cravings and hunger throughout the day.

As any endurance athlete or adventurer quickly learns, most of your energy comes not from what you eat for breakfast but from your dinner the night before. The more nourishing and substantial your evening feast, the more you can do or longer you can go without eating the next day. Eating the *right* breakfast can help regulate your blood sugar, but it's not actually burned for fuel that day. Since the body takes eight to sixteen hours to process your meals, the majority of each day's fuel comes from the dinner you ate the evening before. Eating your most substantial meal in the evening can help release endorphins, improve sleep quality, reduce next-day hunger, and provide energy to fuel activities the next morning.

When I began fasting regularly, I learned that I tend not to get hungry until I start eating. Hunger pangs and cravings pass quickly, usually dissipating after just a few minutes. Once you fast for a few hours, your body moves carbohydrates out of glycogen stores in your muscles and liver to provide energy to fuel your brain and hunger is reduced.

According to our circadian rhythm, melatonin rises after sundown to help us sleep, and cortisol—a stress hormone—rises in the morning hours to wake us up. If you eat in the morning when blood cortisol is high, however, high-glycemic carbs cause insulin to spike and decrease sensitivity to insulin. That's one of the reasons you might be starving a couple of hours after a big, carb-y breakfast. Eating from dawn to dusk, while it certainly works for some people (especially those who eat real food), can also provoke an insatiable urge to keep eating. How often have you stared at the clock, eager for the next mealtime? Frequent snacking trains your body to be hungry. Fasting does precisely the opposite.

The more you adapt to burning fat by eating fewer carbs and occasionally fasting, the less you think about food. When you can get through your day without the distraction of constant hunger, you can get a heck of a lot more done. Enjoy the energy that comes with digestion-free workdays as your peers look on in awe.

When you graze on frequent meals throughout the day, your body assumes that you live in a time of plenty and spends energy readily. A steady supply of glucose leads your cells to divide readily to perform bodily functions, store fat, and build muscle—you can think of this as "build" mode. Cell division is biologically expensive, however; research suggests that constant grazing may accelerate the aging process by decreasing the length of telomeres. Fasting, however, signals your cells that it's time to focus the body's energy on conserving, restoring, and repairing your body's internal machinery. You can think of fasting as "cleanse" mode, where your cells scavenge your body for free radicals, agents of disease, and damaged cells and recycles them to conserve energy. The trade-off is that too much fasting can stress the adrenals, so occasional luxurious feasting can actually help keep the body in balance.

HOW TO BEAT FALSE HUNGER

True hunger is generally experienced in the body and brain, not in the stomach. If you get light-headed or weak, or your workout suffers, you're probably fasting too much. It may take some practice, but once you reconnect with the feeling of true hunger, you can follow your body's lead and eat whenever the feeling strikes.

Whenever you get hungry, ask yourself:

• Am I thirsty? Drink water and cravings may subside.
• Have I had my fill of greens and fiber today? Go for a salad, veggies, or a green smoothie.
• Am I emotional or bored? Wait twenty minutes, go for a walk, or exercise.
• Did I drink alcohol recently? Your body is probably tricking you into thinking you're hungry because your insulin is out of whack.

- Have I eaten my fill of protein today? Grab some.
- Did I eat sugar, grains, fried food, or other "carbage"? Your insulin and blood sugar are unstable. You probably don't need more food. Wait it out.
- Have I exercised today? Try it and you might find you're not hungry anymore.
- Am I fasting too much? Go ahead and eat. Bonus if you make raw green veggies the first thing to hit your belly.

What If I Really Need Breakfast?

No problem. If you want to lose fat and you prefer not to fast, eat a light, low-carb, high-protein breakfast. If you like savory, farm-fresh eggs are tough to beat. A green smoothie or plain yogurt with nuts and berries is also a filling, nutritious, and convenient breakfast. But remember—eating too many carbs early in the day can make you feel sluggish because the insulin flood shifts your body to "rest and digest" mode, which is great for falling asleep at night but not great when it hits midday. To maximize fat loss, save your carbs (and insulin) until directly after your workout (to build muscle and refuel glycogen stores) and your evening meal. If you eat a particularly large or rich meal (or know you will for dinner), scale back the other meals to avoid overdoing it.

But if you find you are not hungry in the morning, there's no need to force it. Many people find that after their first few tries fasting, hunger doesn't come until you "flip the switch" by eating something.

FREE YOURSELF FROM FOOD

When I started taking fasting seriously, my energy and productivity doubled, I dropped fat while gaining muscle, and I was finally freed from the unrelenting hunger that plagued me for most of my life. Interestingly, I also learned that I don't tend to get hungry until whenever I choose to have my first meal, usually in the afternoon. Many of my listeners are surprised to learn that I record my weekly hour-long shows on the same day back-to-back, often eight or more without a meal. When I'm finished with work in the evening, I'm ready to *feast*.

But wait—why would you get more energy from eating less often? As anyone who's just polished off a slice of birthday cake knows, digestion takes energy. Bloating, brain fog, that banal, empty feeling where you just want to take a nap—this is "rest and digest" mode, when your body redirects the energy that otherwise would have been used to fuel the brain and body to try to make use of whatever the heck was in that corn dog. Ugh.

"WHAT'D YOU HAVE FOR LUNCH?"

When Alyson and I showed up at the photo shoot for the cover of this book at one thirty in the afternoon, my photographer asked cheerfully, "So, what'd you guys have for lunch?"

"We haven't really eaten yet, actually," Alyson replied.

The photographer turned to his wife and smiled. "And *that's* why they're so lean!"

Mentally, I enjoy the freedom that comes with eating later in the day. While everyone else is feverishly trying to figure out what the heck they should eat for their next meal, I'm sipping tea and thinking about something else. If I skip breakfast to get straight to my morning routine and plan for a larger meal later in the day, I find that I'm full of energy until the afternoon or evening without a substantial meal. This affords me an extra couple of hours a day during which I would have otherwise been finding, preparing, or eating breakfast, lunch, and snacks.

So, what do you do while everyone else is eating breakfast and lunch? Anything you want. All the time it normally takes you to find, prepare, and eat extraneous meals has just been transformed into 100 percent free time. If finding, preparing, and eating breakfast and lunch once took a total of two hours a day, that's what you've got. Enjoy that extra two hours to do whatever you please. Think about it . . . an extra two hours of free time every day for the rest of your life. Take that, *4-Hour Workweek*.

Here's how the Fasting and Feasting eating pattern stacks up against a standard American eating schedule.

STANDARD AMERICAN EATING PATTERN

MORNING	Meal 1	Breakfast
	Meal 2	Snack
MIDDAY	Meal 3	Lunch
	Meal 4	Afternoon snack
EVENING	Meal 5	Dinner (and dessert)
	Meal 6	Evening snack

Total: 6 meals. Time to find, prepare, and eat meals: 2 to 3 hours.

FASTING AND FEASTING

MORNING	Beverages	Water, coffee, tea, herbal tonics
MIDDAY	Meal 1	Raw veggies, fruits, nuts, and light snacks
EVENING	Meal 2	Glorious feast (and dessert)

Total: 2 meals. Time to find, prepare, and eat meals: 45 to 60 minutes.

The Fasting Phase: Foods to Eat During Daylight Hours

When I "fast" during the day, I don't always go without *all* calories. I start most mornings with heavy cream in my coffee (pure fat), and I might snack on raw nuts, veggies, or fruit whenever it feels right. Most days, I prefer to eat at least one light meal before my evening feast, usually at midday or in the afternoon. One way I think about Fasting and Feasting is that I eat raw foods during the day and cooked meals at night. Since we spend as many days as we can hiking, mountain biking, or adventuring, we don't cook our first meal until we get back to base camp as the sun sets (a cooked feast is also great for morale). If I get real hunger during daylight hours, I eat light foods that won't steal too much energy for digestion—salads, green smoothies, or even raw vegetables like celery, cucumbers, or carrots for a snack.

Here are a few examples of low-calorie, low-carb, light foods I might eat during "fat-fasting":

- Raw green vegetables like cucumbers or celery
- Grass-fed butter, ghee, or cream (in coffee or melted on leftovers)
- Green smoothie
- Carrots
- Avocado
- Coconut
- Nuts
- Jerky
- Sardines
- Bone broth
- Bone marrow
- Soup
- Plain yogurt
- Raw cheese
- Whole apple or citrus

While undereating during the fasting phase, drink plenty of water and enjoy as many naturally calorie-free drinks such as coffee, tea, and seltzer as you like. When you get hungry, eat freely from the snacks above, but do your best to save your largest meal until the evening feast.

Fasting on a Whim

If you're not hungry at mealtime or just can't find clean food, go ahead and skip a meal every once in a while. Just have a glass of water or an herbal tea. This often happens when I'm traveling, when I didn't plan to skip a meal but it just feels right anyway. Great! This temporary "fasting" will allow your body to burn fat and direct its energy to repair and recovery instead of digestion.

Fasted Exercise for Rapid Fat Loss

If you want to drop fat as quickly as possible, work out fasted. Research suggests that the effects of eating Wild and exercising in a fasted state are synergistic; eating low-carb boosts the body's responses to human growth hormone, while fasted exercise boosts its production. If you're looking to gain muscle, improve recovery, and upgrade performance, this is exactly what you want.

When Not to Fast

Fasting and Feasting is completely optional on the Wild Diet. Fasting is easy when life is good, but it doesn't work for everyone. If you're stressed, sleepless, or someone who burns through calories with reckless abandon with a high metabolism or tons of exercise, you don't need the added stressor of going without food, which can actually increase the risk of overtraining. If you feel dizzy, weak, or confused while fasting, it's time to eat. Food is fuel, so make sure you get enough. The first few times you try fasting, make sure you have plenty of healthy snacks ready when the going gets tough. Take it slow and let your body adapt.

Fasting isn't advisable during pregnancy, while nursing, if you're diabetic, or if you have a history of eating disorders. As mentioned earlier in this part, some women find that skipping meals can lead to weight gain, mood swings, disrupted sleep, and worse. You may find that skipping meals simply isn't for you. That's great—now you know that. If you feel differently in the future, go ahead and try it again to see if you feel the same way. But if going without food for part of the day truly makes you miserable, there's no need to force it.

Before you start fasting, I suggest that you avoid processed carbs, sugars, and starches for a few weeks and fill up on high-protein foods to let your body adapt to running on fat. Once the fat-burning mechanisms of your body are firing on all cylinders, you can learn to trust your hunger and appetite. In a healthy body, you can listen to your instincts and simply eat until you're full.

How to Break Your Fast: The Anabolic Effects of Feasting

If you're worried you'll waste away if you don't suck down a protein shake every two hours, don't be. When I started my experiments with fasting, I was afraid that I would get weak and all of my hard-earned muscles would fall off. But instead, I hit a personal best in my dead lift and gained 10 pounds of lean muscle while consistently skipping breakfast.

My approach to Fasting and Feasting involves eating a generous meal later in the day; usually in the afternoon between noon and three p.m., or whenever I get hungry. This tends to work out to sixteen to twenty hours a day of undereating—running on nothing but fat—and four to eight hours of feasting. When I can, I feast after an intense workout to maximize anabolism (a fancy word that means muscle building and repair).

Each fast concludes with the promise of a big anabolic payoff. To make the best of the surge of growth hormone after sixteen hours of fasting, work out during the last few hours of your fast. Your post-workout feast breaks the fast, and the circulating growth hormone acts to partition the nutrients from your meal to your glycogen stores and muscle fibers. It's natural to crave carbs following exercise because you burned through muscle and liver glycogen during your workout. Eat some, but make sure you go for natural options—such as sweet potatoes, bananas, whole-grain rice, dairy, or coconut water—instead of processed products marketed to athletes. Protein powders are convenient, easy choices for post-exercise feeding, but real fresh food like sweet potatoes, eggs, and dairy are usually better for you.

Fasting and Feasting can also be applied at the macro level by cycling your intake of food on a weekly or monthly basis. Since overeating sometimes happens naturally, I often treat vacations and holidays as an extended feasting phase. Like a bodybuilder in a "building phase," I exercise more frequently and with heavier weights than usual in an attempt to use the extra carbs and calories to grow muscle. When I return to my normal habits, I treat the following few days as a "cleansing" phase. To compensate for overeating during the feasting phase, I fast more often in the days after; drink plenty of teas, tonics, and liquids; and consume smaller meals, primarily green and fibrous vegetables.

Get Started Now: Fasting and Feasting Plan

How do you start? Simple. Tomorrow, make lunch your first meal. If you stop eating at eight p.m. and don't eat until noon the next day, that's sixteen hours of fasting—perfect for stimulating growth hormone, which boosts metabolism, builds muscle, and slows aging. The fact that you sleep through the majority of your fast makes it relatively painless.

If you've trained your body to expect food every two hours, then you might feel hungry the first few times you try fasting. But it will all be in your head. Running just on the fat stored in their bodies, most Americans could walk from New York to Florida without actually needing a bite to eat. Give yourself a week or two for your body to re-learn how to run on fat, and you'll find fasting gets easier.

Fasting shouldn't feel like *forcing* yourself not to eat food. While fasting, you're liberated from having to think about food so you can spend your energy elsewhere. That little voice that usually nags every few minutes, *"Hey, is it time to eat? I think it's time to eat!"* now has a response that works every time. "There's an epic feast coming tonight," you might say. "No need to bother me until then." After all, you have important things to do today.

The best day for your first fast is your day off, perhaps Sunday, so you won't fall prey to the stress of the workday. Do your best to get plenty of sleep and have a satisfying feast the night before your first fast to keep cortisol in check.

YOUR MENU:

9:00 a.m.—Fatty Coffee (page 249): 1 cup of coffee with 1 tablespoon heavy cream, coconut milk, butter, or other real-food fat

Noon—Meal 1: Giant salad with avocado, cucumber, and feta over mixed greens drizzled with olive oil and balsamic

6:00 p.m.—Meal 2: Beef Tenderloin with Buttered Onions, Horseradish, and Arugula (page 181)

7:00 p.m.—Dessert: Strawberries and real grass-fed whipped cream

If you get hungry between lunch and dinner, eat freely of the snacks listed on page 305. Remember to drink plenty of water and spice it up with a bit of herbal tea or club soda with a slice of citrus if you're in the mood for a tasty drink. Good luck—I'll see you on the other side.

WATCH OUT—FASTING MIGHT MAKE YOU SUPERHUMAN

I don't really know how to explain it, but there is a fascinating phenomenon that often kicks in when people try fasting. Once you find that you *can* in fact go without food for some or most of the day with great energy, you ask yourself: "What else am I capable of?" That's where life gets interesting.

I'll offer my own example. In my first two years of regular fasting, I went from a struggling musician with a desk job to a multiple-award-winning talk show host, bestselling author, and millionaire at the reins of the hottest food app publisher in America. With the extra time, clarity, and confidence you get from fasting, you might find that the entire trajectory of your life changes. Get in touch at wilddiet book.com and let me know how it goes.

RECALIBRATE YOUR CIRCADIAN RHYTHM

Have you ever spent all night looking at the ceiling, cursing yourself for not getting a wink of sleep? Me too. I was always a terrible sleeper, lucky to get six hours of restless sleep at most. I'd count hundreds of sheep, take drugs, write, have sex, perform full-body muscle relaxation, meditate, try breathing exercises—nothing seemed to work. Now I sleep like a baby—working on this book, I'm usually conked out by nine thirty p.m. What changed?

Nearly all organisms are programmed to honor cycles of light and dark. We call these cycles circadian rhythms. Our blinding and noisy world of electronics and artificial lights, many of which are bright enough to mimic the sun, upset these rhythms. When your biology is out of sync with your environment, a circadian "mismatch," you pay the price with disrupted sleep, agitation, digestive disorders, constipation, chronic fatigue, chronic cravings for sweets and carbs, fat gain, and decreased resistance to stress.

Your circadian rhythm affects your eating pattern, but few people realize that what you eat and when can recalibrate your circadian rhythm. Habitually eating too much in the morning and throughout the day works against our natural eating patterns and saps energy. Big, heavy, carb-filled meals put our bodies in "rest and digest" mode, when nutrients and energy are diverted to digestion.

Large feasts in the evening can help you fall straight to sleep, so it's best to save heavy meals and carbs until dinner if you want to maximize energy during the day. If you have trouble waking up or falling asleep, consider catching at least fifteen minutes of sunlight in the morning and avoid artificial lights after sundown to reset your circadian rhythm.

Contrary to popular belief, sleeping for eight hours at a time is not necessarily the best way to sleep for everyone. Sleeping this way popped up only within the last hundred years—post industrialization—when artificial lights made it possible to keep working after sunset. But before that, human beings slept more like animals: in two short segments—a long sleep just after dusk, followed by quiet waking time in the middle of the night, and then a return to bed for a morning nap. Don't be afraid to take naps or sleep in—we've been refreshing our bodies and brains with siestas for thousands of years.

When you fall asleep shortly after the natural darkness of the night and wake with the sunrise, without an alarm, feeling rested, you are in sync. If you're thinking that requires more time in your bed, you're right, and you're welcome. Like Benjamin Franklin said, "Early to bed, early to rise, makes a man healthy, wealthy, and wise."

THE BIG SECRET THE TABLOIDS WON'T TELL YOU

Want to know how superstars, fitness models, and professional athletes stay so lean and become superhuman? They sleep. A lot.

No, it's not some sexy new thigh-sculpting machine, fat-blasting wonder drug, or superfood from a country you've never heard of. These specimens of mankind probably just sleep more than you. If you want to cure yourself of nearly any affliction known to man or feel like a rock star, you need more sleep. How do you know when you've had enough? Sleep until you reliably can wake up without an alarm (hopefully somewhere in the neighborhood of the sunrise).

Not only will getting a good night's sleep help to reduce your risk of disease, but it will improve your focus, sharpen your reflexes, and give you the energy you need to rock it. Remember that muscle isn't built in the gym—it recovers and grows while you sleep. Sleep and rest is also prime territory to burn fat. So be honest with yourself—is your four a.m. workout really improving your performance or just stressing you out? A simple rule: If you don't get solid sleep, don't overdo it in your workout. Sounds crazy, but if you exercise smart, you can get away with far less time sweating than you'd expect.

If you have trouble sleeping, try this:

- Get fifteen minutes of sunlight early in the day to reset your circadian rhythm.
- Eat a large feast after sundown and let your "rest and digest" mode trigger an early bedtime.
- Avoid artificial light and electronics after sundown (or use blue-blocking lenses).
- Drink chamomile or kava tea, natural plants that relax the body and mind.
- Supplement 0.5 to 1 mg of melatonin after sundown.
- Carry an eye mask and earplugs in your overnight bag for noisy or bright environments.

- Use heavy, light-blocking shades in your bedroom.

- Avoid strenuous exercise in the hours before sleep.

- Keep your bedroom cool; most people sleep best at less than 70°F.

- Go to bed at the same time every night, even on the weekend, to avoid disrupting hormones.

- Avoid alcohol, which prevents the body from entering deep, restorative sleep (one or two drinks with dinner is fine).

PART III

Wild Movement

> If you're not having fun, you're doing something wrong.
>
> —*Groucho Marx*

The modern world seems like it's built to prevent us from using our bodies. Today, many of us spend the majority of our waking hours seated in front of a desk or steering wheel. Your body doesn't know quite what to make of this, given the fact that humans moved constantly for millennia. We've never *needed* to exercise—physical movement was simply a requirement of life.

Imagine a jaguar stalking silently through the jungle, muscles rippling under its coat. This beast is capable of exploding into action with blinding speed, but all that power is channeled into smooth, fluid, effortless movement—beautiful to watch. This is how humans are meant to move, too: with grace, power, and economy. For the vast majority of human existence, we spent all day moving: walking, running, pulling, pushing, and lifting. These lean, hard bodies—male and female—were required for work and survival.

One of the first Europeans to explore the American Southwest was Álvar Núñez Cabeza de Vaca. He lived among the Native Americans for eight years in the sixteenth century and witnessed their legendary strength and vigor firsthand. Impressed by their epic feats of athleticism during the hunt, he wrote: "The men were happy, generous, with amazing physical prowess. . . . One Native American ran down a buffalo on foot and killed it with his knife as he ran by its side. . . ." The natives were also notoriously difficult to kill: "Traversed by an arrow, he does not die but recovers from his wound. . . ." Cabeza de Vaca continued, "They go naked in the most burning sun, in winter they go out in early dawn to take a bath, breaking the ice with their body."

Our bodies are capable of much more than most of us realize. Remember this the next time you're dreading your workout or standing on the shore of a lake afraid it's too cold to jump in. Your body is meant to withstand hot and cold, and stimulating the biological machinery to adapt to the seasons is good for you. But don't worry—you don't need to live like Tarzan to get as lean and fit as a wild animal.

WHY GRINDING ON A TREADMILL IS NOT THE BEST WAY TO BURN FAT

The diet industry tells us that we need to "burn off" calories if we're to have any hope of dropping a few pounds. Trainers might tell you to spend an hour on an expensive machine that measures all the calories you burn off down to the last Tic-Tac. "Eat less and exercise more!" they declare.

But you don't need to grind it out on the StairMaster all day or powerlift with greased-up meatheads to get in shape. Exercise is not about "burning off" your burger or punishing yourself—it's about your well-being. To put calorie burning into perspective, you'd need sixty minutes on the treadmill to "burn off" the amount of calories in one Starbucks muffin. There's a better way.

In this chapter, you'll learn how to perform simple exercises that drive hormonal and metabolic changes to burn fat, build muscle, and improve performance. You will be amazed at how much you can achieve with a few short, intense bursts of exercise that take just minutes a week.

A "DOSE" OF EXERCISE

There is common assumption that more exercise is better, but it isn't that simple. Some types of exercises are much more effective for fat loss, and they might not be the ones you think.

The best use of exercise isn't for burning off calories but for setting off a hormonal cascade in your body that results in an adaptive response. This process is called hormesis, which is a biological response to low doses of a stressor that improves the ability of the body to handle stressors in the future.

While homeostasis seeks to bring the body to a normal state, hormesis brings the body to a better-than-normal state. For example, when an athlete lifts weights, the stress of the heavy load damages the muscles by overloading them. The body reacts with inflammation and an immune response—in small doses, these otherwise problematic processes are beneficial to the body, as it uses inflammation and stress to rebuild and grow stronger. Whenever your body faces a challenge and you give it what it needs to recover, you come back bigger and better every time you push yourself.

Your body needs to be constantly challenged in order to become stronger and leaner. For most people, it takes a few weeks to adapt to a routine and reach the point of diminishing returns. Doing the same exercises over and over can cause burnout and repetitive stress injuries. Keeping your body guessing and unable to adapt by ensuring variety is part of your exercise routine. If you'd like to build and tone your muscle, prioritize strength-training sessions. If you want to lose fat quickly, prioritize interval training. Once you're strong enough to breeze through your workout, it's time to add to the weight and change it up.

WHY DO I *HAVE* TO EXERCISE?

You can accomplish a lot just by eating Wild. You'll burn fat, build lean muscle mass, and boost your metabolism. Bodybuilders often say that six-packs are carved by spoons—meaning that what you eat (and don't eat) will determine how much fat you carry—and they're right. If you want to drop fat, you need to eat right. But if you want to step it up a notch, you'll have to move your body. With an effective exercise plan, you can kick off a hormonal cascade that moves your physiology toward being lean. You can achieve spectacular fat loss and body composition with far less exercise than the fitness industry would lead you to believe. And it's not only possible but essential that you find exercises and activities that you love.

When someone asks for my secret to six-pack abs, I tell them that it's as much about how I live as how I train. Here's the truth:

I eat clean and fast several times a week. I spend most of the day with my core engaged—standing, moving, or sitting cross-legged. I schedule intense full-body workouts in my calendar and stick to them like I booked a flight.

Exercise isn't about your vanity; it's about your well-being. The flood of endorphins and other raw materials that your body releases during and immediately following exercise literally helps you get stronger and smarter.

An enormous amount of brainpower is dedicated to the countless feats of movement we achieve without even thinking about them. Recent science has shown that the brain can actually grow, adapt, and rewire and repurpose itself—this is known as neuroplasticity. Actively moving and training your body helps your brain *grow* and has been shown not just to improve your body but increase your intelligence as well. This mental and physical training is what allows amateurs to become Olympians, and it's not just their bodies but their brains that adapt to the incredible demands of the professional athlete.

THE POWER OF FULL-BODY, FUNCTIONAL MOVEMENT

There's a reason that Mickey trained Rocky for his fight against Apollo Creed by jumping rope, sprinting up stairs, and chasing chickens through the alley—each task takes an efficient nervous system, quick reflexes, and economical, balanced movement. In the cult wrestling classic *Vision Quest*, while Louden Swain's hopeless competitors train on pegboards and machines, the camera cuts to the freakish, undefeated farm boy adversary who's slogging up the bleachers in the pouring rain with a tree on his shoulders. That's functional movement, and you don't need fancy machines when you train like that.

When you work out, use your whole body. Studies have found that explosive full-body movements like squats, dead lifts, and pull-ups increase our anabolic hormones like growth hormone and testosterone while decreasing circulating cortisol, a stress hormone. On the flip side, isolated exercises like bicep curls aren't a great use of time if you want to lose fat. These one-muscle-at-a-time moves don't stimulate enough muscle fibers to build lean muscle or expend enough energy to maximize your calorie burn, and they lead to only incremental gains in the exact muscles you isolate. Whole-body exercises that target the large muscle groups in the legs and back are a better strategy for fat loss.

WHAT ABOUT MY AB ROLLER?

Despite what the late-night infomercials and checkout-aisle magazines tell you, ab-crunching, -rolling, and -shocking gadgets won't give you a six-pack, and doing traditional ab exercises such as crunches and sit-ups don't cause fat loss on your stomach any more than bicep curls would. The key to getting sculpted abs is to burn off the fat that covers them. This is best achieved by full-body movements that incorporate the large muscle groups—like squats, presses, dead lifts, pull-ups, and kettlebell swings—which set off a hormonal cascade to boost fat metabolism. Once your abs are visible, ab-targeted exercises like planks, crunches, bicycle kicks, and even pull-ups can increase definition.

Aim for balance in your movements to create symmetry in your body. For example, if you're stuck in one position for most of the day, do your best to exercise in the opposite position. If you spend most of the day crouched forward for your job, take on a sport like kayaking that incorporates a full range of motion to open up your back and shoulders. If you've done a few too many push-ups, make sure you strengthen the opposite muscles in your back with rows or another equal-and-opposite movement. (I'm actually writing this on the floor in a "Sphinx" position right now to stretch my back.)

These days, you can learn just about any exercise for free with a search on Google. To ensure you learn correct form for lifting heavy weights or high-intensity exercises, however, I suggest you find a well-respected trainer. Ask him or her to construct a proper high-intensity interval workout with a complementary full-body strength-training program tailored to your specific goals. There are a lot of bad trainers out there—ask friends, check reviews, and don't be afraid to shop around to find a trainer who will motivate you to achieve more than you could on your own.

Poor form leads to injury, and getting hurt will kill your progress. Learn the movement, start slowly, prioritize proper form, and reexamine your movements from time to time to ensure you're not getting sloppy. If a trainer isn't in your budget, spend five bucks and grab a jump rope. Jumping rope provides an awesome full-body workout that will tone you up quickly with minimal effort. And if you think jumping rope is for little girls, it's time to rewatch *Rocky*.

CASE STUDY: HOW TO LOSE FAT BY EXERCISING LESS

When I first studied the science that suggested I could exercise for just minutes a week and lose fat, I had to see it for myself. At the time, I was running 50 miles a week, often for several hours a day. After finishing in the top 3 percent of runners in my previous marathon, I assumed that I was in tip-top running shape. I figured that running less would make me slower and fatter. The results are far more interesting.

By switching from endurance to sprints, I gained 10 pounds, but I actually *lost* body fat! The muscle that came on from my new sprint routine combined with the fat loss increased definition and size in my shoulders and abs. My body regained healthy color and a more masculine shape, and my running speed and strength increased dramatically. I felt *tons* better. Even my face changed from hauntingly thin to healthy and full—all from exercising much *less*.

Have you ever noticed that most endurance athletes are rail-thin, pale, and look a little unhealthy? But what about athletes who are required to perform short bursts of maximum output, like sprinters, linebackers, soccer players, and wide receivers? They're lean and mean!

When it comes to getting lean and fit, your body responds to quality over quantity. Exercise is beneficial only up to a point, after which you start wasting muscle instead of building it, retaining fat instead of burning it, and flooding your body with stress hormones that throw your metabolism out of whack. This is known as overtraining.

If you're overtrained, your body doesn't know you are running a marathon or if you've just been run over by a truck. Your nervous system simply knows that it is experiencing trauma. So, your hormones go wacky, your fight/flight response is heightened, and your body pumps out stress hormones. For long-term training, fat loss, and health, this is all bad news. Because it's always trying to recover from what you just did to it and protecting itself from whatever might happen next, your befuddled body never has a chance to heal. Due to the presence of stress hormones, you readily store fat—the opposite of what you're hoping for when you're putting in all those miles. Give your body time to recover and it will reward you with improved performance and a leaner physique. Remember: You build muscle and burn fat while you sleep, not when you're in the gym.

If you live for endurance athletics like marathons and triathlons, more power to you. Finishing such an event is a tremendous accomplishment. But know that endurance exercise isn't the best solution to fat loss. Intensity trumps endurance when body composition is concerned, so don't skimp on intervals even if you are an endurance athlete. Besides, running is more fun when you pretend you're being chased by a tiger.

THE 7-MINUTE WILD INTERVAL WORKOUT

A word of caution: Intervals are extremely vigorous. If you are a beginner, get your doctor's clearance before attempting any type of high-intensity exercise such as high-intensity interval training.

Want more bang for your buck? If you're short on time, try a 7-minute Wild Interval Workout. A Wild Workout session consists of 20 seconds of maximum output followed by 10 seconds of rest repeated 10 times without pausing for a total of 5 minutes. Each session begins with a 60-second warm-up and ends with a 60-second cooldown.

The Wild Interval Workout results in unique changes in skeletal muscle and endurance capacity that were previously believed to require hours of exercise each week. While moderate aerobic exercise improves only aerobic systems, the interval training actually improves both anaerobic (intense, muscle-building) and aerobic (slower, oxygen-consuming) body systems.

If you want to look and feel like an athlete, the following workout will help you train more like one. This routine is based on science developed by the Japanese Olympic Speed Skating team in the 1970s, finding that a work session followed by even shorter periods of recovery dramatically improved speed, power, and performance as compared to endurance cardio.

Hill sprints are a fantastic interval workout for beginners and veterans alike. Steep inclines reduce impact on your joints and require more power from the large muscle groups in the legs. Give yourself 7 minutes, and you'll get more out of this workout than most people do in 2 hours on a treadmill.

All you have to do is find a hill with a steep incline and run as far and as fast as you can for 20 seconds—give it absolutely everything you've got. There are two alternating phases to the Wild Workout—a work phase and a recovery phase. For a 7-minute workout, you will perform 10 sets of 20-second sprints with 10 seconds of recovery between each set. It looks like this:

Warm-Up: 60 seconds of light cardio, mobility, and dynamic stretching.
Work Phase: Sprint for 20 seconds as fast as you can without stopping.
Recovery Phase: Rest for 10 seconds. Catch your breath and get ready for the next round.
Repeat: 9 times for a total of 5 minutes.
Cooldown: 60 seconds of light cardio, mobility, and dynamic stretching.

Before you begin, shake out your joints and get your juices flowing with a quick warm-up. To begin your workout, start your timer and sprint as fast as you can up the hill. After 20 seconds, take 10 seconds to catch your breath before your next sprint. You should be huffing and puffing as soon as your 5 minutes starts and completely out of juice by the end. The last few rounds should be almost impossible. Remember, you get out of exercise what you put in, so don't let that whiny voice that sometimes pops into your head psych you out of a great workout.

Don't have a hill for your workout? Any high-intensity exercise will do—sprinting, bicycle sprints, jump rope, jumping jacks, burpees, rowing, swimming, and anything else that gets your blood pumping. The 7-minute workout is a great place to start, but if your level of fitness requires more rest, go ahead and take it. When I'm without my timer, I often sprint at a slightly lower intensity for as long as a minute, counting in my head. I follow longer work intervals with more rest—if I sprint for a minute, then I rest for longer than 10 seconds. Feel free to use this workout as a template to customize as your fitness improves with more sets and shorter rest.

Everybody else loves to hate it, but my favorite full-body interval workout while traveling or limited on space and time is the infamous burpee. Professional athletes, CrossFit trainers, and elite military forces swear by the dreaded burpee, which just might be the ultimate full-body exercise. It's viciously efficient and uncompromisingly effective. You're probably sweating just by thinking about it. If you don't know what a burpee is, hold on to your hat.

HOW TO PERFORM A BURPEE

1. Begin in a squat position with hands on the floor in front of you (leapfrog position).
2. Kick your feet back, while simultaneously lowering yourself into the bottom portion of a push-up.
3. Return your feet to the squat position, while simultaneously pushing up with your arms (perform the push-up while returning your feet to the squat position).
4. Leap up as high as you can from the squat position and extend your arms above your head, reaching toward the ceiling.
5. Move as quickly as possible back to the first position.
6. Repeat. No wussing out.

STRENGTH WORKOUT

Regardless of your gender, if you want a sexy body, get your lift on and build some muscle. High performers focus on intensity, explosive movements, and muscle adaptation, not "face time" in the gym. If you want to burn fat, boost your metabolism, tone your muscles, and strengthen bone mass, then lifting weights is far more effective than cardio. Lifting heavy things increases lean muscle tissue, one of the body's most powerful mechanisms for burning fat. The more lean tissue you have, the more calories you burn, which increases your resting metabolic rate.

To maximize hormonal response, perform full-body exercises that stimulate as many muscles and expend as much energy as possible at the same time. My favorite full-body exercises include:

WARM-UP

- ☐ Jumping jacks
- ☐ Shadowboxing
- ☐ Dancing
- ☐ Jogging

BODY WEIGHT

- ☐ Sprint
- ☐ Squat
- ☐ Push-up
- ☐ Pull-up
- ☐ Burpee
- ☐ Handstand push-up

MINIMAL EQUIPMENT

☐ Kettlebell swing
☐ Jump rope
☐ Resistance band pulls

GYM EQUIPMENT

☐ Weighted squat
☐ Dead lift
☐ Row
☐ Bench press
☐ Leg press
☐ Lat pull-down

ABEL'S STRENGTH-TRAINING TIPS

Exercise your entire body during each workout—the legs, trunk, core, arms, and shoulders.

Focus on symmetry, form, and balance to avoid injury.

Lift heavy—use a weight that you can only lift 5 to 15 times before compromising form. If only lighter weights are available, focus on bursting into the movement and continue until exhaustion.

Use a steady cadence for each lift to eliminate momentum and ensure constant load.

Aim for 2 sets of 5 to 15 reps for each exercise. As soon as you can't make it through a movement with good form, it's time to stop and rest.

Rest at least 30 seconds between sets, longer for monster lifts with heavy weights like dead lifts and presses. You want to rest long enough for your muscles to recover enough to make it through your second set, but not so long that you start to cool down.

Aim to finish your workout in 45 minutes or less.

If building strength or size is the goal, overload your muscles with increasing weight. Once 10 to 15 reps can be performed with perfect form, increase the weight by 10 to 20 percent.

WHERE TO START?

If you're not ready for a high-intensity workout or monster lifts, that's okay. Everyone starts somewhere. Building the habit of moving your body on a regular basis is far more important than any short-term fitness goals, so know that the most important step is to consistently show up for your workout. Make the space for consistent exercise sessions or outdoor adventures in your schedule and stick to them like you booked a flight.

If you're out of shape, start with low-intensity aerobic exercise like walking and strength training. You can start interval training once your fitness level improves in the weeks ahead. Here's the good news if you're carrying extra weight: You have more muscle than you think, mostly in your legs and thighs to support your trunk. The muscles in your thighs are little fat-burning factories, and yours are likely already developed. Start with some squats and you'll have a huge head start on the skinny people.

WILD WORKOUT PROGRAM

1. Break a sweat every day.
2. Walk often, preferably outside in the sun at least once a day.
3. Complete one strength workout a week.
4. Complete one interval workout a week.
5. Rest at least one day a week.

I'll conclude this section with my best piece of fitness advice:

Break a sweat every day doing something you love.

You don't need to, and shouldn't, force yourself to do anything miserable for the sake of your health. Active, unstructured fun is an integral component of a good life. If you don't like anything in particular yet, try a bunch of things. Cross-training, or training for more than one activity at once, is best for balance. My favorites are outside in the fresh air—hiking, trail running, mountain biking, backcountry skiing, swimming, and bouldering. My mom loves daily walks and teaches Zumba at church. My brother Mark stays in great shape tilling dirt as an organic farmer. You might like golf. Cool! Fun is the most important part. Make that happen and your health will take care of itself.

THE SPRINTING ANGELS

For years, I thought I had a useless superpower—I could finish a marathon. But being able to run long distances at a moderate pace doesn't seem to bring much of a competitive advantage in a world swirling with planes, trains, and automobiles. My daily runs were a form of meditation—a bit of "me" time to reconnect with my body and clear my mind. Being able to run quickly was merely a nifty side effect without much tangible benefit.

But while outside for lunch at fellow author and friend Danny Dreyer's ChiRunning workshop on March 29, 2014, I saw a passerby collapse facedown on the sidewalk. His skin was purplish, his tongue was swollen, and he was gasping for air. As another passerby called 911, I sprinted for a quarter mile across the school lot into the school gym to find an emergency responder (incidentally, also a listener to my show) who remarkably had an oxygen tank in the back of his car. We sprinted back to the victim and the EMT administered advanced CPR and used the oxygen tank to keep him breathing. Though weak, the man had a pulse when the ambulance arrived a few minutes later. One of the police officers said that if it weren't for our quick sprinting across the school grounds, the man likely wouldn't have made it.

A few weeks later, I received an e-mail from a TV reporter in Dallas who said a man named Doug had recently survived a heart attack and was searching for the "three angels" who had saved his life. Now recovering from a quadruple bypass, Doug says that he is "living proof that CPR works." Being in great shape isn't just for you, it's part of being a good Samaritan.

PART IV

The Wild Diet

Famished and thirsty on a sunny afternoon in a small village in Thailand, we happened upon an open-air restaurant. We sat down, saw that *everything* looked good, and ordered an enormous feast, our first meal of the day. A moment later, the cook sprinted out the back of the kitchen with an empty basket. After five minutes, he reappeared with eggs from his neighbor's chickens, veggies from the garden, and spices to make curry from scratch. That's fresh food, and it's the way the healthiest people on earth eat every day.

Once food is picked or packed, it enters a state of rapid decomposition that destroys essential vitamins, minerals, and phytonutrients. When I go back to where I grew up on the old farm in New Hampshire, we make salads and smoothies from the weeds, herbs, spices, fruit, flowers, vegetables, and other plants growing in our backyard. That's what freshness is all about—food that was very Recently Alive and Well (RAW). That means the cow that produced your cheese grazed happily on pasture, your eggs come from chickens eating their natural diet of insects and worms in the backyard, and your seasonal veggies were just picked from an organic garden.

Food is more than the sum of its nutrients. When eaten the right way, according to the laws of nature, food is medicine. Before the Civil War, most families in America were treated by women who collected remedies from nearby woods and streams or grew them in their gardens. One of these women, Martha Ballard, offers a glimpse of what healers like herself believed medicine to be. She writes,

Nature offers solutions to its own problems. Remedies for illness can be found in the earth, in the animal world, and in the human body itself.

Food is the foundation for life. It's meant to nourish and bring your body to its optimal state of health—burning fat, building muscle, and bringing peace of mind. The closer you can get to a food's source—straight from the ground, tree, or carcass—the better.

Is all modern, post-agricultural food harmful, fattening, or unhealthy? Not necessarily, but the Wild Diet follows this principle: Eat plenty of whole and naturally edible foods; and be skeptical of manipulated, processed, and invented food products. This way, your body will burn fat as its main fuel source, returning you to the lean human body that's already a part of your genetic code.

WHAT'S ON THE MENU

Over hundreds of thousands of years, nature has fine-tuned human physiology to thrive on a diet of plants and animals—vegetables, meat, and occasional fruits, nuts, and seeds—which are naturally high in fat, protein, and fiber and relatively low in carbohydrates (also known as carbs). Plants (vegetables, fruits, nuts, seeds, and herbs and spices) and animals (meat, fish, fowl, and eggs) will make up the lion's share of your meals. Nutrient-dense vegetables, fruits, herbs and spices will represent your main source of fibrous carbohydrates and micronutrients (vitamins, minerals, antioxidants, anti-inflammatory agents, and phytonutrients). Raw nuts, seeds, their derivative butters, and animal foods provide nutrient-dense sources of energy, stimulate minimal insulin production, offer the quality forms of healthy protein and fat, and will represent the bulk of your caloric intake.

One of the benefits of Wild foods—especially vegetables, meats, and fruits—is that they are difficult to overeat. Vegetables and fruits provide considerable bulk, fiber, and water, which fill up our stomachs and supply us with energy throughout the day. Protein and fat from meat are also extremely satisfying and keep hunger at bay. Because these foods are digested slowly, they provide steady energy over the day and normalize blood glucose and insulin levels. Aim to eat at least two to three times more plant food by weight as you do eat meat . . . and look forward to feeling very full and satisfied.

One of the best things about eating fresh foods is that they don't take much time, effort, or creativity to taste great. You can eat many vegetables raw—it doesn't get much easier than that. It's hard to screw up fresh, high-quality foods even if you are a hopeless cook.

But please don't take this to mean that you can eat fatty foods *and* lots of quick-burning carbs. If you want to lose fat, you'll want to avoid starches and sugars—pasta, biscuits, toast, hash browns, fries, sweets, and everything else that raises your blood sugar. Don't worry, you still get one "free" meal a week where you can eat whatever you want. And if there is such thing as a "free lunch," it's directly after your workout. After all, cheesecake is good for the soul.

HOW TO BURN FAT WITH WILD FOOD

It's time to return your body to the fat-burning machine it was meant to be. When you burn more energy than you consume, your body releases hormones and enzymes that signal your fat cells to release stored fat (adipose) for energy. The fat cells then empty their contents (called triglycerol) into the bloodstream as free fatty acids. These free fatty acids are then transported through the blood to whatever tissues need energy—including the liver, kidneys, and muscles. Then the glycerol and fatty acids are further broken down within the tissue cells by chemical processes that ultimately produce energy for your body.

Eventually, all that remains from your stored fat deposits is water and carbon dioxide, which your body excretes as urine, sweat, or exhaled air. Pretty cool, right?

If you want to understand fat loss, there's good news and bad news. Which do you want first? Okay. Here's the bad news.

Sugar becomes fat.

And the good news.

Fat becomes energy.

When you follow the Wild Diet, we're going to help your body adapt from a fat-storing "Sugar Burner" to a lean and mean "Fat Burner." How? By avoiding sugar and grains, and eating plenty of delicious veggies, meats, nuts, and legumes instead. I transformed my flabby belly to lean, sculpted abs by eating butter, heavy cream, animal fat, bacon, cheese, nuts, avocado, coconut, and even chocolate. You can, too.

HOW OUR BODIES STORE FAT

From parsnips to pot roast, all food is made up of macronutrients, micronutrients, and water. Macronutrients—proteins, carbohydrates, and fats—provide energy (measured as calories, but only for convenience's sake) to sustain life. While some of each macronutrient is necessary for normal function, each plays a very different role in fat metabolism. Let's get one thing straight: It's not fat that's making most of the developed world store fat—it's carbs. While fats tend to burn clean and provide steady energy for the body, carbs and sugar burn dirty, creating free radicals, accelerating aging, feeding pathogens, and taxing the liver and pancreas in the process.

All carbohydrates break down in your system into glucose (a simple form of sugar), producing a rapid increase in blood sugar. When your blood sugar is elevated from overconsumption of carbs, your pancreas secretes insulin to clear glucose (which is damaging to organs and tissues in excess) from your blood and store it in liver, muscle, or fat cells.

The body can handle only so many carbs at a time. Once the glycogen storage cells in the liver and muscle are full—as they are nearly all the time in sedentary people since they don't use them as energy for exercise—the remainder of the glucose is converted to and stored as fat.

Your body can either store or burn fat, but not both at the same time. The level of the hormone insulin in your blood dictates whether your body will burn fat (called lipolysis) or store it (called lipogenesis). Specifically, when insulin is elevated, your body is unable to release fat from your fat stores. Keeping carbs low and fasting are the main tools I use to keep insulin levels in check, which allows me to burn stored body fat as well as dietary fat for energy instead of sugar. While fasting and eating low carb enables you to burn fat with ease, chowing on carbs does precisely the opposite.

The primary role of insulin is the storage of nutrients, for better or worse. Insulin also regulates the level of sugar in the blood, induces fat storage, and performs thousands of other tasks within the human body. In excess, insulin can make you hungry, moody, sleepy, bloated, or light-headed. It can also elevate cholesterol, raise blood pressure, cause your body to retain fluid, wreak havoc on your arteries, and convert sugar into fat.

Have you noticed that some people around you tend to gain weight every year even though they haven't changed their diet or exercise habits? In most cases, their weight gain occurs because they are on their way to insulin resistance syndrome (also known as metabolic syndrome or syndrome X), an increasingly common condition that results from long-term overconsumption of carbohydrates and other lifestyle imbalances out of sync with our biology.

Insulin resistance occurs as the body's constant battle to regulate your skyrocketing blood sugar with floods of insulin eventually causes the system to malfunction. (You know that groggy, achy, gross feeling you get just after the sugar high? That's what too much insulin feels like.) Once desensitized, insulin essentially stops working and your body requires *more* of it to properly clear glucose from the bloodstream. As a result, the pancreas pumps out more and more insulin, which creates the constant state of elevated insulin levels in the blood (known as hyperinsulinemia) and low blood sugar (hypoglycemia). This abundance of fat-storing insulin causes people to become fatter and fatter despite eating the same foods they have for years.

This partially explains why some couch-strapped teenagers can drink gallons of soda and eat all the pizza, chips, and donuts they want without gaining weight: Their insulin sensitivity is still intact. As the body ages and insulin resistance eventually kicks in, they suddenly start gaining weight. Some of us can withstand the onslaught of carbs longer than others, but at some point the body just gives up. Eventually, the cells that produce insulin (which are called pancreatic beta cells) burn out.

Once burnt-out pancreatic beta cells are unable to produce sufficient insulin, the body officially has type 2 diabetes, which often leads to nerve damage, blindness, kidney failure, heart attack, and stroke. Type 2 diabetes was once a rare affliction, diagnosed in less than one-tenth of one percent of the population at the turn of the twentieth century. Now, type 2 diabetes is a full-blown epidemic affecting 10 percent of the population and quickly increasing with a price tag of $245 billion a year as of 2012. The good news is this: If you catch it in time, resistance to insulin is reversible.

Insulin isn't all bad. You can even use it to your advantage to shuttle amino acids and glucose to build muscle after an intense workout. In fact, many athletes, bodybuilders, models, and movie stars drop weight by carefully controlling insulin through a cyclical ketogenic diet. You'll see how to use this same strategy to improve body composition on page 311.

Fat

The biggest problem with fat is that it's called "fat." The fact that the fat you eat and the fat that's stored in your body are called by the same name is misleading. The human digestive system is a work of art, and the attempt to explain any whole food in terms of macronutrients often misses the point. While the world of nutrition likes to make things complicated, deciding what to eat for lunch shouldn't be.

You can think of fat as "concentrated energy," providing twice as many calories per gram as protein or carbs. But eating fat isn't *fattening*; in fact, the overwhelming majority of independent studies support a high-fat diet for humans. Compared to those who restrict themselves to a low-fat diet, dieters who eat more fat experience a leaner body composition as well as reduced cholesterol, triglycerides, blood pressure, and other heart disease risk factors. Fat is a fat-burner's best friend.

If food marketers and backward government recommendations have frightened you away from fat, here are some reasons to fall back in love with it. Fat-friendly plans like the Wild Diet increase fat-burning hormones, promote lean muscle growth, inhibit muscle breakdown, and boost production of youth-restoring growth hormone. Short-chain fats, found in coconut oil, promote weight loss and are associated with a decrease in body weight, waist size, and blood triglycerides. Fats protect your body, promote proper cell function, support the release of fat-burning hormones, aid in the absorption of vitamins and minerals, and add flavor to foods. Fats are found in animals, fish, eggs, milk, nuts, and some vegetables and fungi.

During my high-fat experiments on the *Fat-Burning Man* show, I'd drink a cup of heavy cream, fry up eight egg yolks in bacon fat for breakfast, and down full-fat coconut cream by the can. Interestingly, the same biomarkers of health that the fat-phobic might say would go haywire—specifically cholesterol, triglycerides, and C-reactive protein—each came back normal or even improved. I've even been spotted eating grass-fed butter by the stick in a pinch, and I carry around packets of fat as snacks while working or adventuring, which are wonderful for your skin and brain. Fat really isn't as scary as it might seem.

The Truth About Saturated Fat, Cholesterol, and Heart Disease

For decades, Americans have been told that eating saturated fat and cholesterol (found in butter, beef, and other animal fats) clogs arteries and causes heart disease. The justification for the anti–saturated fat propaganda is misguided, however, based upon Ancel Keys's doctored data from the 1950s. In fact, research shows that some saturated fat can actually *decrease* cholesterol, blood pressure, risk of heart disease, and risk of obesity. We've been eating saturated fat safely for thousands of years, as has much of the animal kingdom. It's not fat that's the problem; it's *processed* saturated fat and trans fats that we need to worry about.

Cholesterol, in and of itself, isn't actually bad for you. In fact, almost every cell in the body produces cholesterol. Cholesterol is nature's repair substance and is vital to the function of the brain and nervous system. Many important hormones are made of cholesterol, including the sex hormones testosterone, estrogen, and progesterone, hormones that regulate mineral metabolism and blood sugar, as well as hormones that help us tolerate stress. Cholesterol even acts as a powerful antioxidant that protects us against free radicals and cancer. Suffice it to say that when you eat real food, mostly plants, you don't need to study the science of cholesterol, count calories, or steer clear of eggs to avoid heart disease and achieve great health.

If you're worried about heart disease, know that *eating* cholesterol doesn't necessarily clog your arteries, either. In fact, you're just as likely to have a heart attack with low cholesterol as you are with high cholesterol. And in some studies, high cholesterol is associated with a longer life-span.

Most excess cholesterol is made by the body itself, rather than consumed in the diet. In fact, most Americans consume only about one-third of the amount of cholesterol every day that the body already makes on its own. And much of the cholesterol we consume doesn't even make it into the bloodstream, so if worries about cholesterol have been keeping you away from delicious food, it's time to bring bacon back to breakfast.

The Good Fats We Crave

Our native diet was extremely high in fat—primarily the much-maligned saturated fat. The Inuit enjoyed lives free of heart disease despite sourcing 90 percent or more of their daily calories from fat. Native Americans favored meat from healthy, older animals because they had built up layers of nutrient-dense saturated fat along their backs, which was rendered and stored to provide concentrated energy during the meager seasons.

Our ancestors coveted natural fats and oils like they were liquid gold. Before modern oil processing, our fat was sourced from animals, including butter, lard, tallow, marrow, and from fatty plants like coconut and olive. Unlike polyunsaturated fat, these saturated and monounsaturated fats store well in your pantry and resist oxidization and rancidity.

Our Favorite Fats

Cooking Fats

Cook low and slow and keep the drippings.

- Butter and ghee (particularly from grass-fed cows)
- Animal fats from grass-fed/pastured/wild animals (lard, tallow, duck, etc.)
- Coconut oil

Fats to Eat Cold

Since they have a low smoke point and contain delicate omega-3s, eat these fats cold.

- Olive oil*
- Avocado oil
- Fish oils
- Nuts and nut butters
- Flaxseed oil
- Other whole, natural fats

Healthy fat is perfect for curbing the appetite. When I'm hungry or need a boost of energy, I reach for high-fat foods like nuts, eggs, avocado, coconut, and full-fat dairy. At 9 calories per gram, fat is more calorically dense than protein or carbs. That makes it easier to overeat than protein, fruits, or vegetables. Mindlessly pounding sticks of butter, chugging whipping cream, or slurping bacon fat by the spoonful won't do you any favors. Adjust your consumption of fat based on hunger, energy, and exercise levels to find a healthy balance. If your weight begins to drift, you may find that eating more protein or non-starchy vegetables and scaling down your fat intake is more effective for fat loss in your body.

*You *can* cook with olive oil, but it's not good to fry or grease a skillet with olive oil because those cooking methods are high temp—and you'll notice because you'll fill the house with smoke!

OMEGA-3s

When you eat Wild foods, you'll be getting plenty of brain-boosting, fat-burning omega-3s, a polyunsaturated fat that occurs naturally in oily fish, grass-fed meats and eggs, nuts, seeds, and leafy green vegetables. Omega-3s are anti-inflammatory agents involved in producing energy from food substances and then moving that energy throughout your system. Omega-3s also encourage fat metabolism by regulating insulin levels.

Healthy sources of omega-3s include:

- Wild-caught fish and seafood, especially cold-water fish such as salmon, mackerel, halibut, and herring
- Pasture-raised poultry and their eggs
- Pasture-raised ruminant animals, such as cows, bison, and lamb
- Pasture-raised liver and organ meats
- Flax- and chia seeds and their oil, which can be used as an ingredient in salad dressings, poured over vegetables, or used as a supplement
- Walnuts and macadamia nuts
- Leafy green vegetables

Fats to Avoid

Avoid anything that is processed, packaged, or fried—especially processed foods containing newfangled trans fats, hydrogenated fats, and polyunsaturated oils. This includes shortening, margarine, and industrial seed oils (e.g., corn, cottonseed, soybean, safflower, and canola). It's not just processed vegetable fats that cause problems, though. Industrial animal fats are best avoided, as well.

While fat from healthy animals is nutrient dense and beneficial for your health, fat from sick animals isn't. Since cows, poultry, and fish are fed high-carb, GMO, non-native diets in industrial feedlots and fish farms, its best to avoid fat from conventional meat. Like humans, animals store antibiotics, feed pesticides, synthetic growth hormones, and other toxins in their fat stores. If you're eating conventional meat that may come from a sick animal, trim or drain off any excess fat to avoid toxins.

PROTEIN

Protein will be one of your best weapons to reach and maintain your ideal body composition. If you want to curb hunger and lose weight rapidly without feeling deprived, eat more high-quality protein—up to 1 gram per pound of your ideal body weight daily. Consuming plenty of protein does more than just keep you feeling full, it actually helps build your muscles, organs, and brain. As the only food constituent containing nitrogen, protein forms the basic building blocks of human matter and is essential to growth and repair of the body.

Eating protein propels anabolism (muscle-building), decreases risk of catabolism (muscle-wasting), and actually increases your resting metabolic rate by producing body heat (known as thermogenesis). Protein also boosts your overall health by improving immunity and antioxidant function and enhancing insulin function. Protein is found in many foods, notably meats, fish, seafood, eggs, and dairy, as well as vegetables, beans, nuts, legumes, and fungi.

You can eat as much protein as you'd like, but make it high quality. Don't be afraid of eating too much protein as long as it's in the form of whole food. Go for grass-finished, pastured, wild, local game, and organic meats over conventionally raised and processed meats. In a pinch, unsweetened protein shakes or bars can help get the protein you need, but it's always best to go with real food.

During digestion, your body breaks food down into energy. In order to access this energy, the body must *expend* energy. Protein requires two and a half to three times more energy to digest than carbohydrates or fat. This means that the same caloric intake of protein burns more energy than an equal amount of fat or carbs, resulting in rapid fat loss. This is known as thermogenesis, and it's one of the reasons you'd need to eat twice as much protein to get the equivalent caloric energy in the same amount of fat.

Is it possible to eat too much protein? Theoretically, yes. The protein ceiling falls somewhere around 40 percent of your caloric intake. However, since protein is very filling and only contains 4 calories per gram (as opposed to 9 calories per gram in fat or 7 calories per gram in alcohol), unless you're drinking a lot of protein shakes, eating protein bars, or overdoing supplements, that 40 percent of your protein intake is nearly impossible to overreach.

If you are physically active or trying to build muscle, eat at least 50 to 100 grams of protein a day and up to 1 gram of protein per pound of ideal body weight. This amount of protein will help you increase your lean muscle, especially if you are engaging in high-intensity training as recommended.

The protein in a palm-size portion of meat adds up quickly:

- 6 ounces of lean beef or turkey has upward of 50 grams of protein
- 6 ounces of tuna has 40 grams of protein
- 1 cup of cottage cheese has 28 grams of protein
- 1 cup of lentils has 9 grams of protein
- 1 egg has 6 grams of protein

When you prepare a meal, build it around pastured, grass-fed, or wild-caught animal protein and fibrous vegetables and boost your energy intake and add flavor with nutrient-dense fat. Try to get at least a few bites of a protein-rich food in each meal. It may go against your habits and conditioning, but I cannot overemphasize the importance of eating plenty of protein for fat loss; building strong, toned muscle; and a lean body composition. Fear steak no longer.

CARBOHYDRATES

Most people overeat carbs, especially the bad kind. Anthropologists estimate that many of our hunter-gathering ancestors consumed fewer than 100 grams of net carbs a day, primarily from fruits and vegetables. In stark contrast, the typical American consumes *350 to 600 grams a day* primarily from various sugar and grain products. As carbohydrates are primarily responsible for enabling fat storage, it is not difficult to see why many of us are overweight.

Imagine filling two cups with pure, white sugar and spooning it into your mouth one bite at a time. Believe it or not, that's the amount of simple sugar your body metabolizes every day if you source 60 percent of your calories from carbs, as most of us do. Bread, pasta, cereal, potatoes, rice, fruit, dessert, candy, and so many more: They are all carbohydrates that your body converts to a simple form of sugar called glucose to be readily stored in muscle or as fat.

As far as your body is concerned, processed carbs *are* sugar. Since sugar rots your teeth, accelerates aging, and feeds cancer cells, it's best not to have too much of it. If there is anything worth counting, it's carbs. Limiting carb intake maximizes fat burning and helps to regulate blood sugar and insulin levels. But all carbs are not created equal.

There are three main categories of carbs:

Sugar: Found in concentrates, powders, syrups, and fruit
Starch: Found in roots, tubers, cereals, and grains.
Fiber: Found in roughage, vegetables, fruits, nuts, seeds, and whole grains. Roughage is essential to keeping your digestive tract in good working order.

The total number of carbohydrates listed on nutrition labels is not the whole story. It's *net* carbs that really matter, since total carbs includes fiber. Fiber from fruit and veggies is beneficial—fiber feeds your probiotic gut bacteria, detoxifies your digestive tract, and gives you steady energy throughout the day.

Count your *net* carbs, not your total carbs. To calculate net carbs, simply subtract the dietary fiber content from the total carbs.

Carbs – Fiber = Net Carbs

Limiting net carbs to 50 to 100 grams per day accelerates fat burning for most people. For what it's worth, for bodybuilding, Arnold Schwarzenegger recommended consuming just 60 to 100 grams of net carbs a day, with the rest of calories coming from fat and protein. Hard to argue with the Terminator.

As long as you limit starches, sugars, and fruit, it's difficult to exceed 100 grams of net carbs in a day even if you eat generous amounts of colorful vegetables and a few servings of fruit.

"HAVE YOU CONSUMED RICE TODAY?"

On a visit to the small Indonesian island of Bali, our guide brought us to paddies and plantations to sample numerous strains of ancient rice. Our favorite, red rice, is a long grain with a deep reddish-brown hue on the outside and a white center. When you cook it just right (low and slow), this chewy and wholesome rice adopts the fluffy texture of old-fashioned whole-grain oats.

Like other grains, many modern strains of rice have been domesticated and bred for characteristics that have little to do with your health. Low-quality rice even contains "troubling" levels of arsenic, a known carcinogen and poison. However, many healthful ancient strains of rice are readily available at health food stores, Asian markets, in some supermarkets, and online.

Wild rice (actually an edible grass) is relatively easy to find and tastes more nutty and substantial than the overcooked mush that comes out of an ice cream scoop at many restaurants in America. Unlike processed white rice, whole-grain rice—like brown, black, and red—leaves the bran intact, making for a more nutritious grain. Both brown and red rice can be long-, medium- or short-grain. Long-grain rice is drier and fluffs when cooked. Short-grain rice has higher starch content and is sticky when cooked.

In most of the world, rice isn't just a side dish, it's a part of life. In the Thai language, "How are you?" translates roughly to "Have you consumed rice today?"

As we whizzed through the magnificent rolling rice paddies while touring through Bali, our guide and driver explained: "Almost all of our rice is still grown by hand, not machines. Many farmers here." More than food, rice is considered sacred and often plays a fundamental role in Balinese offerings and ceremonies.

"How do Americans grow rice?" our driver inquired, glancing in the rearview mirror as we narrowly escaped a head-on collision with a speeding truck hauling hand-woven baskets.

"With big machines, cheap oil, and lots of pesticides," I admitted. "But we're working on that."

How Many Carbs Should I Eat?

For most people, the best range for healthy fat loss is 50 to 100 grams of net carbs a day, perhaps more if you're especially physically active. But you don't need to "count carbs" because it's easy to stay well within 50 to 150 grams on the Wild Diet—even when you eat loads of colorful vegetables and a fair amount of fruit. It's difficult to stay in this range, however, when you consume modern foods such as grains, processed foods, or sugars.

In modest amounts, carbs are not your enemy. Consuming carbs from fruits and vegetables is necessary to achieve optimal body function and balance—especially if you are physically active, have a high metabolism, or have a low tolerance for fat or protein. Moderate consumption of slow-burning carbs and starches promotes healthy body function by providing your brain with glucose (brain fuel) and your liver and muscles with glycogen (muscle fuel) and helps regulate circadian rhythms to help you sleep, especially when you eat carbs at night.

The more active you are, the better your body can utilize and dispose of carbs. So if you have a very active metabolism or you are an athlete, don't be afraid of fueling up with slow-burning starches and carbs like boiled sweet potatoes, whole-grain rice, quinoa, and other whole Wild foods. But be careful—eating carbs in excess of your glycogen stores will risk fat storage, despite large amounts of exercise. This is easy to do when you come back from your long runs and eat a whole pie. Been there, done that.

SLOW-BURNING VS. QUICK-BURNING CARBS

The Glycemic Index (GI) is a rating system that evaluates how different foods affect blood sugar levels—essentially, it's a rough indicator of the likelihood that eating that food will make you store fat, with lower numbers being more favorable for fat burning. High-GI carbohydrates, such as white bread, sugar, cereal, and most other processed food, burn quickly, spike your blood sugar, and cause a flood of insulin that triggers your body to store fat and become hungry again within an hour or two.

In contrast, slow-burning starches and lower-GI foods, such as vegetables, cut your appetite and keep you satisfied for hours on end. These slow-burning carbs are more efficient at keeping glucose levels stabilized and insulin in check. The Wild Diet prioritizes slow-burning carbohydrates with low GIs to ensure more consistent and long-lasting energy and reduced fat storage.

When to Eat Carbs

The best time to eat carbs is in the evening, as carbs cue your body to enter "rest and digest" mode and help you fall asleep. Most people lose the most fat when avoiding carbs in the morning in favor of a high-fat or high-protein breakfast instead. Think "gatherer" by day—light snacking on low-glycemic veggies, nuts, and fruit—and "hunter" by night, with a hearty source of protein, plenty of fat, and slow-burning carbs like whole-grain rice or sweet potato. For example, I might snack on raw carbs like veggies and fruit during the day, but tend to avoid cooked carbs until late afternoon or evening.

Consuming carbs within sixty to ninety minutes immediately following intervals, strength training, or other intense physical activity will aid recovery and refuel glyco-gen stores for your next session. After an intense workout, your body is primed to absorb nutrients, and insulin helps shunt extra carb calories to help replenish and grow muscle tissue. I often work out fasted and eat a carb- and protein-heavy meal directly after. See the "Fasting and Feasting" section on pages 55 to 69 for more details.

VITAMINS

Vitamins have an essential role not only in maintaining the health of the body but in protection from illness and disease. Science has discovered more than 40 different vitamins, of which about a dozen are essential for humans. Vitamin D can be synthesized by the skin when exposed to sunlight, and gut bacteria can synthesize vitamin K, but many vitamins must be obtained from food.

A well-nourished person generally carries a month's supply of vitamins in their body. Of those, vitamin C is the first that needs to be replenished (lest you get a mean case of scurvy like a sea-weary pirate, or my roommate in college who subsisted almost exclusively on ramen noodles). The second vitamin to replenish is vitamin A, which aids vision and prevents eye disease. Eat a wide variety of herbs and spices, and fresh seasonal fruits and vegetables to ensure you get the full spectrum of nutrients you need to thrive.

MINERALS AND TRACE ELEMENTS

Minerals have vital roles in body functions. We require a steady quantity of certain minerals to function normally, including magnesium, calcium, sulphur, phosphorus, sodium, and potassium. Other minerals are required in smaller amounts, including iodine, iron, and flourine.

Unfortunately, decades of unsustainable farming practices have caused the amount of minerals in our soil—and our food—to plummet. We counter this lack of minerals in our soil by consuming bone broth weekly and supplementing with bulkier minerals such as magnesium in powdered form. To improve taste and nutrition, add a few drops of trace minerals to your drinking water.

VARIETY, THE SPICE OF LIFE

Many fat-loss programs recommend that you eat the same meals every month, every week, or even every day, often because they want to sell you their microwave dinners, protein bars, and shakes. Gym rats might argue that it's "easier to hit your macros" when you eat the same thing every day. But that's terrible advice, and here's why.

Not only will eating the same thing every day bore you to tears, but you'll also be missing out on the wide spectrum of nutrients naturally found in seasonal foods. When you let what naturally grows during the season dictate what you put on your plate—tomatoes in the summer and apples in September, for example—your fresh produce will be more satisfying and filling because the harvest contains the cycle of nutrients your body needs to thrive. The more you incorporate variety into your nutritional habits, the healthier and happier you'll be.

While hunter-gatherers in the Australian outback today live on eight hundred varieties of wild plant foods, Americans live principally on three industrial crops: corn, soy, and wheat. Since we're missing out on the majority of foods that our ancestors once ate, many of us are deficient in critical vitamins and minerals, including vitamin D, vitamin K, magnesium, and zinc, to name a few.

What gave hunter-gatherers perfect teeth, lean frames, and disease-free bodies? They relished in nutrient-dense delicacies like beaver tail, stewed bonemeal pudding, and fermented caribou intestines stuffed with organ meats. You don't have much use for multivitamins when you eat food like that.

Fortunately, fermented caribou intestine isn't the only nutrient-dense food out there.

One of the easiest ways to get more variety in your diet is by looking at your traditional family recipes. What did your grandparents eat? Were there strange soups, cod livers, or fermented vegetables fizzing in the cupboard? Perhaps you'll find old family recipes for nutrient-dense meals like liver and onions, sausage, or haggis. Get in touch with your relatives and dust off that family cookbook to see what you can bring back to life.

The body's ability to absorb nutrients is dictated by the presence or absence of cofactors, critical substances that "unlock" the nutrition in food to be utilized by the body, and many traditional food preparations and dishes are designed to keep our bodies healthy. For example, eating cheese with eggs can increase uptake of vitamin D; eating wasabi and ginger with raw fish protects against bacteria, viruses, and disease; and soaking and sprouting nuts, seeds, and grains, as our ancestors once did, reduces antinutrients like lectins and phytates that can damage the gut and releases enzymes that help our bodies gain access to their nutrients.

Nutrients from real food are vastly superior to synthetic and added vitamins and minerals—it's difficult, expensive, and some would argue impossible to compensate for a poor diet through supplementation. As such, it's essential to aim for fresh, high-quality foods that are naturally high in micronutrients to achieve optimal health.

THE CURIOUS CASE OF POTTENGER'S CATS

Dr. Francis Pottenger Jr. was a veterinarian who worked in a lab that produced adrenal hormones and tested them on cats. The death rate of Pottenger's cats was high, but he noticed when the offal portion of their diet—liver, tripe, sweetbreads, brains, and heart—was served raw rather than cooked, the health of the cats improved markedly.

Beginning in 1932, Pottenger conducted a remarkable ten-year experiment that evaluated five diets over four generations, including nine hundred cats. He found that cats fed raw milk, raw meat, and offal maintained health throughout four generations of breeding. However, the cats that ate only cooked meat and pasteurized, evaporated, or condensed milk experienced steadily deteriorating health.

- First-generation cats developed degenerative diseases late in life.
- Second-generation cats developed degenerative diseases in midlife.
- Third-generation cats developed diseases, allergies, and soft bones and succumbed to parasitic infections early in life. Most of the cats could not produce offspring.
- Not a single fourth-generation cat could reproduce. Fourth-generation cats suffered almost all of the medically documented human degenerative diseases.

It's now generally accepted that the decline in health of Pottenger's cats was due to nutritional deficiencies induced by cooking and processing, which destroys taurine, an essential nutrient for cats. High-temperature processing techniques like pasteurization and homogenization destroy nutrients in a similar manner. For tips on how to feed your pets their native diet, see page 316.

GO FRESH, LOCAL, ORGANIC, AND IN-SEASON

Go organic when you can—remember, all food was once organic. Today, certified organic crops have a higher standard of quality and are required to be grown in safe soil, have no modifications, and must remain separate from conventional products. Organic farmers are not allowed to use synthetic pesticides, bioengineered genes (GMOs), petroleum-based fertilizers, or sewage sludge–based fertilizers. Organic foods have fewer pesticides, synthetic fertilizers, growth hormones, and antibiotics, and contain higher levels of nutrients than conventional foods. Conventional growers make no such promises.

As such, it is important to go for fresh, organic plants and animals when you can. Honor the natural cycles of the seasons and save a few bucks by purchasing foods that are local and fresh, like cucumbers in the summer, apples in September, and corn in late spring.

Why Heirloom Produce and Heritage Livestock Are Better Than Conventional

Have you ever sliced into a deep pink tomato with white stripes? Perhaps you've eaten carrots that are nearly blue, or a small spiky, bulbous cucumber with a long, spindly vine? If so, you probably know that heirloom varieties of fruits and vegetables are not only beautiful, they're delicious. By definition, heirloom varieties come from seeds that have been passed down from generation to generation and have been allowed to reproduce naturally (think "the opposite of dwarf wheat and GMOs"). Generally speaking, these varieties of fruits and vegetables are more nutritionally dense (you can tell by their deep and varied coloration) than their conventional counterparts. Plus, they are usually locally grown and have been allowed to ripen on the vine, making them more tasty and nutritious.

Heirloom livestock are also quite different from the cows, pigs, and chickens you find on a factory farm. Heirloom chickens are beautiful—speckled red and brown, sleek black with dapples of gray, or maybe a deep chocolate brown—and they come in countless colors and look nothing like the pure white, extra-large-breasted chickens packed into factory-farm cages. These poor conventional animals, such as the enormous turkeys many of us eat during the holidays, are bred to have breasts so large that their feet would break if they attempted to walk during adulthood.

Heritage livestock, however, from chickens and pigs to cows and sheep, are more capable of withstanding the elements and have a stronger immune system, making it so they do not need antibiotics to survive and thrive like their conventional cousins. Heritage livestock is often raised organic and fed their natural diet, making their eggs, dairy, and meat more nutritious than conventional. Remember: The healthier the animal you eat, the healthier you'll be.

After trying some truly strange exotic fruits and vegetables in distant lands, I've learned this: The weirder it looks, the better it tastes. Get your tomatoes ugly.

EAT LIKE THE LOCALS

While sampling raw cacao, fresh heirloom chile pepper, local tobacco, and cat poop coffee at a plantation on the Indonesian island of Bali, I chatted with two locals about how they eat at home. Despite the fact that nearly every restaurant, villa, and resort brings visitors a whopping glass of tropical fruit juice, the locals don't bother.

"We're too lazy to make juice!" our friend Nyoman says. "Fruit turns to juice in stomach anyway. We just eat fruit," he says, smiling. "We sometimes take two meals a day, with no breakfast. But usually we eat fried banana with Bali coffee in the morning."

"How about lunch and dinner?"

"We cook vegetables, rice, and maybe meat or fish. We only need a few bites. Not like the Americans who eat half a chicken. . . . A little chicken leg feeds our whole family!" Nyoman exclaims as our guide, Wayan, nods in approval.

As any local will tell you, the heavy, rich meals offered at the restaurants are meals that you wouldn't find at home in daily practice. They cook one meal a day—vegetables, rice, and meat—and eat it around noon. In the evening, they don't use microwaves. Like the fresh eggs at their village markets, they eat their food at room temperature with the rest of their family. We found that cooking meals in advance and eating food at room temperature saves time and takes the stress out of family dinners.

"What advice would you give someone who gets fat here to lose weight?" I ask, now crying from the chiles.

"Always give them fresh food," Nyoman explains. "Anyone who eats too much food from boxes gets fat."

GREENS: THE ONE THING EVERY HEALTH EXPERT AGREES ABOUT

Although health experts squabble about everything else, there is one thing about which almost every health expert worth his or her salt agrees—that we should all eat more fresh green vegetables. Above all else, healthy people make it a priority to get their greens every day, and you should, too.

I eat an enormous amount of vegetables, as often as I can—usually several times a day, which takes deliberate effort. Raw veggie addiction is much like beer, coffee, and smoking: I crave greens every day and get cranky without them. That's where you want to be. Push through the first few days of salad eating until you're hooked.

HOW TO MAKE A GREEN SMOOTHIE

It's a versatile, delicious, nutritional powerhouse that is incredibly easy to make. The most effective fat-burning breakfast on the face of the Earth is the green smoothie.

The nutritional equivalent of eating a salad and then some, green smoothies are packed with vitamins and minerals, water, satiating fiber, and raw food enzymes to aid digestion. Green smoothies are detoxifying and alkalizing, which restores balance within your body to burn off fat and restore health.

Store-bought "green smoothies" from the bottle are almost always devoid of fiber and packed with preservatives and sugar. Avoid them and make your own—it will taste better, be better for you, and save you money.

Combine the following four categories of ingredients to taste:

- Green vegetable (use one or more): kale, spinach, bok choy, collard greens, cabbage greens, Swiss chard, beet greens, sprouts, cucumber, broccoli, celery, avocado
- Liquid (use one): water, tea, almond milk, coconut milk, coconut water, raw milk, kefir. Add ice if you like your smoothie chilled.
- Fruit (use one or more, fresh or frozen): strawberries, blueberries, bananas, apples, cherries, coconut, carrots, beets (top and root), lemon, ginger root, pumpkin, tomatoes
- Add-ins: protein powder (with no added sugar), flax meal (for omega-3s), cinnamon (regulates blood sugar), stevia, spirulina, chlorella, hulled hemp seeds, chia seeds soaked in water, olive oil, powdered vitamin C

Do you *need* to drink green smoothies? Absolutely not. Really, if we would just *eat* our daily salads, we wouldn't have to blend them up in some ridiculous contraption. But green smoothies are great if you're in a hurry or if you don't find yourself eating a daily salad. If you'd rather drink your salad than eat it, give it a whirl.

MEAT, FOWL, AND EGGS

While drifting down a river in Fiji where *Anaconda* (the movie about enormous man-eating snakes) was filmed, Alyson and I spotted giant beast was scrambling down a cliff. Muscular and graceful, this magnificent animal bounded to the riverbank and burst through the jungle below. It was . . . a cow.

"I've never seen a cow like that," I said to my Fijian guide. "It's like a supercow."

He chuckled. "Yes, wild cow. We let them loose in the jungle when they're babies and they live in the jungle. When they're big enough, we call them back and have a feast. Our cows have good lives here."

Meet Your Meat

If you believe that the animals your chicken nuggets are made from have ever seen the light of day or felt grass under their feet, you are living a fantasy of bygone times. Today, factory-farmed animals are not treated humanely, but Big Food does its best to keep that a secret. As shoppers, we're encouraged to distance ourselves from the animals we're eating as much as possible. But if you take the time to befriend a backyard cow, you'll look at your burger differently.

When you eat beef, you're not just eating the cow, you're consuming the entire food chain. If the cow that became your burger lived on food it's not meant to eat, like the corn fed to conventional cattle to fatten them quickly, and survived on a steady dose of antibiotics and growth hormones, you're eating the meat of a sick animal. The toxic, marbled meat from blubbery feedlot cows, for example, bears little resemblance to meat from the powerful aurochs (wild cows) and buffalo our ancestors ate in the natural world.

Meat from wild animals typically carry little external fat, nearly no fat between the muscles, and contain very few toxins. In stark contrast, feedlot animals are fat and sick, with several inches of white fat covering their bodies. Despite the fact that the FDA has known about the health risks for nearly fifty years, it's common for factory farms to feed their cows industrial poultry litter (yes, bird poop) as a staple of their diet. When you eat conventional meat, these toxins, chemicals, and hormones in the meat transfer their negative effects to you.

Production lines often move too quickly for the limited staff in conventional slaughterhouses. Hiccups and minor mishaps in the rapid assembly-line disembowelment of conventionally raised cattle often leads to feces in the meat. This is the root cause of food poisoning from E. coli contamination, which is a daily occurrence across America and one of the principal reasons our meat is banned in other countries. In addition, while the fat from wild or pasture-raised animals is healthy and high in brain-boosting omega-3 fatty acids, the fat of conventionally raised animals is toxic.

Always buy the cleanest and highest-quality meat (free of hormones, additives, preservatives, artificial coloring agents, etc.) you can find and afford. Game meats and pasture-raised organic animals raised in their natural environment are best. If you eat factory-farmed meat, know that the fat is where the majority of the animal's toxins are stored. Go for a lean cut and trim off the fat before cooking.

One of our favorite things about eating Wild: We save money on grass-finished meat by eating the whole animal, nose to tail, as our ancestors once did. The cuts with the highest nutrient density are actually the organs, not the muscle meat. In fact, many hunter-gatherers, after claiming their kill, ate the prized organs like the liver raw in the field to replenish their energy, accessing its vast spectrum of nutrients after a long hunt. If there was too much to carry, hunters often left the muscle meat, the least nutrient-dense part of the animal, behind in favor of fatty cuts and organ meats.

In the animal kingdom, this is referred to as the "high-grading" of food. During salmon runs in Alaska, grizzly bears do the same, eating only the livers and leaving the rest of the fish on the riverbank. According to the National Park Service,

If you see bears only eating the skin, brains, and eggs of a salmon, they are practicing good energy economics. At these times, a bear's profit margin in calories is so high that it can ignore some excess fish. As a bear fills up on salmon, it can "afford" to not eat certain parts of the fish. This behavior has been nicknamed "high-grading." Like miners looking for high-grade ore, bears try to consume high-grade fat.

Salmon are a high-calorie meal for a bear. A sockeye salmon contains about 4,500 calories, but the fattiest parts of the fish contain the most calories proportionally. Bears know this and prefer to eat the skin, brain, and eggs—the fattiest parts of a salmon—when fish are in abundance.

If you're looking to save a buck at the farmers' market, this is great news for you. While you might get sticker shock from premium cuts of grass-fed meat, many farmers are willing to part with their fatty offcuts and organ meat for less than half of the price of their steaks. When you learn how to prepare offcuts, like stew meat, meaty bones, and organs, supply and demand often works in your favor. To get the most bang for your buck, ask for marrow bones (for soup and for the dog when she's good), roasts, liver, heart, chicken feet, fish stock bones, and offcuts that you can throw in chili or a stew.

Eggs

Whole eggs from healthy fowl are among the most nutritious foods on earth. Within the walls of its shell, an egg contains enough nutrients to transform a single fertilized cell into a chirping chick in twenty-one days.

In spite of that, the fat-free fad misled nutritionists and doctors into telling us to give up eggs since they contain cholesterol and saturated fat. But as we learned on page 97, cholesterol in food is not at all the same thing as the cholesterol that clogs arteries. One Harvard study found that healthy men and women could eat seven eggs a day with no increased risk of heart disease. That's a lot of quiche.

Eggs are an excellent source of high-quality fat and protein, making them an economic and healthful staple. At 75 calories apiece, eggs are a fat burner's best friend. Scrambled, poached, hard-boiled, Benedict, or baked into homemade desserts, we usually eat several eggs a day in one form or another. If you're bored with chicken eggs, branch out and experiment with quail eggs (tiny and tasty) or duck eggs (big and buttery).

For best nutrition, choose eggs from free-roaming poultry in pasture on their natural diet of insects, seeds, and fruits. The better the diet of your chicken, the more nutrients in your eggs. Pastured eggs are particularly high in choline, an essential nutrient critical to brain function that 90 percent of Americans don't get enough of. Egg yolks are also the richest sources of lutein and zeaxanthin, antioxidants that keep eyes healthy and protect them from the leading cause of blindness, macular degeneration. Eggs are loaded with other vital nutrients, including folate, riboflavin, selenium, and B vitamins.

How to Choose Your Eggs

Buying eggs is confusing, isn't it? Which is better: organic, pasture-raised, or omega-3 enriched? Are farm-fresh eggs really more healthful than conventional? While each

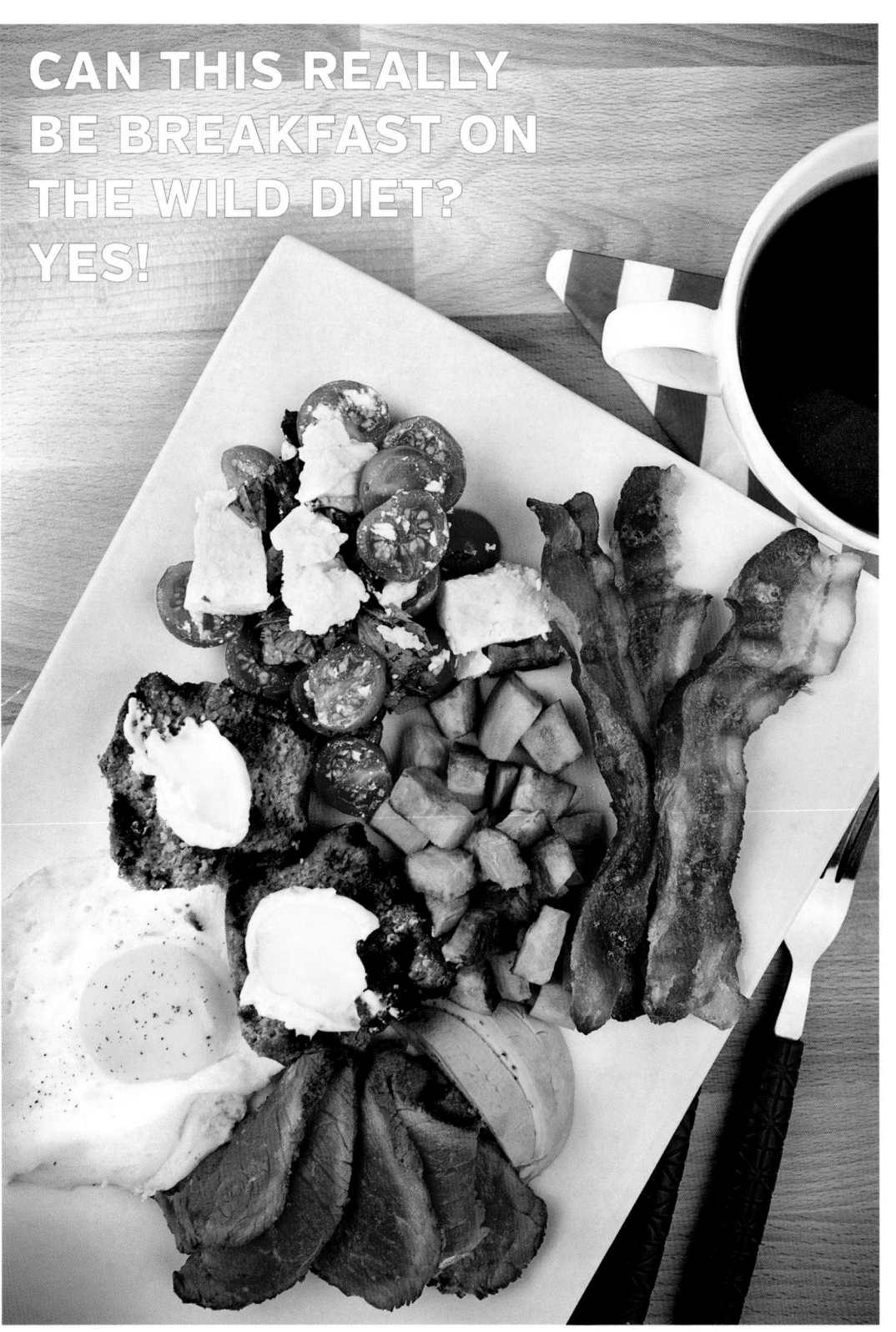

CAN THIS REALLY
BE BREAKFAST ON
THE WILD DIET?
YES!

Many diet and fitness gurus have always been skinny and fit. They never show you pictures of themselves flabby and miserable, because they've never been that way—they don't have "before and after" shots. But I've been there.

I followed a "heart-healthy," low-fat diet for years and exercised three to five times a week. According to conventional wisdom, I should have been lean, fit, and healthy. But that wasn't the case.

I was sluggish, overweight, and had borderline hypertension. My skin was pale and puffy, my gut was constantly bloated, and I rarely slept through the night. I thought that my health problems, moon-shaped face, and double chin were just genetics. After all, I came from a long line of barrel-chested, big-boned, burly mountain men who loved to eat. I assumed that, as I got older, the changes happening to my body were things I couldn't change.

A few weeks of the Wild Diet and one six-pack later, I realized I had been completely wrong. This book will show you exactly how I got there.

Abel before the Wild Diet

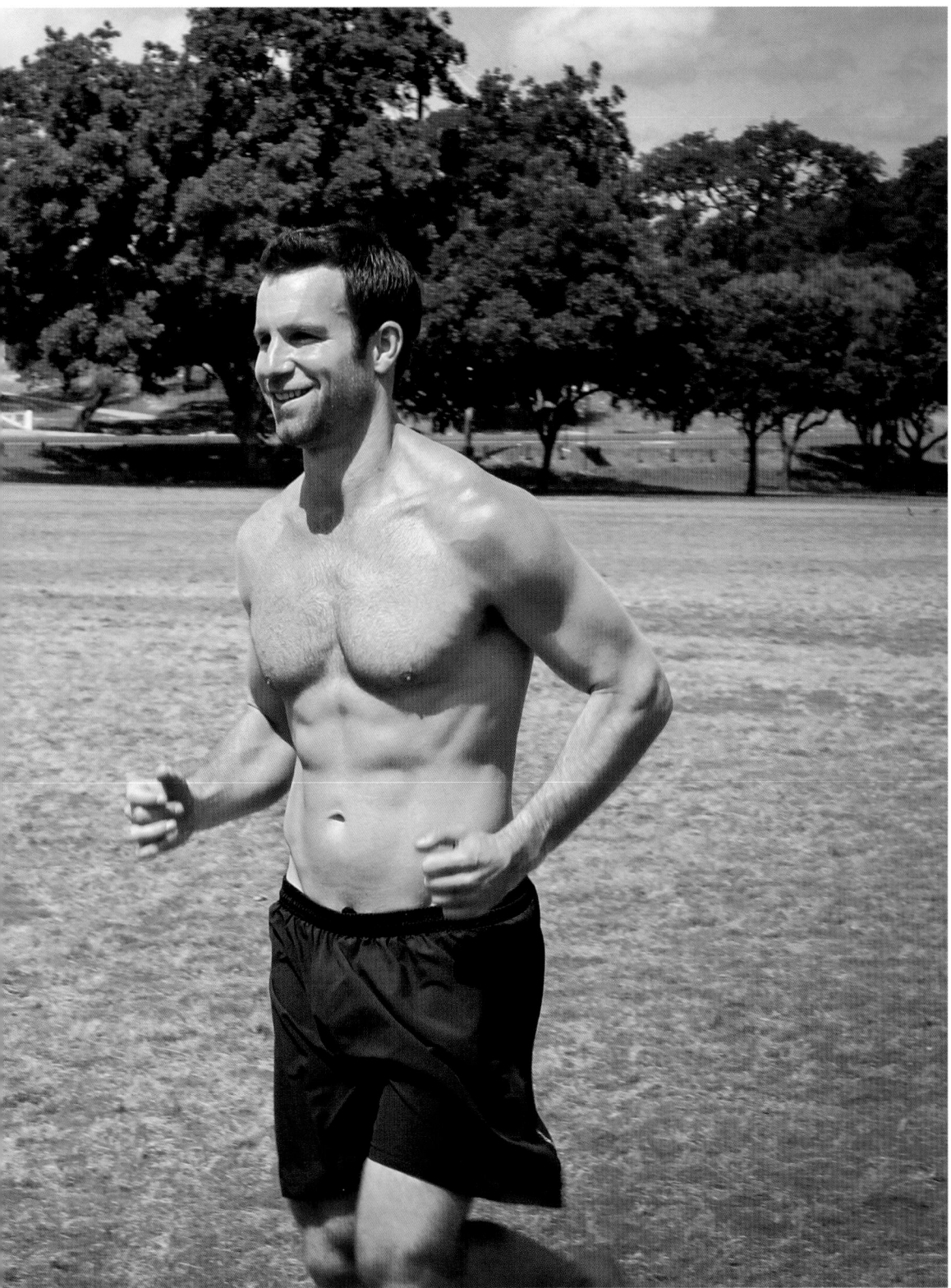

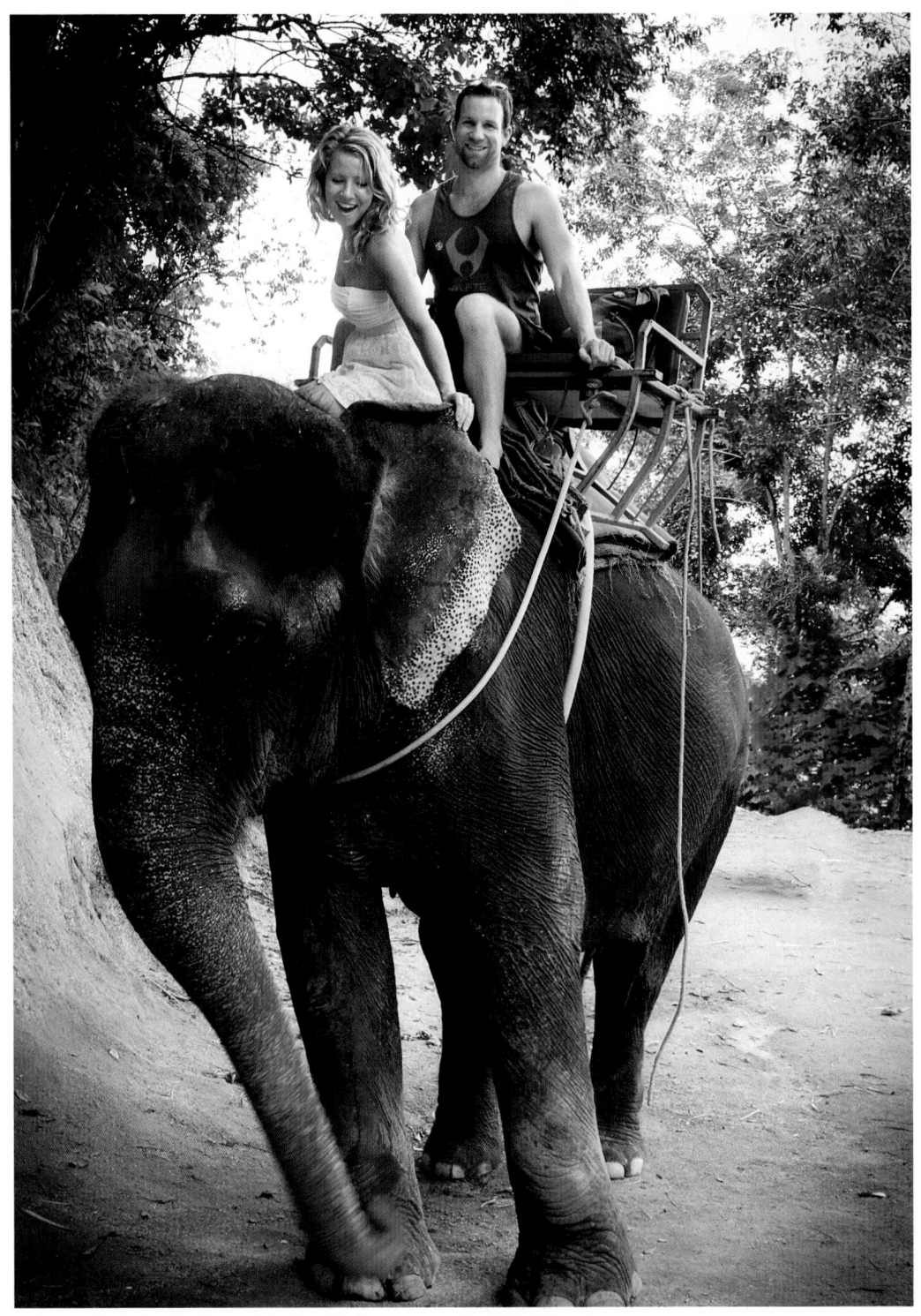

Abel and Alyson commuting in Thailand

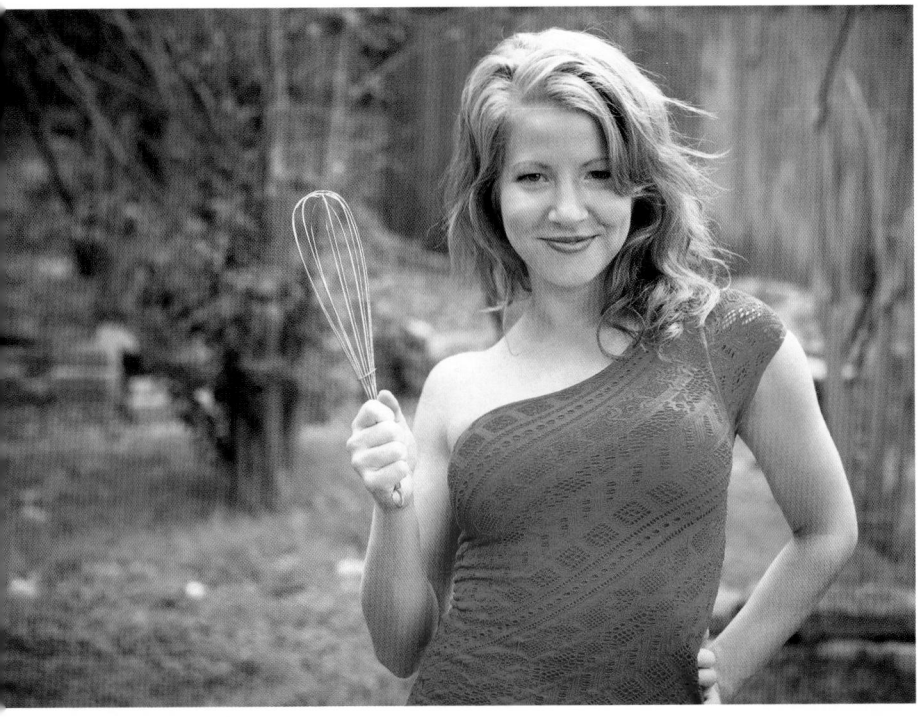

Meet Alyson, Abel's
kitchen copilot
(and wife)

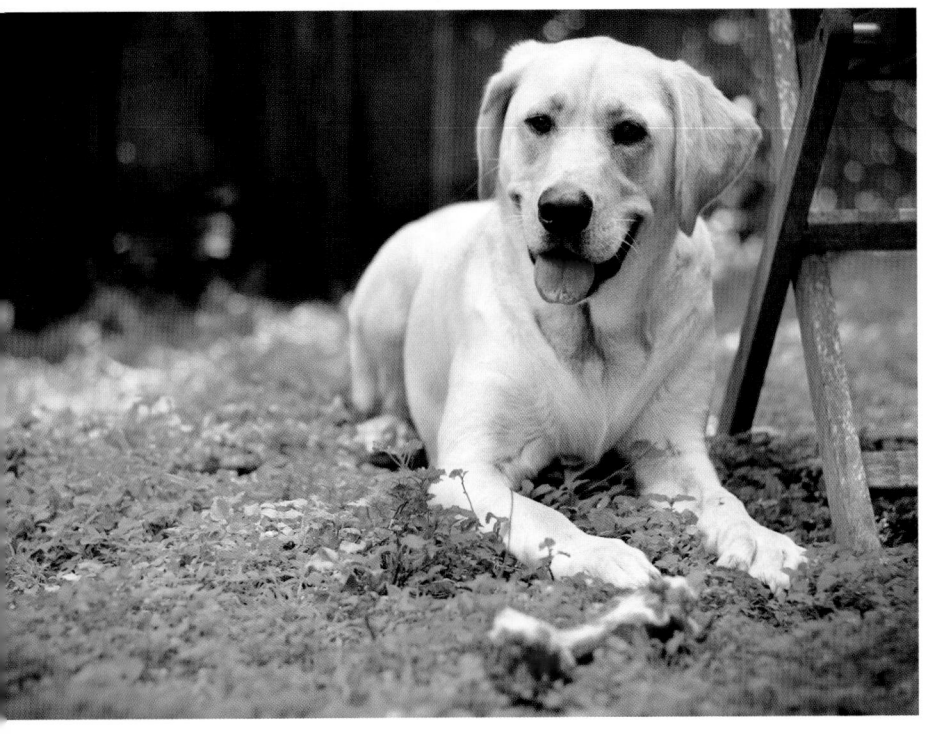

Bailey enjoys a raw,
meaty bone from the
farmers' market

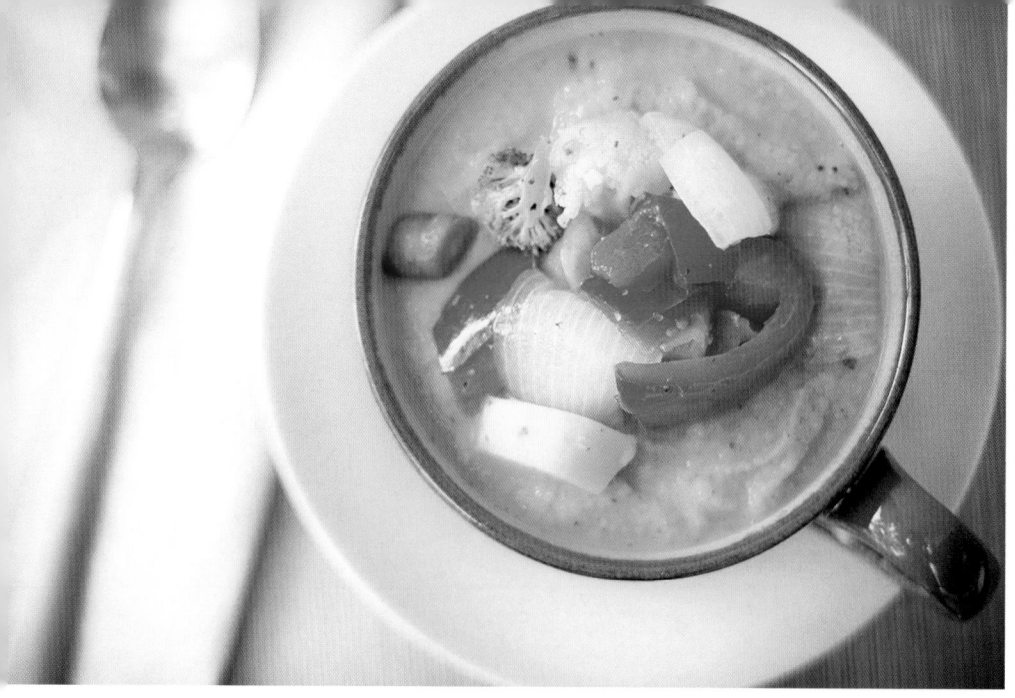

Creamy Roasted Vegetable Soup

Page 217

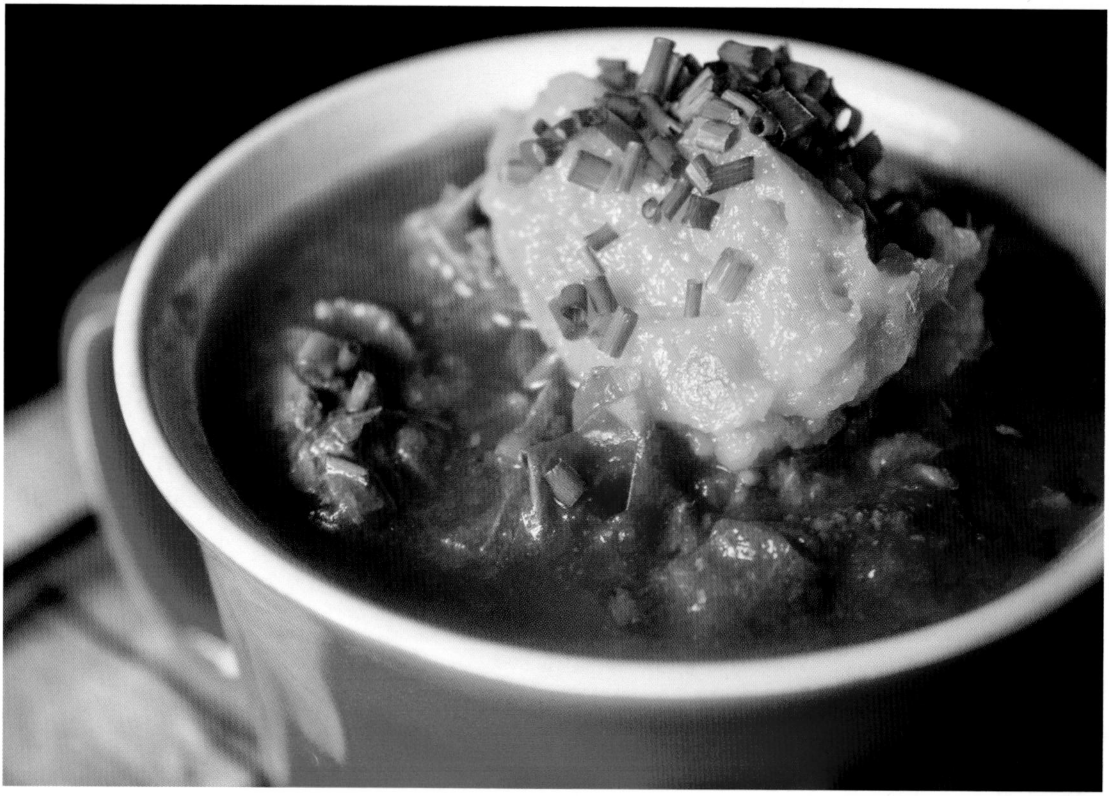

Spicy Beef Chili with Mashed Sweet Potato

Page 179

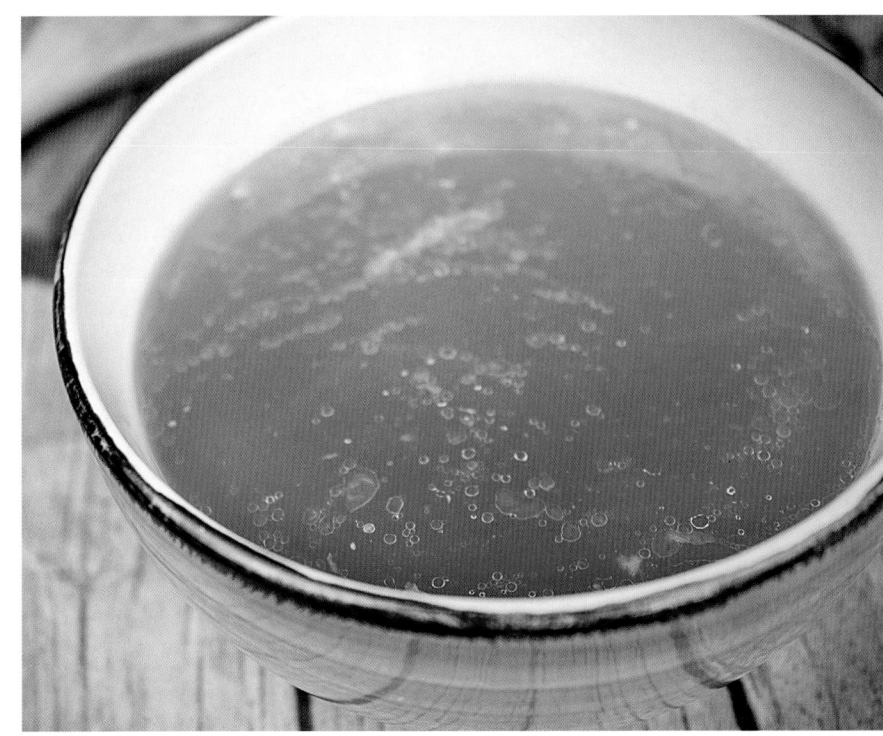

Bone Broth

Page 337

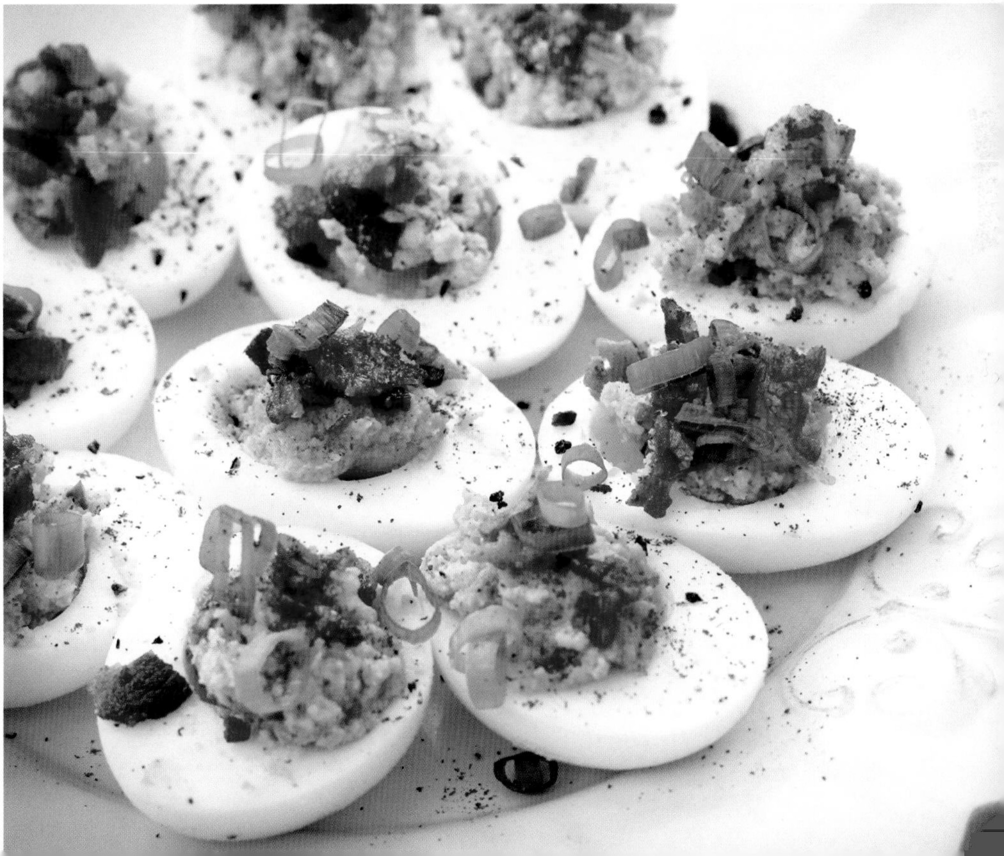

Bacon Deviled Eggs

In the Wild Kitchen app

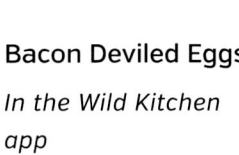

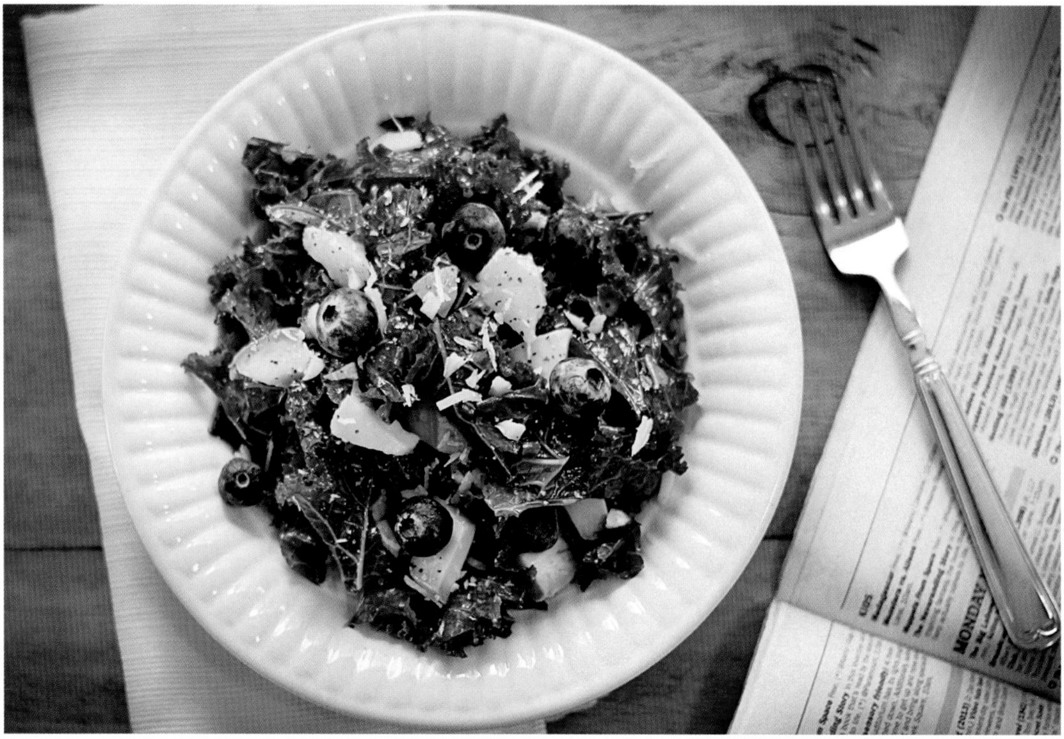

Blueberry, Avocado, and Kale Salad

In the Wild Kitchen app

Green Monster
Frittata with
Bruschetta

Page 213

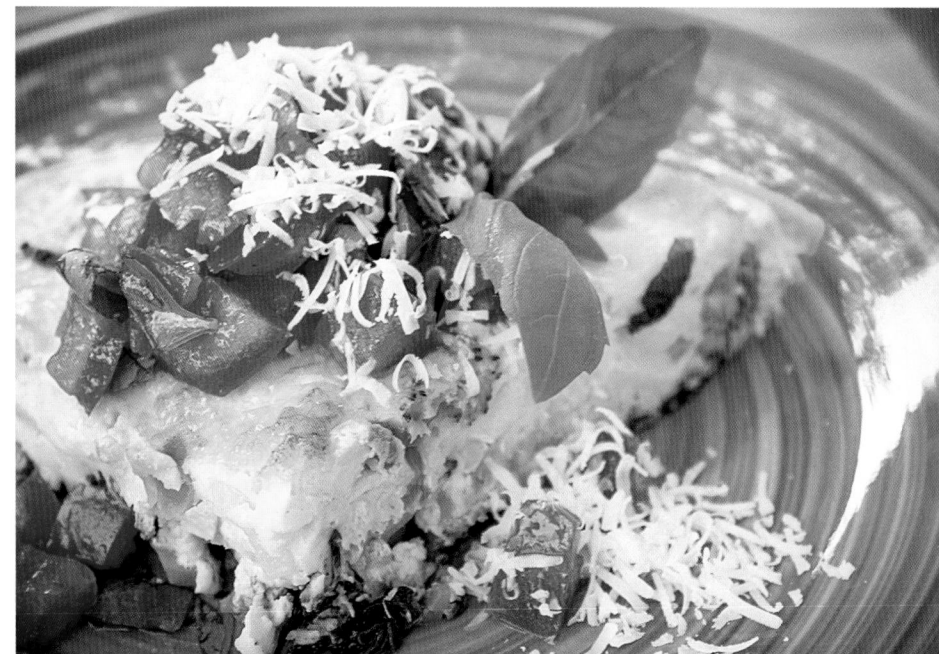

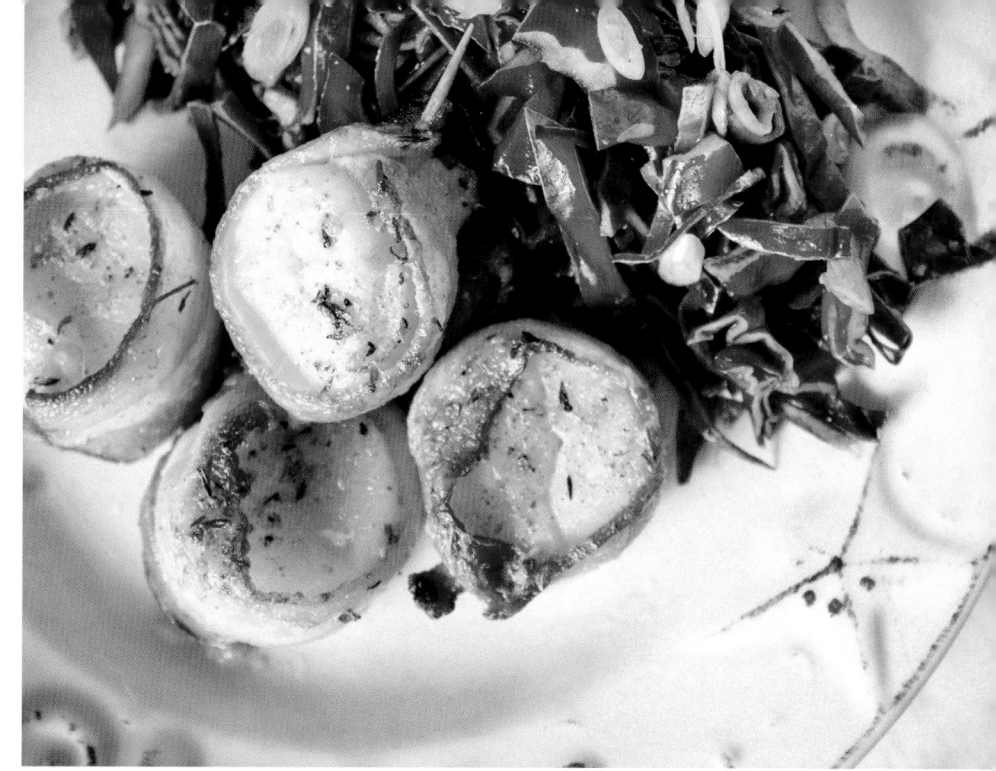

Bacon-Wrapped Scallops and Sweet Slaw

Page 200

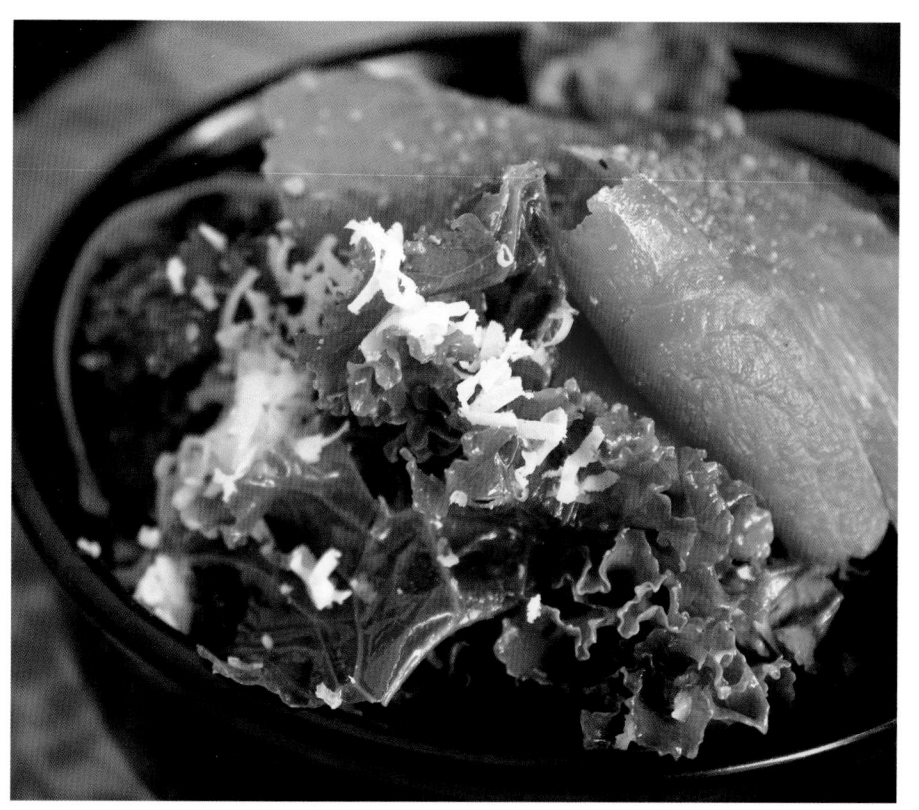

Smoked Salmon and Kale Salad

Page 211

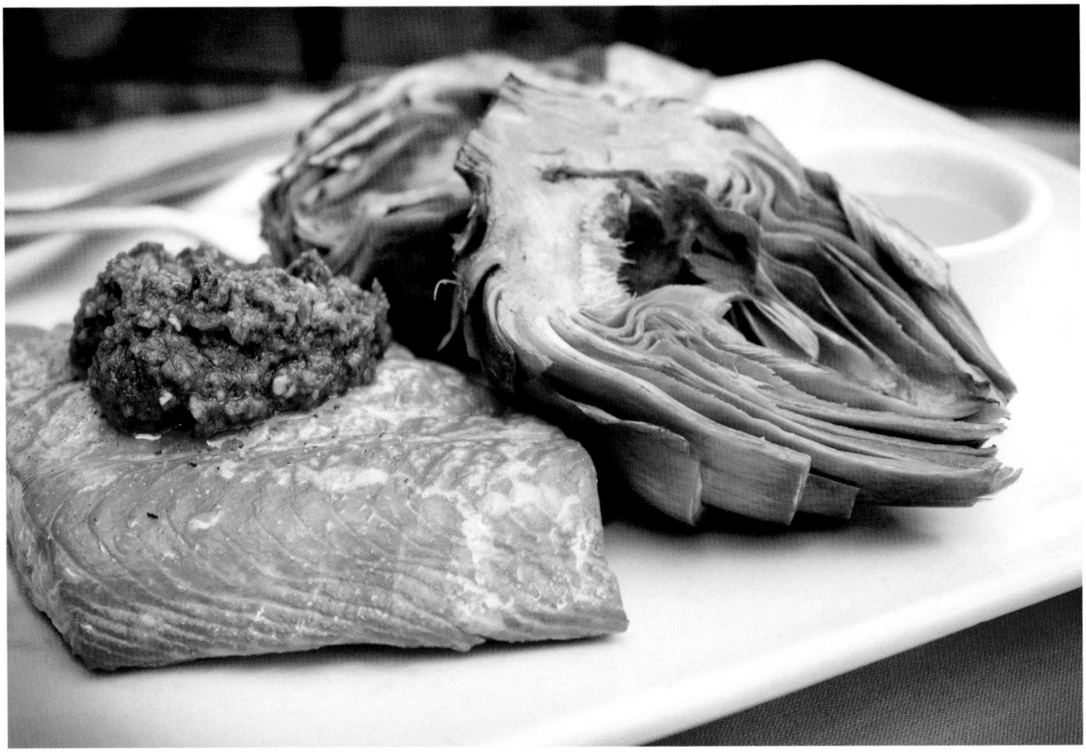

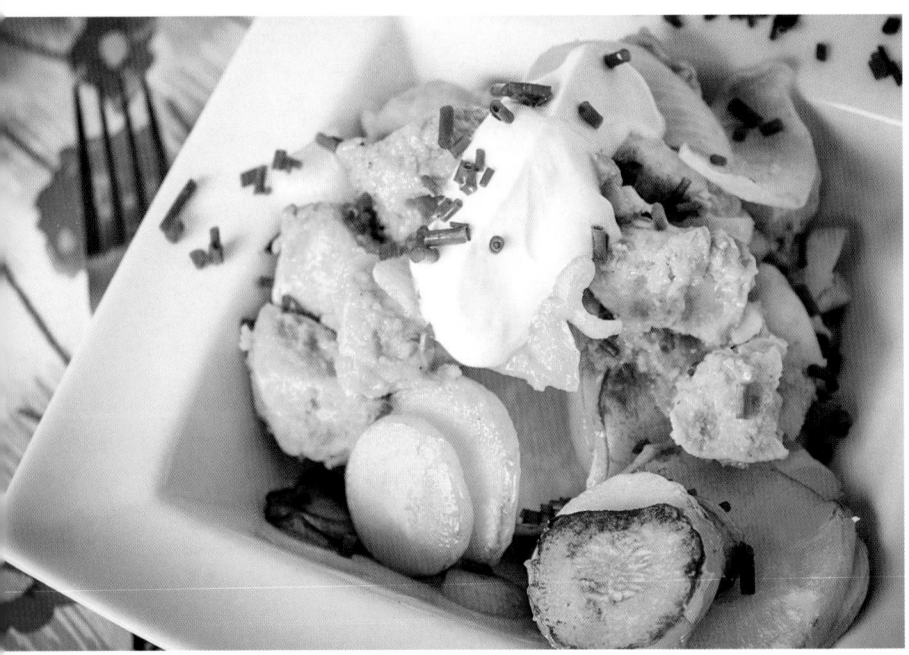

Baked Pesto Salmon with Roasted Artichokes

Page 197

Curried Chicken
and Onions with
Butter-Fried Parsnips

Page 152

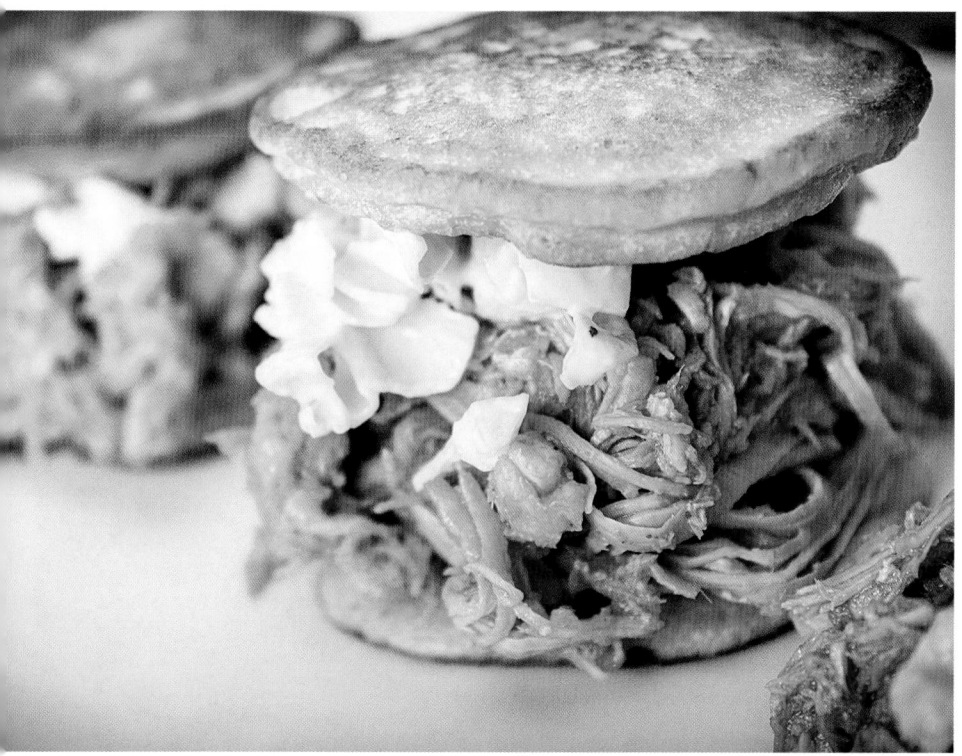

Pulled Pork Sliders

Page 159

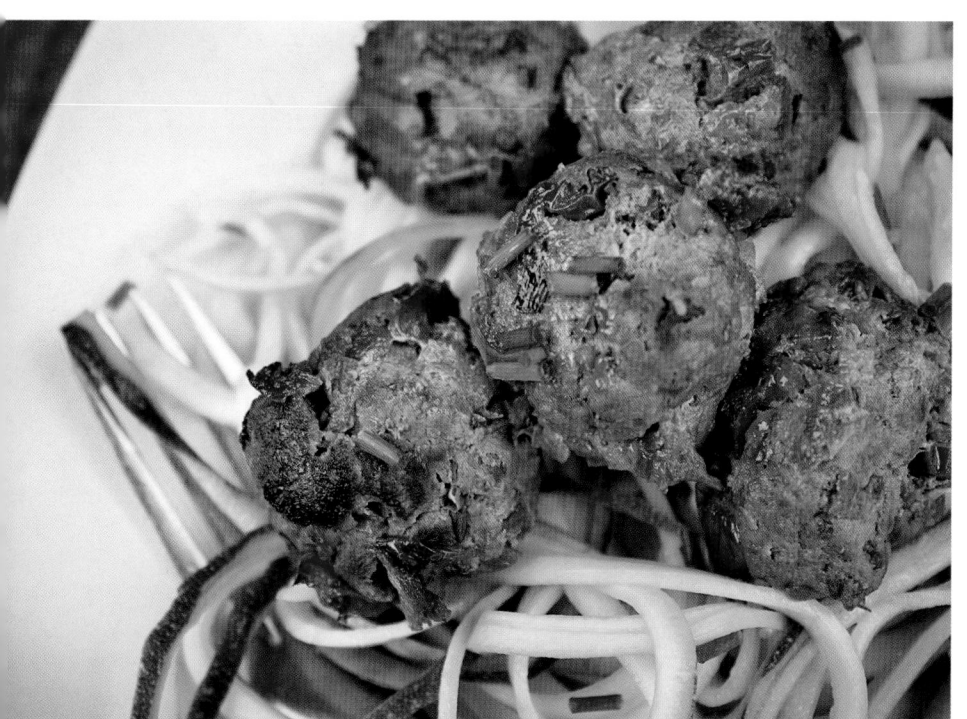

Sun-Dried Tomato Meatballs with Zucchini Noodles

Page 188

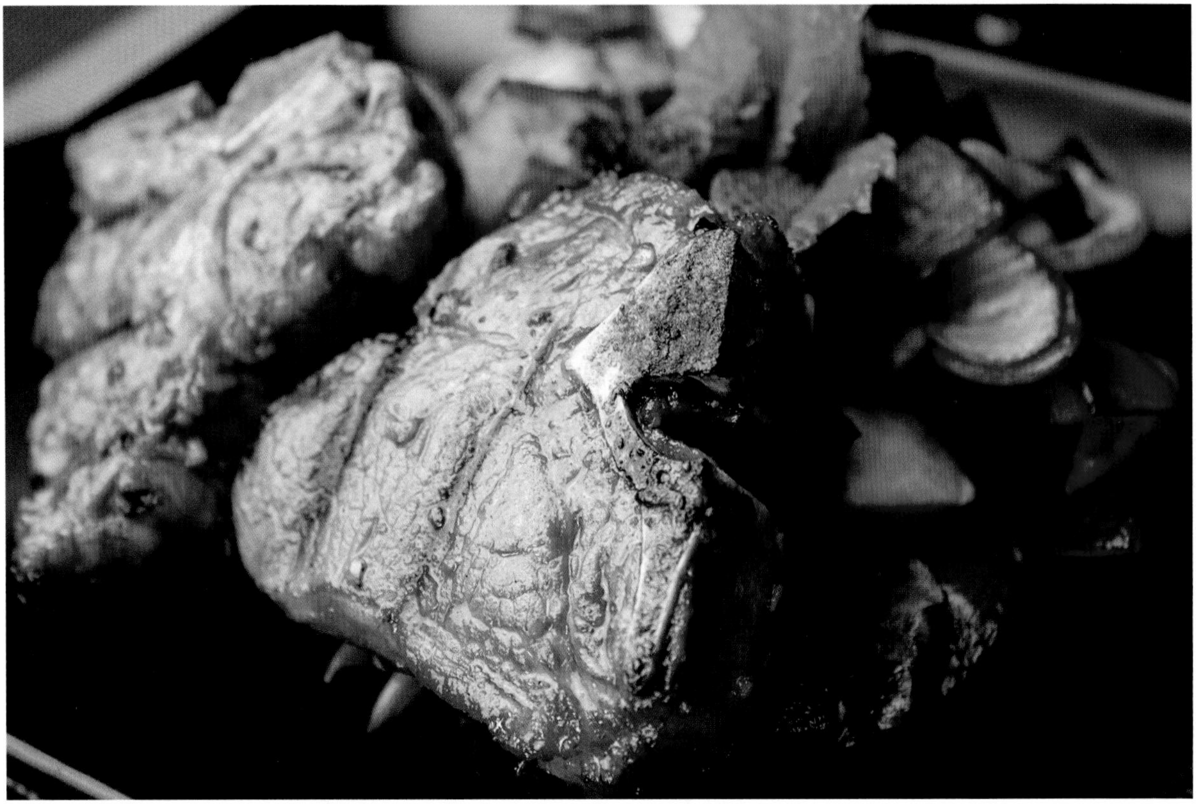

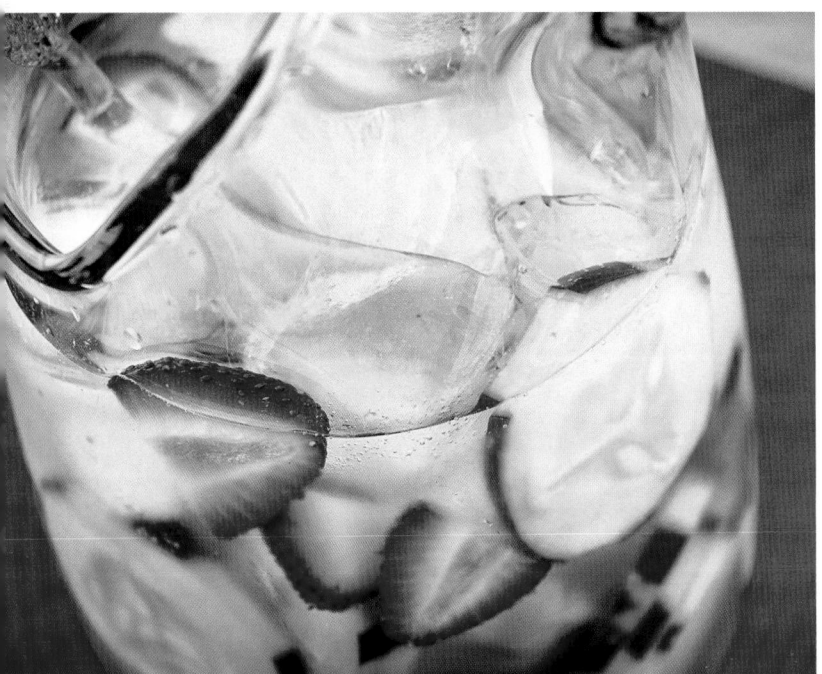

Ginger Lamb Chops with Roasted Vegetables

Page 185

Cucumber-Strawberry
Spa Water

Page 244

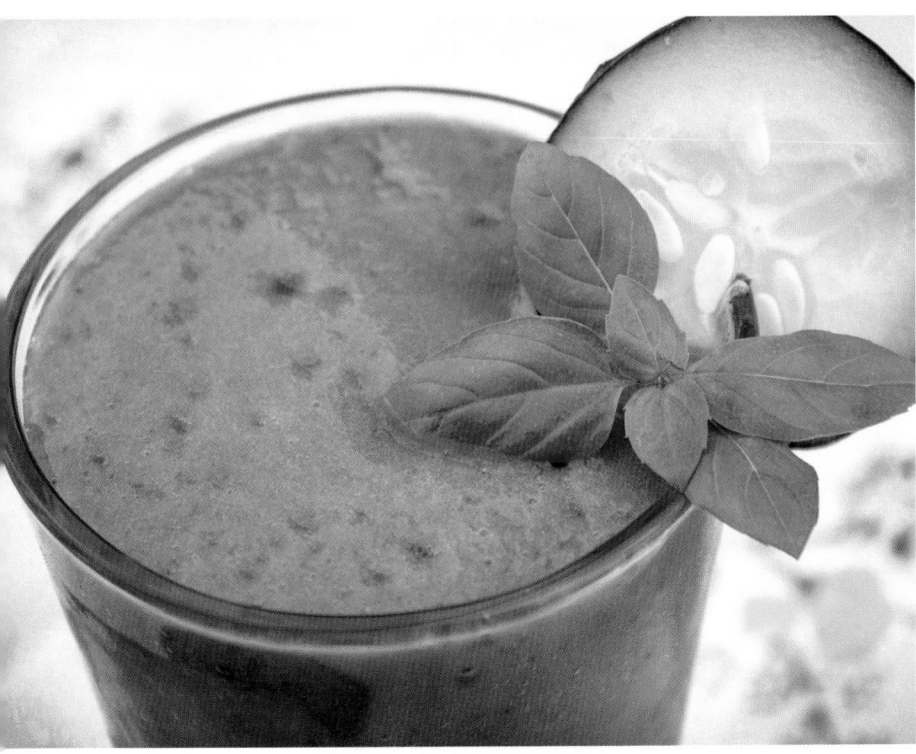

**Cucumber-Basil
Smoothie**

Page 236

**Fudgey Carob
Peanut Butter Bars**

*In the Wild Kitchen
app*

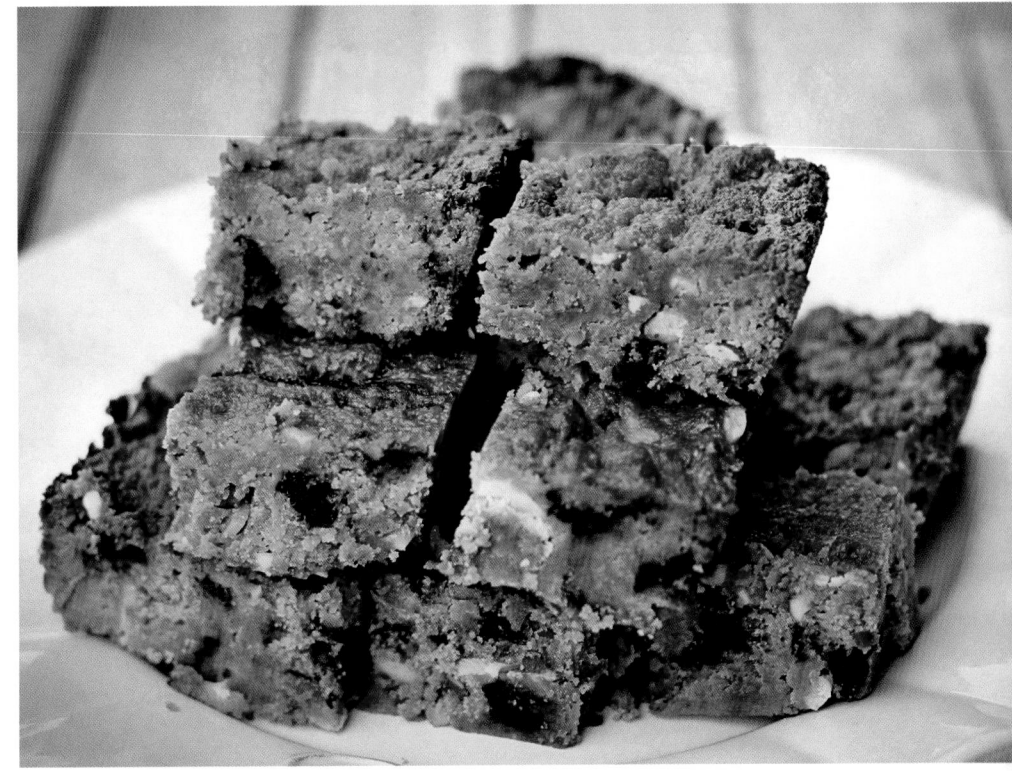

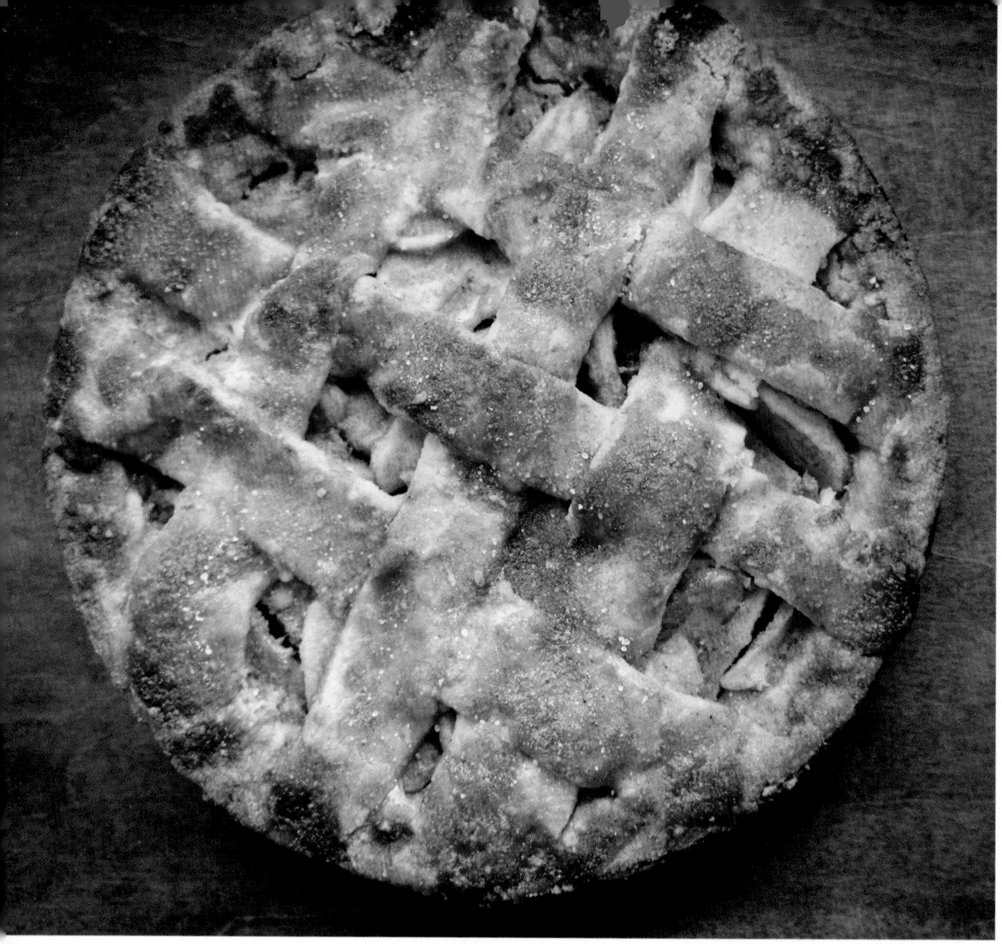

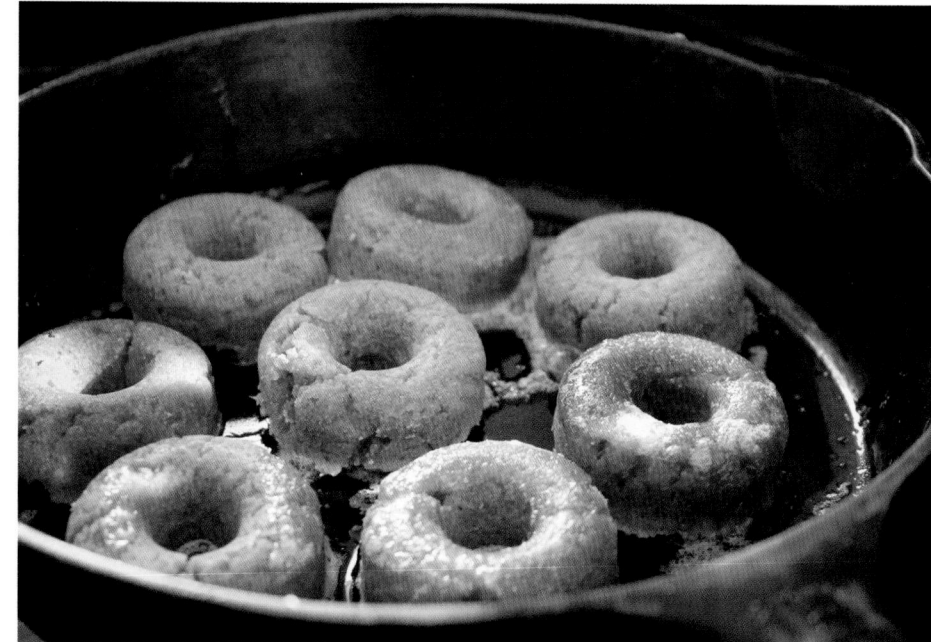

**Old-Fashioned
Apple Pie**

Page 262

Apple Cider Donuts

Page 255

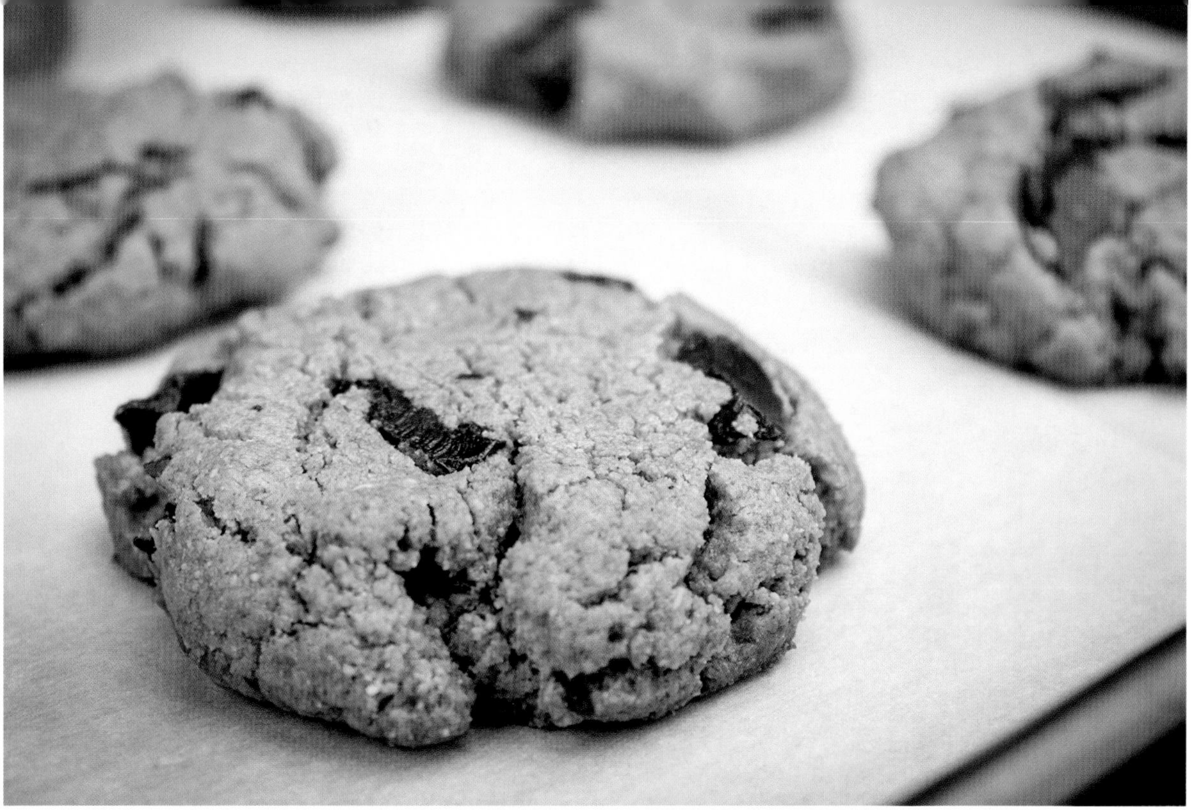

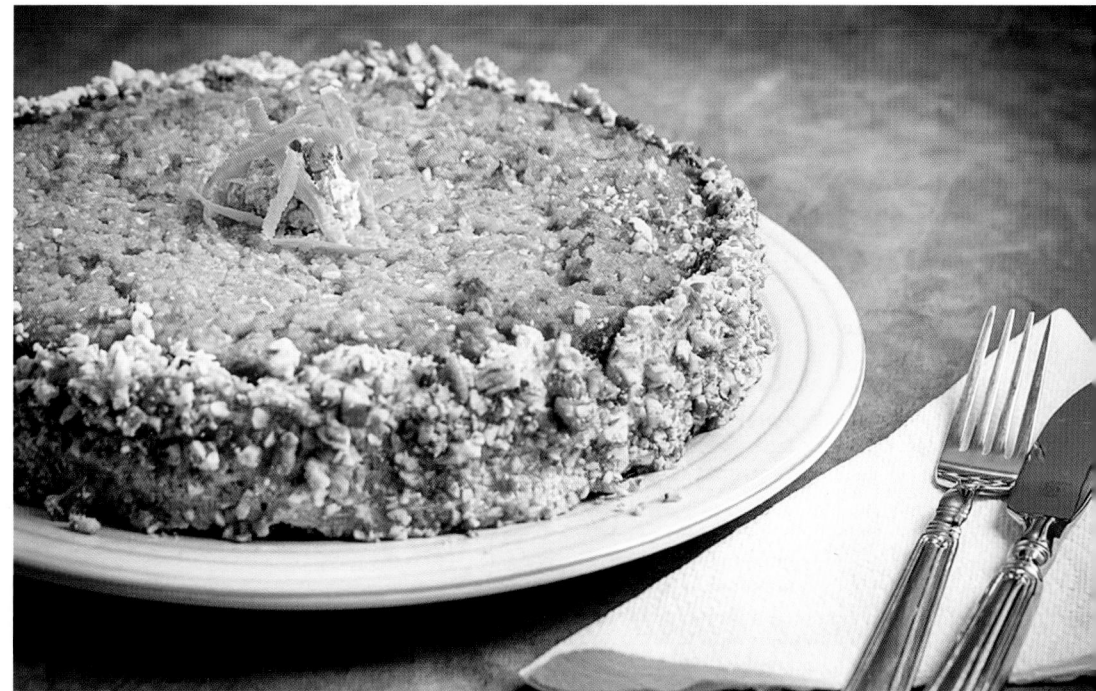

Peanut Butter Chocolate Chunk Cookies

Page 253

Carrot Cake

Page 257

THE WILD DIET PLATE

1. Most of your plate should be covered with fresh leafy vegetables such as kale, spinach, arugula, collards, or other greens. Raw is best, but steamed or lightly cooked veggies count, too. Fresh organic veggies are preferable, but flash-frozen works well in a pinch. When eating out, ask for extra greens or other colorful veggies instead of a starch.

2. Proteins such as grass-fed beef, chicken, turkey, pork, eggs, or seafood should make up about a quarter of your plate. A generous serving of protein is the size of the palm of your hand. If you're still hungry, feel free to eat protein and green veggies until you're satisfied.

3. Eat whole fruit as a snack or use to sweeten other foods. Limit to 1–2 servings of whole fruit a day to maximize fat loss.

4. Add energy to your meals with nutrient-dense fat. Fat should come from grass-fed meat, butter, coconut oil, avocado oil, olive oil, or unsalted nuts such as almonds, pecans, macadamias, or walnuts. Avoid processed oils.

5. If you are particularly active, have a high metabolism, or are less tolerant of fat or protein, consider a side of starch such as boiled sweet potato or whole-grain rice with lunch or dinner. If you find that carbs slow your fat loss, skip the starch and eat extra protein, veggies, or fat instead.

might come from a chicken, the conventional eggs you find for 99 cents at the supermarket are best avoided.

Pastured—Hens are allowed to roam free, eating plants and insects (their natural food). Depending on the farmer or how the carton is labeled, these chickens may also be fed with commercial feed.

Organic—The hens are not treated with antibiotics or hormones and received organic feed, but may have limited access to the outdoors.

Free-range—The hens live in a house with a small window that allows them the *option* of going outside.

Omega-3 enriched—These hens live lives similar to those of conventional chickens, but their feed is supplemented with an omega-3 source like flaxseeds. The hens may have had some access to the outside.

Cage-free—This term is relatively meaningless, as the chickens could still be raised in a foul, filthy, overcrowded henhouse.

Conventional—These chickens never see the light of day and are usually raised in an overfilled henhouse with cages. They are fed on GMO feed and kept alive with antibiotics.

Pastured > Organic > Omega-3 > Free-range/Cage-free > Conventional/Factory-Farmed

Best-case scenario, your eggs are local, organic, and come from happy, healthy hens that roam free on pasture. Eggs from your local farmer's free-roaming chickens might not be "certified" organic, but they're just as good if they were raised according to organic principles even if they aren't officially certified. Farm-fresh eggs from free-range hens are higher in vitamins A and E and omega-3s than conventional eggs. Although they might cost more than conventional eggs, the additional nutrients in pastured eggs provide more bang for the buck.

FISH AND SEAFOOD

Eating fresh seafood off the line is one of the greatest pleasures in life. I've had many meals of fresh fish, oysters, mussels, clams, and more that have left me with a tangible head buzz from sea nutrients that we probably haven't even discovered yet. Fish are a fat burner's best friend—if you're looking to eat fewer calories to lean down quickly, choosing a grilled fish entrée can fill you up on roughly half the calories of a steak.

Swordfish, shark, tuna, and other large fish should be eaten sparingly since they carry high levels of mercury and other toxins in their meat from living in polluted oceans. Generally, smaller fish like sardines, anchovies, and trout carry fewer toxins. One of the advantages of eating smaller fish and shellfish is that you eat the whole animal in one bite. While organ meats like liver, kidney, or heart can be intimidating at first, eating nose to tail is easy when you chow down on oysters, mussels, clams, or other shellfish. Eating the whole animal ensures that you maximize your intake of vitamins and minerals that are difficult to source from muscle meats or vegetables.

When it comes to fish and seafood, always buy wild. Farmed fish is easy to come by, but you should know that the standards of quality and regulation at international fish farms are troubling. Like commercial cattle operations, many fish farms will feed their fish whatever is cheapest and fattens the fish rapidly—including processed GMO soy, poultry feces, and worse. I do my best to avoid farmed fish and recommend you do the same.

Make an excuse to feed yourself seafood, even if you need to use supplements to get there. Since I spend most of my time living in the mountains where fresh fish can be difficult to source, I start most days with fermented cod-liver oil or omega-3 fish oil. Nutrient-dense fat from seafood fuels the brain, eases hunger pangs, and frontloads the day's nutrition by supplying your body with critical vitamins like A and D.

DAIRY

Take it from a dairy lover—it's difficult to get high-quality milk and dairy in America these days. But when you can, it's worth it. My grandfather, an organic dairy farmer, made yogurt the old-fashioned way, by leaving raw, warm milk from a grass-fed cow in the barn to ferment. The natural probiotics in the milk begin to predigest the lactose in milk and—voilà—you have a mason jar full of plain, raw yogurt. These days, what most people call "yogurt" is more like a syrup or custard, with many packaged yogurt products containing as much sugar as a can of soda.

From an anthropological perspective, dairy is a unique food—humans are the only animal to drink the milk of another species. But several thousand years ago, about 40 percent of us adapted the ability to digest lactose, the main sugar in milk. Since milk is meant to spur growth in developing mammals, it's great for adding muscle, but it isn't going to help much with burning fat. In fact, dairy stalls fat loss in many individuals, most likely due to its high carbohydrate/lactose content and insulin-elevating effects. For most people, limiting or avoiding most dairy gets them the quickest fat loss.

However, the legends of using saturated fat in dairy and eggs to build muscle are epic. Vince Gironda, the "Iron Guru," declared that nutrition was 85 to 90 percent of bodybuilding, advocated eating thirty-six eggs a day and was known to slug heavy cream by the cup. Casey Viator, who became Mr. America as a teen, consumed two dozen eggs and two gallons of raw milk a day. So if you want to bulk up, go ahead and try the Gallon of Milk a Day diet. But don't blame me when you clear the hallways.

Cow's milk contains substances that are difficult for some people to digest, including lactose, casein, and whey. Those who are lactose intolerant have trouble digesting the main sugar (lactose) found in milk. When the undigested sugars reach the colon, they begin to ferment, producing gas that can cause cramping, bloating, nausea, flatulence, and diarrhea. If you experience any of these symptoms, dairy may be responsible.

If you have trouble digesting high-temperature pasteurized dairy, it might not be because you're lactose intolerant, but because the high temperature and processing destroys the cofactors and enzymes that are critical to effective digestion and absorption of nutrients. Fermented dairy, such as aged hard cheese, yogurt, and kefir, is generally easier to digest than milk.

If cow dairy continues to cause problems, try goat milk. Structurally and nutritionally, goat milk is one of the closer corollaries to human breast milk, making it arguably more suitable for human consumption than cow dairy. Goat milk fat does not clump together, keeping it more homogenized and also aiding digestibility. It also has less casein, less lactose, and more easily digestible protein content than cow dairy.

For optimal fat loss, it's best to not drink milk very often since it can raise insulin. But if you do choose to drink milk, always go for full fat—the fat slows your absorption of simple sugars. Besides, the cream is the best part!

If dairy sits well with you, go for fermented options such as plain yogurt, raw cheese, cottage cheese, sour cream, or kefir. The cultures in these foods are healthy probiotics and also predigest some of the lactose in the milk for you, which makes them easier on your gut. I drink milk in small quantities as a treat or as a post-workout recovery drink. Coming from a family of dairy lovers, I eat grass-fed butter, heavy cream, ghee, yogurt, cheese, and cottage cheese often, especially after a hearty workout.

Choose your dairy carefully and vote with your food dollar in favor of happy cows on pasture. Avoid high-temperature pasteurized and homogenized milk from conventional feedlots and do your best to find raw, organic, pasture-raised, grass-fed, and full-fat dairy.

NUTS AND SEEDS

Raw, soaked, sprouted, or roasted, nuts are a reliable snack for the aspiring hunter-gatherer. If you're looking to lose fat, limiting nuts to a handful a day is a sensible max. Since nuts and seeds are calorie dense and usually come shelled for you, they're easy to overeat. When you eat nuts, imagine that you need to shell each nut by hand, enjoying them one at a time like humans once did.

To avoid spoilage and rancidity, nuts should be stored in the freezer or, at the very least, sold and stored in a cool, dark place. Watch out for packaged nuts, which are usually fried in industrial oil and often contain gluten and MSG.

Peanuts (technically a legume) are one of the cheapest and most-sprayed crops on earth, often slathered with chemical pesticides. Go organic and limit your consumption since they're easy to overeat. As peanuts are a common allergen, watch for any signs of inflammation like achy joints or upset stomach, which could indicate intolerance, sensitivity, or allergy.

FRUIT

Think of fruit as nature's candy—meant to be enjoyed as a seasonal treat. Fruit contains a significant amount of sugar, primarily fructose. In small quantities, this isn't a problem, but to achieve optimal fat burning, it's best to enjoy most fruits infrequently. Many fruits, such as the domesticated apples, pears, and bananas you might find at a convenience store, have been bred for sweetness and size and contain many times the amount of sugar that would have been found in older, native varieties.

Tropical fruit like cantaloupe and watermelon tend to be high in sugar, as are pineapples, mangoes, papayas, bananas, and grapes. Think of these fruits as treats, not staples, especially if you want to lose fat. Dried fruit, such as dates, figs, raisins, apricots, and prunes, should be eaten sparingly or used as a sweetener—they go wonderfully with cheese and nuts for a satisfying dessert. We often blend fresh or dried fruit with our desserts instead of using sugar, which adds unique flavor and substance to our pies, cakes, yogurt, ice cream, and other homemade treats. But keep in mind that dried fruit is quite sugary and easy to overeat.

If you want to lose fat, one to two servings of fruit a day is a sensible maximum. If you're highly active, you can handle a bit more—let your hunger and energy dictate how much you eat, but know that too much fruit can slow fat loss.

STARCHY VEGETABLES

When you eat starches, cook them low and slow—boiled, steamed, or in a slow cooker—which can cut the glycemic index of a starch in half when compared to high-temperature cooking like baking, grilling, or frying. When you do eat quick-burning carbs and simple sugars, you can reduce their glycemic effect by limiting quantities or combining them with fat, fiber, and/or an acid such as vinegar. To limit spikes in blood glucose, always consume your carbs with fiber (this happens automatically when you eat vegetables, fruit, and grains whole).

The timing of carb consumption is important, especially if your goal is to lose weight. Since too much starch can slow fat loss, eat starchy vegetables in small quantities as part of your evening feast and avoid them earlier in the day. Eating one to two servings of starch with your evening meal can help you sleep, reduce cortisol, and replenish glycogen in your muscles and liver. If you're physically active, you may also choose to consume starches in the hours before or immediately following exercise, which will help shuttle nutrients to your hungry muscles.

The glycemic index of individual foods and glycemic load of meals are not perfect measurements, but both are useful tools as you explore the vegetable world. Stick to low-sugar, slow-cooked, fibrous, heritage, heirloom, and whole foods, and eat slowly to keep the glycemic effect of your meals to a minimum. Starchy veggies like sweet potatoes, yams, and colored heirloom potatoes are nutritionally superior to the white-fleshed domesticated potatoes and stimulate a more favorable insulin response.

HOW TO PICK YOUR PRODUCE

When you're picking your produce, remember that the eye can be deceiving. Many foods are doctored so that they will appeal to you on the grocery shelves. Take, for instance, the humble apple. You may shun the slightly dull-looking local, organic apple and reach instead for the sparkling, perfectly proportioned "delicious" apple from some country across the world.

This apple, however, has some dirty little secrets. It was grown in chemical fertilizer, picked before it was ripe, sprayed with forty-two toxic pesticides, gassed with ethylene, and sprayed with wax to enhance its appearance, and, after being shipped from across the world in the belly of a tanker, has been dead and decomposing for weeks before it even reaches the shelf in front of you. The local organic apple, in comparison, was picked by your neighbor just days earlier.

Say you lay the sparkling apple next to the organic apple on the ground. A worm approaches. Which apple do you think the worm will choose to eat, the decomposing apple slathered in chemicals and wax or the fresh organic one? Smart worm.

Most cities have farmers' markets or health food stores that carry local produce. If you're stuck shopping at a chain grocery, then look for the produce that has traveled the shortest distance to reach you. Not only will you be getting more nutrient-dense produce, but it'll taste better, too. If you can't find fresh produce that fits your budget, flash-frozen works fine in a pinch.

BEANS, LENTILS, AND LEGUMES

Beans are an economical source for slow-burning carbs, fiber, and satisfying protein. Legumes like beans and lentils are not as nutrient dense as vegetables, fruits, tree nuts, seeds, and animal fats, but they're handy because they're cheap and store well on the shelf.

At most restaurants, beans and legumes are often prepared incorrectly or incompletely. Since legumes contain lectins, a protein that can damage the gut, improperly prepared legumes have been implicated in irritable bowel syndrome, arthritis, peptic ulcers, autoimmune conditions, allergies, and type 2 diabetes. Lectins aren't a problem for most people, however, when grains and legumes are prepared according to the healthful traditional techniques of our ancestors—soaked overnight in an acidic medium (see page 271).

THE 90/10 RULE:
YOU DON'T HAVE TO BE PERFECT

While eating clean can be challenging at times, it is an important part of your health. Organic is good, pasture raised and grass finished is great, and adding local to the mix is as good as it gets. If you can, visit local farms or farmers' markets, pick your favorite, and stock up on their meat, eggs, and produce. When it comes to taste and nutrition, nothing beats fresh, high-quality food.

That said, you don't have to be perfect. Your body doesn't adapt to your occasional missteps; it adapts to what you do habitually every single day. The most effective thing you can do is build those automatic habits so you don't have to rely on willpower to eat right. If you eat Wild 90 percent of the time, go ahead and have some fun with the other 10 percent. (What does fun look like? Well, the night before the photo shoot for the cover of this book, my after-dinner treat included three slices of homemade cheesecake and two peanut butter cookies.)

If you eat clean most of the time but your beef isn't grass fed, your eggs aren't pastured, and your vegetables are conventionally raised, you will still get great results and be light-years ahead of where you started. The Wild Diet is about opening your palate to new tastes and experiences, so don't create the unnecessary stress of having to only eat from farmers' markets and health food stores. Do the best you can.

YOUR "FREE" MEAL

If you've tried our recipes, you're already aware that I eat more than my fair share of homemade cookies, ice cream, breads, cheesecake, pies, puddings, and other delights. If you have to avoid your favorite foods for the rest of your life, then why in the world would you ever stick to any diet? Take it from a former fat kid—indulging from time to time is good for the soul.

Cultivating a healthy relationship with food and taking pleasure in what you eat is far more important than any short-term weight-loss goals. Not only will indulgences satisfy cravings and help prevent you from bingeing, but varying your daily caloric intake can help you boost your metabolism and burn fat.

So here it is: You have permission to indulge and eat whatever you like for one meal a week. Anything you want. Really. Pizza, pastries, grilled cheese, ice cream . . . the world is your oyster. The most important thing is to enjoy yourself—the benefits of "free" meals are psychological as much as they are physiological. Consider your "free" meals as a well-deserved treat for building healthy habits. Forget the guilt and savor every second of your indulgence.

If you need more convincing, know that fasting or undereating for too long can not only be detrimental to fat loss but actually cause weight gain. I almost always break my fast after twenty-four hours, as fasting more than that often makes me feel cranky, drained, and weak. As a result of extended caloric restriction, your body may drop your metabolic rate and jack up your appetite due to a decrease in leptin, a fat-burning hormone. This, in turn, increases production of cortisol (a stress hormone), which makes losing fat difficult. To prevent this drop in leptin from occurring, your "free meal" keeps your metabolism on its toes. Especially if you're fasting during the day, make sure that you eat enough during your evening feast to fuel activities the next day, The more you eat the night before, the longer you can go the next day until your first meal.

STAY WILD

For the sake of your overall health and sanity, do yourself a favor and get the highest-quality food you can find for your "free" meals. If you love donuts, don't get them from the gas station—go to the best bakery in town. If you love pizza, get it fresh from a legendary Italian restaurant, not from Pizza Hut. While a few slices of buttered whole-grain gluten-free oat sourdough might be a worthy indulgence, a single slice of store-bought bread made with domesticated "dwarf" wheat could ruin the weekend.

Don't waste your free meals on junk food—get the good stuff. There's no need to eat whatever's in front of you—plan ahead and make your "free" meal a celebratory feast with people you love. If you can, exercise on the same day as your "free" meal to use those extra calories for good, not evil.

My favorite treats? Ice cream covered in melted chocolate, blueberry cheesecake, flourless sweet potato pancakes slathered in fresh butter and my cousin's local maple syrup, and homemade pumpkin pie with whipped cream and raw milk to wash it down.

Make your "free" meals your only outlet for eating unhealthy foods, and do not let any of these eating habits creep into your daily routine. If you cheat by accident, wait until the following week for your next "free" meal.

TIPS FOR "FREE" MEALS

- Keep a "food craving notepad" throughout the week. Every time you get a craving for something, add it to the list of foods for your "free" meal. This way you can acknowledge your craving and remind yourself that you will have permission to indulge during your meal.
- Indulge on a regular day off, as you will have more control over when and where you eat.
- Plan ahead and eat out at your favorite restaurants. Make your free meals fun.
- Drink plenty of water, in excess of 8 ounces eight times a day, to help your body process excess salt and carbohydrates.
- If you choose to eat carb- or sugar-heavy foods, do your best not to eat high amounts of fat at the same time.
- Never eat dessert alone. Sharing dessert will help you enjoy your treat more slowly and is always better than eating that whole brownie by yourself.
- Minimize insulin surges by blunting jumps in blood sugar.
- No matter what, throw out all "indulgent" food before the next morning. Yes, even leftovers.

Still not convinced? Okay, you don't *have* to use the "free" meals. If you can stick to the plan without them, and you are looking for maximum fat loss, then there's no need to force indulgences. However, if you have a tendency to cheat habitually or you constantly want to quit because you feel deprived of your favorite foods, then by all means— use the free meal! It's best to cram all your bad habits into one or two meals than to deny them and binge later.

If you find that you would rather follow the 90/10 rule by enjoying "free" treats ad hoc and unscheduled, that's great. Take great pleasure in them, but don't let the treats sneak into your habits.

TROUBLESHOOTING

If you "accidentally" munch on a bread roll at dinner, don't guilt yourself into being unable to enjoy your juicy, grass-finished tenderloin. The Wild Diet is a template—it contains sensible guidelines for healthy fat burning and health, but it's not uncompromising. If you drop the ball and polish off a slice of your boss's birthday cake, roll with it. We're all human.

That said, if you're not consistently sticking to the plan, make sure you aren't making excuses. Genetics are not an excuse. The past is not an excuse. Your present condition is not an excuse. You can either make excuses or get results, but you can't do both.

If you find that cheating "happens" during the week, don't fret, but skip your "free" meal. If you indulge regularly, it's not really indulging anymore—it's just poor decision-making and a lack of commitment to success. So do your best to squeeze your indulgences into one or two meals a week.

If you fall off the wagon, dust your butt off and hop back on. No one will remember or care that you ate a cupcake. Retraining your body and your mind is a process, and as long as you're improving your habits, the results will come.

PART V

Wild Cooking, Meals, and Recipes

> Woe to the cook whose sauce has no sting.
>
> —*Geoffrey Chaucer*

Want to hear something a little nuts? Despite hosting my show, blogging about health for a decade, and writing several bestselling books on the subject, I'm not really that into fitness and nutrition. I'm just really into great food.

Sure, I can teach you how to get lean by choking down skinless chicken breast and steamed broccoli for the next forty days. But that doesn't sound like any fun at all. Actually, after years of dedicated research, trial and error, and guinea pigging, I've learned that obsessing over the macronutrient content of food, carb-timing, or an intensive exercise program is not the key to staying fit, strong, and healthy. One of the best things you can do to improve your health is to think of cooking as a gift to yourself and others. Fumbling your way around the kitchen and learning how to prepare your own meals will do more for your health than any exercise routine, miracle drug, or fad diet in existence. I don't know of any other single activity that can make such a tremendous positive change in the quality of your life. The only way to guarantee you and your family get the quality of food you deserve is by preparing food yourself.

Sharing a home-cooked meal not only means more nutritious food, but it also fills a fundamental need for real, live, social interaction. It relieves the stress of our fast-paced lifestyles and solidifies the bond of family and friendship. It's a time to actually laugh out loud, talk, share, relax, and nourish your body.

Learning how to cook may just change your life. My wife, Alyson, gave up a career as one of the top professional gamers in the United States because she had more fun in the kitchen once she started cooking (if you're as big a nerd as we are, then you may have seen her on Season 1 of *WCG Ultimate Gamer*). Now she cooks for a living, with bestselling apps and many of the recipes in this book to her name. My dad, a master of the cast-iron skillet, paid his way through college by becoming a short-order cook. My friend George, injured during his time as a Marine, learned how to cook at home to help heal his body, losing 100 pounds in the process. Two years after creating the Civilized Caveman blog to share his recipes, George is now a full-time chef with a *New York Times*-bestselling cookbook and #1 app to his name. It all started with scrambled eggs.

If you want to know our secret to maintaining beach-ready bodies year-round without pain, misery, or restriction, it's all about alchemy in an apron. Learn how to create your favorite foods and share them with people you love. When you master the art of sourcing and creating mouth-watering meals that nourish your body and mind, you can quite literally manifest the body and health that you deserve by eating ridiculously well.

Crunchy zucchini pasta, juicy bacon burgers, homemade pumpkin pie, and much more await in the pages ahead. In creating meals for *The Wild Diet*, my extended family, Alyson, and I brought some of the tastiest recipes from our kitchen and community together to help you enjoy the best food you've ever tasted. I sincerely hope that these recipes help you in your journey. By all means, experiment and inject variety into your meals. Making them your own is part of the fun.

Hungry yet? Let's get cooking.

WILD DIET STAPLES

We used to microwave
Now we just eat nuts and berries.

—*Talking Heads*

Eat as many non-starchy vegetables and as much protein as you like, and round out your meals and snacks with nuts, seeds, oils, and fats. My favorites from each list are in **bold**.

Green and Non-Starchy Vegetables

Vegetables are extremely versatile: You can eat most of them raw or lightly steamed as a snack, side dish, pasta substitute, or main dish. You can also add them to soups, chilis, stews, roasts, salads, stir-fries, and casseroles. Nutritionally, leafy greens are as good as it gets.

Aim for organic, local, and farm fresh when possible.

- Artichoke
- Arugula
- Asparagus
- Avocado
- Beet greens
- Bell peppers
- Bok choy
- **Broccoli**
- Brussels sprouts
- Cabbage
- Carrots
- Cauliflower
- **Celery**
- Collard greens
- **Cucumbers**
- Eggplant
- Fennel
- Fiddlehead ferns
- **Garlic**
- **Jerusalem artichokes**
- Jicama
- **Kale**
- Leeks
- Mushrooms
- Mustard greens
- Olives
- Onions
- Parsnips
- Peppers (all kinds)
- Pumpkin
- Radishes
- Romaine lettuce
- Rutabaga
- Sea vegetables
- **Spinach**
- Squash
- Swiss chard
- Tomatoes
- Turnip greens
- Watercress

Meats

Prioritize grass fed, pastured, organic, wild, local, and farm fresh when possible.

- **Beef**
- **Bison**/Buffalo
- **Chicken**
- **Duck**
- Elk
- Goose

- **Lamb**
- Pork
- **Turkey**
- Veal
- Venison
- **Wild boar**

Fish

Prioritize wild caught and local when possible.

- Catfish
- Cod
- Flounder
- Haddock
- Halibut
- Herring
- Mackerel
- Pollock

- **Salmon**
- **Sea bass**
- Snapper
- Swordfish
- Trout
- **Tuna**
- Other wild fish

Crustaceans/Mollusks

Prioritize wild caught and local when possible.

- Clams
- Crab
- Crayfish
- Lobster
- Mussels

- Octopus
- **Oysters**
- **Scallops**
- **Shrimp (wild)**
- Squid (calamari)

Eggs

Prioritize organic, pasture raised, and omega-3 enriched.

- **Chicken**
- **Duck**
- Emu
- Goose

- Pheasant
- **Quail**
- Other bird and fish eggs

Nuts

Buy organic, raw, unsalted nuts and unadulterated butters. Because nuts and seeds are concentrated sources of fat and calories, they have the potential to slow progress if you overeat them.

- **Almonds**
- Brazil nuts
- Chestnuts
- Hazelnuts
- **Macadamia nuts**

- **Pecans**
- Pine nuts
- Pistachios
- Walnuts
- Derivative butters

Seeds

Buy organic, raw, unsalted seeds and unsweetened associated butters. Soaked and sprouted is best. Nuts and seeds are concentrated sources of fat and calories, so they do have the potential to slow progress if you overeat them.

- **Chia seeds**
- **Flaxseeds**
- Hemp seeds

- Pumpkin seeds
- Sesame seeds
- **Sunflower seeds**

Coffee, Tea, and Tonics

Only drink unsweetened beverages and aim for organic.

- **Coffee (organic and fair trade)**
- **Kombucha (less than 5 grams of sugar per bottle)**
- Seltzer water with citrus
- Tea

Fats and Oils

Prioritize virgin, cold-pressed, unprocessed, and UV-protected oils. For animal fats and butter/ghee, always aim for organic and pasture raised. Consume with attention, but make sure you eat until you're not hungry anymore.

- **Avocado oil**
- **Butter**
- **Coconut oil**
- Duck fat
- Ghee
- Lard
- Macadamia oil
- Olive oil
- **Tallow**
- Walnut oil

Digestive Health

Fermented foods promote the growth of friendly gut bacteria, reducing chronic low-grade inflammation and preventing leaky gut syndrome. Gingerroot, lemons, and limes have been used as a remedy for stomach ailments and nausea for centuries.

- Apple cider vinegar
- Ginger
- Kimchi
- Kombucha
- Lemons and limes (and their juice)
- Sauerkraut

Wild Diet Secondary Foods

Eat **no more than two total servings** of secondary foods a day until you reach your body fat goal.

Minimally Processed Meats

Aim for organic, uncured, and grass fed. Avoid added MSG, sugar, nitrates, and nitrites.

- Bacon
- Jerky
- Lean luncheon or deli meats
- Sausage

Canned Fish

Choose wild-caught fish packed in water or olive oil (not soybean oil).

- Anchovies
- Clams
- Crab
- Oysters
- **Salmon**
- **Sardines**
- **Tuna**

Fruit

Aim for organic, local, and farm fresh when possible.

- **Apples***
- Apricots*
- Avocado
- Bananas*
- **Blackberries**
- **Blueberries**
- **Coconut****
- Figs*
- Grapefruit
- Kiwis*
- Melons*
- **Peaches***

- **Pears***
- Prunes*
- **Raspberries**

- **Strawberries**
- **Tomatoes**
- Other whole fruits

*Pay attention to how many of these fruits you consume, as they have a high sugar content.
**Instead of sports drinks, try coconut water, preferably fresh and always without preservatives or added sugar. Otherwise, drink water.

Starchy Vegetables

Aim for organic, local, and farm fresh when possible. If you find you're not making progress with a serving or two of starchy vegetables a day, try avoiding fruit and starchy carbs for a few days to see if cycling carbs helps you through your plateau.

- Beets
- Cassava
- Plantains

- **Sweet potatoes**
- Taro
- Yams

Dairy

Prioritize fermented organic, nonpasteurized (or low-temperature pasteurized), and nonhomogenized. No added sugar.

- **Cottage cheese**
- Cream
- **Farmhouse, aged, artisan, and raw cheeses**

- Kefir
- Plain yogurt

Protein Supplements

Avoid added sugars and artificial sweeteners.

- Brown rice
- Collagen
- Colostrum

- Egg white
- Hemp
- Whey

Beans and Legumes

Ensure that beans and legumes are always soaked overnight and cooked thoroughly low and slow (see how to prepare beans and legumes on page 271). Watch out for BPA canned beans. Organic is best.

- Black beans
- Black-eyed peas
- Garbanzo beans (chickpeas)
- Kidney beans
- **Lentils**

- Navy beans
- Pinto beans
- Split peas
- Sugar snap peas
- White beans

Non-Gluten Whole Grains

Sprouted is best.

- Brown rice
- Buckwheat
- Corn (non-GMO)

- Millet
- Quinoa
- **Wild rice**

Flour

Go for organic, gluten free, and sprouted when possible. Since flour is processed by definition, watch your quantities and back off if you're not making progress.

- **Almond flour**
- Brown rice
- **Coconut flour**
- Flour from ancient grains
- Flaxseed meal

Noodles

- Kelp noodles
- Shirataki (yam/glucomannan) noodles
- Spaghetti squash "noodles"
- Zucchini or squash "noodles"

Sweeteners
Use sparingly.

- Blackstrap molasses
- Dried fruit (chopped or blended)
- 100% maple syrup
- Raw honey
- Stevia leaf or extract
- Xylitol (from birch trees, not corn)

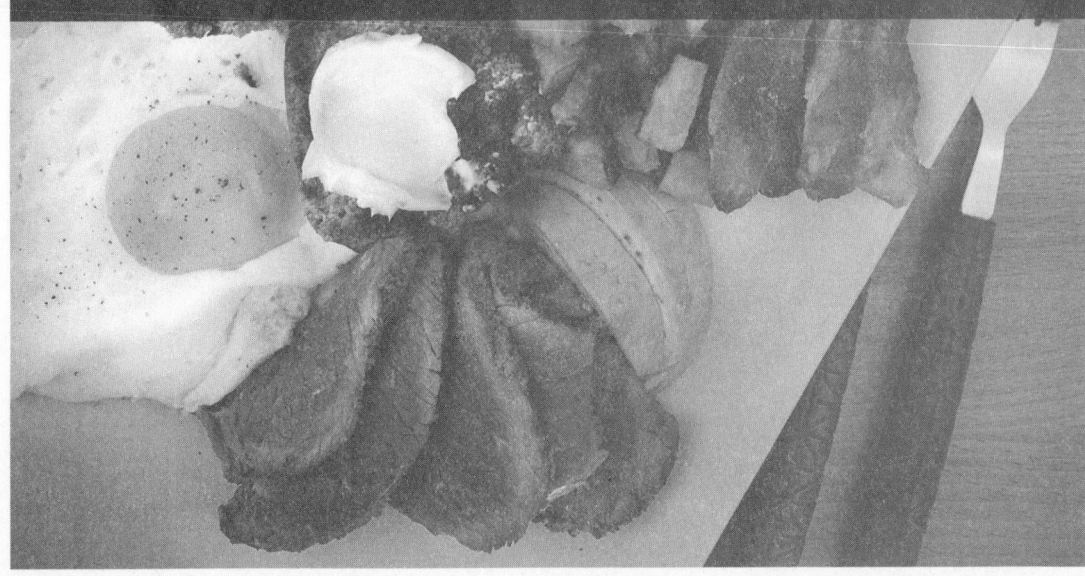

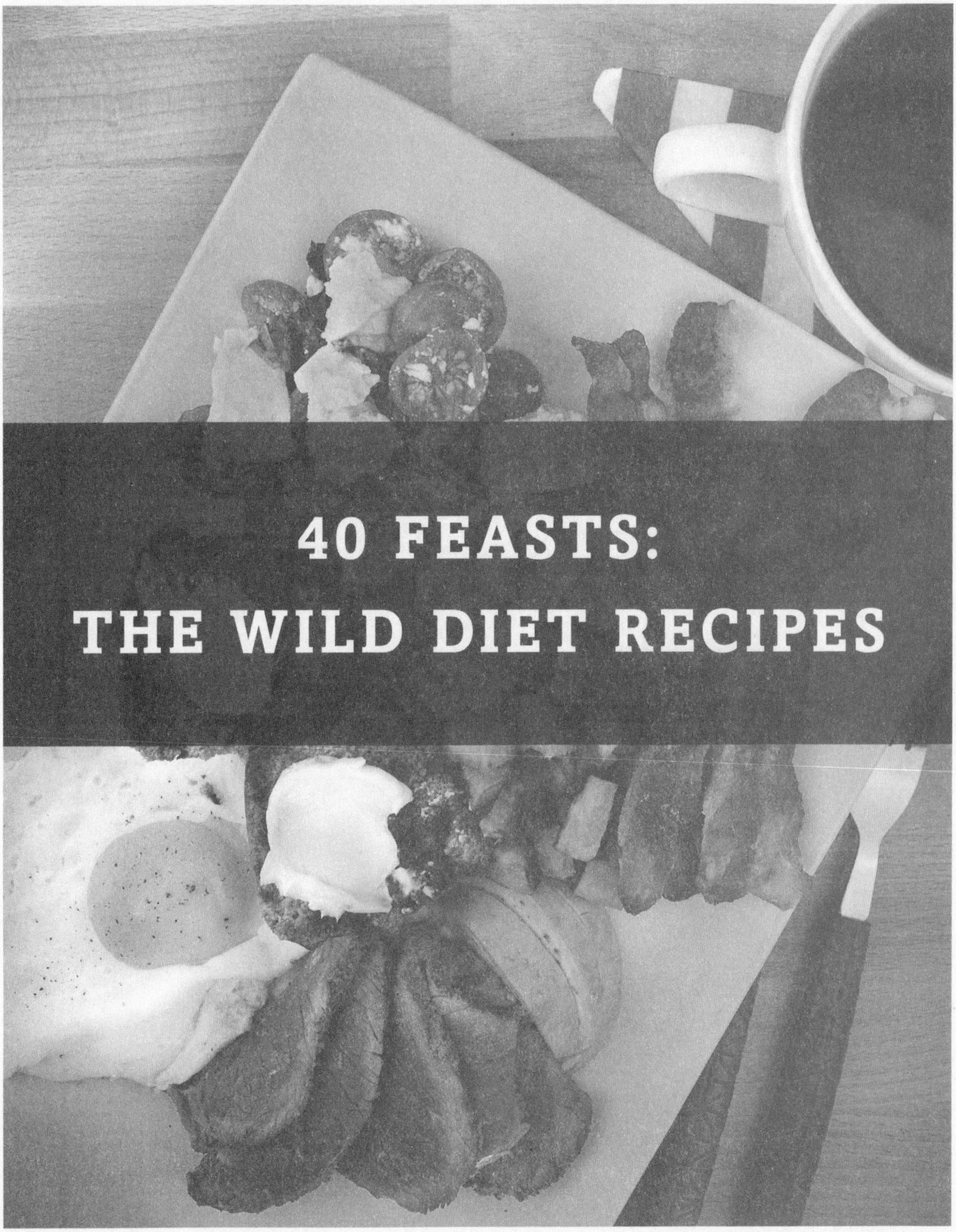

40 FEASTS:
THE WILD DIET RECIPES

CHICKEN AND PORK

Chicken Parmesan with Mixed Greens

So, you thought you had to give up Italian food on the Wild Diet? Think again. This classic dish is so rich and full of flavor that you will never want to go back to a boring old plate of spaghetti and bread again. Fresh tomato sauce, crispy-coated chicken, and melted mozzarella . . . what are you waiting for?

Serves: 4

PREP DAY TIME: 45 minutes

FEAST DAY TIME: 25 minutes

Ingredients

TOMATO SAUCE

1 small onion
3 garlic cloves
¼ cup fresh basil leaves
2½ pounds tomatoes
2 tablespoons grass-fed
    butter or ghee

1 bay leaf
½ teaspoon dried thyme
1 teaspoon dried oregano
1 teaspoon dried parsley
1 teaspoon red pepper flakes
Salt

CHICKEN PARMESAN

3 large eggs
1½ cups almond flour
2 tablespoons onion powder
2 tablespoons garlic powder
1 teaspoon red pepper flakes

1 teaspoon salt
4 boneless, skinless chicken thighs
2 tablespoons grass-fed butter, plus
    more as needed
4 slices mozzarella cheese (optional)

1 bunch mixed greens
Organic extra-virgin olive oil
Balsamic vinegar

Prep Day

TIME: 45 minutes

Tools: Knife, cutting board, garlic press, stockpot, measuring spoons, whisk, 2 mixing bowls

TOMATO SAUCE

1. Peel and dice the onion and mince the garlic cloves. Finely chop the fresh basil leaves. Set aside.

2. Bring a large stockpot half-full of water to a boil. Fill a large bowl with ice and water. Working in batches, cut an "x" on the top of each tomato and drop in the boiling water for 10 seconds. Remove the tomatoes and plunge them immediately into the ice water. Slip the skin off each tomato and remove the seeds. Place the skinned tomatoes into a large bowl.

3. Pour the water out of the stockpot and set it over medium heat. Melt the butter in the bottom.

4. Add onion, garlic, and bay leaf and cook until the onion is translucent, about 5 minutes.

5. Add the tomatoes, basil, thyme, oregano, parsley, red pepper, and salt to taste.

6. Simmer on low until the sauce thickens, stirring occasionally, about 2 hours.

7. Cover and refrigerate for up to 5 days.

CHICKEN PARMESAN

8. Whisk the eggs in a small bowl until frothy. Set aside.

9. In a separate bowl, mix together the almond flour, onion powder, garlic powder, red pepper flakes, and salt.

10. Dip the chicken thighs into the eggs, then dredge them in the almond flour mixture.

11. Melt the butter in a skillet over medium heat.

12. Place the chicken thighs in the skillet and cook until golden brown and the juices run clear, about 3 minutes on each side.

13. Place the chicken in an airtight container, cover, and refrigerate for up to 2 days, or freeze if making later in the week (thaw completely in the refrigerator before cooking).

Feast Day

TIME: 25 minutes

Tools: Medium oven-safe skillet with lid (or 10 x 10-inch baking dish with aluminum foil to cover)

1. Preheat the oven to 450°F.

2. Fill an oven-safe skillet halfway with the tomato sauce and bring to a simmer.

3. Place the chicken thighs in the sauce, cover with a lid, and roast in the oven for 10 minutes.

4. Uncover and top each piece of chicken with a slice of cheese (if using). Bake, uncovered, for 10 minutes more.

5. Serve with mixed greens drizzled with olive oil and balsamic vinegar.

> **NOTES**
>
> Save time by using store-bought tomato sauce. Just be sure it's organic and doesn't include any added sugar.
>
> If you can't find local fresh mozzarella cheese, use Kerrygold cheddar cheese or fresh buffalo mozzarella, or leave the cheese out altogether.

Mustard-Roasted Chicken Legs with Peach Salad

Chicken legs are the ultimate finger food . . . and these happen to be a favorite. Grainy Dijon mustard is one of the few prepared condiments that fits right into the Wild Diet, which is fantastic because it just makes this chicken pop. One of the best things about this meal is that it's easily portable—so go ahead and get your picnic on.

Serves: 4

PREP DAY TIME: 10 minutes

FEAST DAY TIME: 45 minutes

Ingredients

MUSTARD-ROASTED CHICKEN LEGS

2 garlic cloves

¼ cup grainy Dijon mustard

2 tablespoons organic extra-virgin olive oil

2 tablespoons dry white wine (optional)

½ teaspoon sea salt

½ teaspoon freshly ground black pepper

4 whole chicken legs

PEACH SALAD

1 peach

12 Kalamata olives

4 big handfuls of mixed greens

¼ cup shredded Parmesan

Organic extra-virgin olive oil

Balsamic vinegar

Prep Day

TIME: 10 minutes

Tools: Small bowl, garlic press, measuring spoons and cups, storage containers, knife, whisk, cutting board

MUSTARD-ROASTED CHICKEN LEGS

1. Peel and mince the garlic cloves and set aside.

2. In a small bowl, combine the mustard, olive oil, wine (if using), garlic, salt, and pepper. Whisk for about a minute, until everything is incorporated.

3. Evenly distribute the mustard mixture onto the chicken legs, both underneath and on top of the skin.

4. Store in an airtight container in the refrigerator for up to 2 days, or freeze until later in the week (thaw completely in the refrigerator before cooking).

Feast Day

TIME: 45 minutes

Tools: 8 x 8-inch baking dish, aluminum foil, knife, cutting board, cheese grater

MUSTARD-ROASTED CHICKEN LEGS

1. Preheat the oven to 400°F. Line an 8 x 8-inch baking dish with aluminum foil.

2. Place the chicken legs at least 1 inch apart in the prepared dish.

3. Roast the chicken legs for 40 to 45 minutes, until the internal temperature reaches 165°F.

PEACH SALAD

4. Pit the peach and chop the flesh into bite-size pieces.

5. Pit and quarter the olives.

6. Place a big handful of mixed greens onto each plate.

7. Distribute the peaches, olives, and shredded Parmesan over each pile of mixed greens.

8. Drizzle each salad with olive oil and vinegar.

9. Serve with the roasted chicken legs.

Spicy Chicken Thigh Stir-Fry and Cauliflower Fried Rice

Let's be honest: Stir-fries just aren't the same without rice. That's why this spicy chicken stir-fry with a side of Asian-style fried cauliflower "faux rice" is a staple in our kitchen. The "rice" is super easy to prepare, and you get a pile of tasty rice without the carbs.

Serves: 4

PREP DAY TIME: 25 minutes

FEAST DAY TIME: 20 minutes

Ingredients

CHICKEN

2 garlic cloves

1 teaspoon grated fresh ginger

½ cup full-fat unsweetened canned coconut milk

1 teaspoon ground turmeric

1 teaspoon garam masala

1 teaspoon freshly ground black pepper, plus more for seasoning

1 teaspoon sea salt, plus more for seasoning

2 pounds boneless, skinless chicken thighs

½ green bell pepper

½ red bell pepper

Organic unrefined coconut oil, for greasing the skillets

CAULIFLOWER RICE

1 small head cauliflower

1 small onion

1 tablespoon organic unrefined coconut oil

2 tablespoons chopped fresh basil

2 tablespoons chopped fresh cilantro

2 tablespoons coconut aminos (a gluten-free soy sauce alternative) or wheat-free tamari

2 scallions

Sea salt and freshly ground black pepper

Prep Day

TIME: 25 minutes

Tools: Garlic press, peeler, grater, measuring spoons and cups, knife, cutting board, airtight containers, food processor, skillet

CHICKEN

1. Mince the garlic cloves and transfer to a large glass storage container with a tight-fitting lid.

2. Add the ginger, coconut milk, turmeric, garam masala, black pepper, and salt to the container. Shake gently to mix.

3. Cut the chicken thighs into bite-size pieces.

4. Add the chicken to the container with the coconut milk sauce. Close the lid tightly and shake gently to coat. Store in the refrigerator for up to 2 days, or freeze if making later in the week (thaw completely in the refrigerator before cooking).

5. Thinly slice the green and red bell peppers. Place in a storage container and refrigerate for up to 2 days.

CAULIFLOWER RICE

6. Place the cauliflower in a food processor and pulse until the pieces are the size of rice grains. Set aside.

7. Coarsely chop the onion.

8. Grease a large skillet with the coconut oil. Add the onion and sauté over medium heat until softened.

9. Add the cauliflower, basil, cilantro, and coconut aminos to the pan. Stir to combine.

10. Cover and cook until the vegetables are al dente, 5 to 10 minutes.

11. Thinly slice the scallions and stir them into the cauliflower rice. Season with salt and pepper.

12. Store in an airtight container in the refrigerator for up to 1 week.

NOTES

Since you need only half of each bell pepper, you can slice the remaining pepper and store it in the refrigerator for a snack with hummus or to add to salads.

Feast Day

TIME: 20 minutes

Tools: 2 medium skillets, mixing spoon

CHICKEN

1. Grease two skillets with coconut oil and set over medium heat.
2. Add the chicken and bell pepper slices to one of the skillets and cook, stirring regularly, until the chicken is tender and the juices run clear, 10 to 12 minutes.
3. Season with salt and pepper.

CAULIFLOWER RICE

4. Place the cauliflower rice in the second skillet and sauté over medium heat until warm, about 5 minutes.
5. Serve the chicken stir-fry over the cauliflower rice.

Mom's Homemade Chicken Soup

Nothing says comfort like a steaming bowl of chicken soup. When you're a little under the weather, hearty homemade soup made from a whole roasted or raw chicken provides your body with real healing properties from deep inside the bone marrow.

Serves: 6

PREP DAY TIME: 3 hours

FEAST DAY TIME: 15 minutes

Ingredients

1 whole organic pastured roasted chicken	½ teaspoon dried thyme
Filtered water	½ teaspoon dried sage
6 to 8 medium carrots	2 teaspoons sea salt
1 bunch celery (about 12 stalks)	1 teaspoon cracked black pepper
	½ cup chopped fresh parsley

Prep Day

TIME: 3 hours

Tools: Large stockpot, cutting board, kitchen knife, vegetable scrubber (or clean rough sponge), slotted wooden spoon, measuring spoons and cups, small airtight container

1. Place the chicken in the bottom of a large stockpot. Add filtered water to cover the chicken by at least 1 inch. Set on the stovetop, bring to a simmer over high heat, then reduce the heat to low and simmer for about 2 hours.

2. Scrub the carrots and trim off the stems. Cut the carrots into ½-inch chunks and set aside.

3. Trim and wash the celery. Cut the stalks into thin slices. Set aside.

4. When the chicken has simmered for 2 hours, remove it from the broth using a large slotted spoon and place it on a cutting board or rimmed baking sheet. Remove any bones or chunks of skin or fat from the broth and discard.

5. When the chicken is cool enough to touch, remove the skin, bones, and fat and discard.

6. Pull apart the chicken meat into bite-size shreds and return the meat to the stockpot with the broth.

7. Add the carrots, celery, thyme, sage, salt, and pepper. Add more filtered water, if needed. Stir and bring to a boil over medium-high heat. Reduce the heat to maintain a simmer and cook for about 30 minutes, until the vegetables are tender.

8. Cover and refrigerate for up to 5 days, or freeze in an airtight container for up to 1 month.

Feast Day

TIME: 15 minutes

Tools: Ladle, large stockpot

1. Pour the soup into a large stockpot. Bring to a boil over medium-high heat.
2. Reduce the heat to low and simmer for about 10 minutes, or until hot. Stir in the parsley. Serve hot, in soup bowls or heavy mugs.

Curried Chicken and Onions with Butter-Fried Parsnips

This recipe is a favorite from my mom that reminds me of my days growing up in the frosty woods of New Hampshire. During harvest, my brothers and I would huddle around Dad's cast-iron skillet for a snitch of spicy parsnips fried in real butter.

Serves: 2 to 4

PREP DAY TIME: 10 minutes

FEAST DAY TIME: 25 minutes

Ingredients

CHICKEN AND ONIONS

1 pound organic pastured chicken breast

¼ cup whole-milk organic plain yogurt or plain coconut milk yogurt

1½ teaspoons ground cumin

1 tablespoon ground coriander

1 teaspoon ground turmeric

½ teaspoon ground cinnamon

Cayenne pepper

1 medium onion

6 garlic cloves

1 (1½-inch) piece fresh ginger

3 whole cloves

3 cardamom pods

1 tablespoon grass-fed butter or ghee

PARSNIPS

1 pound parsnips

4 tablespoons grass-fed butter

Salt and freshly ground
   black pepper

Prep Day

TIME: 10 minutes

Tools: Kitchen knife, paring knife, cutting board, large mixing bowl, measuring spoons, garlic press, storage container

CHICKEN AND ONIONS

1. Cut the chicken breasts into bite-size cubes. Place in a large bowl.
2. Add the yogurt, cumin, coriander, turmeric, cinnamon, and a dash of cayenne. Mix until the chicken is well coated.
3. Slice the onion and add it to the bowl with the chicken.
4. Peel and mince the garlic cloves and add them to the bowl.
5. With a sharp paring knife, peel the ginger and place the entire chunk in the bowl.
6. Add the cloves and cardamom pods and mix well to completely coat.
7. Cover tightly and refrigerate for up to 2 days.

Feast Day

TIME: 25 minutes

Tools: 2 medium skillets, mixing spoon, tablespoon, sharp chef's knife, cutting board, spatula

CHICKEN AND ONIONS

1. Melt the butter in a large skillet over medium heat. Add the chicken and onion mixture and cook, stirring regularly, until the chicken is cooked through and the onions have softened, 8 to 10 minutes.

2. Cover to keep warm while preparing the parsnips. Remove the ginger, cloves, and cardamom pods before serving.

PARSNIPS

3. Scrub and thinly slice the parsnips.

4. Melt the butter in a large heavy skillet over medium heat. Swirl to coat the bottom and sides of the skillet.

5. Lay the parsnips in a thin layer in the bottom of the pan. Cover and cook for 5 minutes. Uncover and sprinkle with salt and pepper.

6. Cook for 5 minutes more, then flip the parsnips and cook for 5 to 7 minutes more, until both sides are crispy golden brown and the parsnips are very soft in the middle.

7. Serve the parsnips with the chicken and onions.

Lemon Kalamata Chicken Breasts with Caprese Salad

The Mediterranean is well known as a region that relishes real food—fresh-picked tomatoes drizzled with olive oil, bunches of bright green basil, and soft, white cheeses. These moist chicken breasts, paired with a simple Caprese salad, burst with Mediterranean flavor combinations so good you won't even miss the pasta.

Serves: 4

PREP DAY TIME: 10 minutes

FEAST DAY TIME: 45 minutes

Ingredients

CHICKEN
2 large white onions

2 garlic cloves

¼ cup freshly squeezed lemon juice

2 lemons

1 tablespoon grass-fed butter or ghee

4 bone-in, skin-on chicken breasts

½ cup Kalamata olives, pitted

1½ cups chicken broth

Salt and freshly ground black pepper

CAPRESE SALAD
2 ripe large tomatoes

8 ounces fresh mozzarella cheese
   (optional)

8 fresh basil leaves

2 tablespoons organic extra-virgin
   olive oil

¼ teaspoon salt

¼ teaspoon freshly ground black
   pepper

Prep Day

TIME: 10 minutes

Tools: Knife, cutting board, garlic press, measuring cups,
storage containers

CHICKEN

1. Peel and slice the onions into thin rounds and place them in a storage container.

2. Peel and mince the garlic cloves and add to the onion.

3. Squeeze the lemon juice into a separate container with a tight-fitting lid.

4. Slice additional lemons into thin rounds and remove the seeds. Store in a lidded container.

5. Store all the ingredients in the refrigerator for up to 5 days.

Feast Day

TIME: 45 minutes

Tools: Large ovenproof skillet, measuring cups and spoons

CHICKEN

1. Preheat the oven to 350°F. Position a rack in the top third of the oven.
2. Melt the butter in the bottom of a large ovenproof skillet over medium heat. Place the chicken breasts in the skillet skin-side down. Cook for about 4 minutes to brown. Flip the chicken over.
3. Add the onion and garlic mixture and cook for a few minutes, until the onion is just tender.
4. Stir in the lemon juice, olives, and broth. Cover and bring to a simmer. Continue simmering until the chicken is tender, about 15 minutes.
5. Uncover and transfer the pan to the oven. Bake for 15 to 20 minutes. The chicken is ready when the skin is browned and the juices have reduced.
6. Season with salt and pepper.

CAPRESE SALAD

7. While the chicken is baking, prepare the Caprese salad: Cut the tomatoes into ¼-inch-thick slices.
8. Slice the fresh mozzarella to the same thickness (if using).
9. Plate a slice of tomato and top with a slice of cheese (if using) and a basil leaf. Continue layering to make a short "stack" of tomato and mozzarella. Top with a basil leaf, drizzle with olive oil, and sprinkle with salt and pepper.
10. Serve with the chicken.

Cornish Game Hens with Sautéed Green Beans

These fragrant roasted game birds are smothered with a rich garlic pan sauce. Be careful not to overcook—they're best as tender and juicy as possible.

Serves: 4

PREP DAY TIME: 15 minutes

FEAST DAY TIME: 1 hour

Ingredients

CORNISH GAME HENS

4 small Cornish game hens

2 tablespoons organic extra-virgin olive oil

Salt and freshly ground black pepper

1 lemon, quartered

15 garlic cloves

1 cup chicken broth

GREEN BEANS

1 small yellow onion

1 pound green beans

1 teaspoon grass-fed ghee

Prep Day

TIME: 15 minutes

Tools: Measuring spoon, knife, cutting board, 2 storage containers

CORNISH GAME HENS

1. Rub the Cornish game hens all over with the olive oil. Season with salt and pepper.
2. Place a lemon quarter inside the cavity of each game hen.
3. Peel the garlic cloves.
4. Place the hens in an airtight container with the garlic and store in the refrigerator for up to 2 days, or freeze for later use (thaw overnight in the refrigerator before roasting).

SAUTÉED GREEN BEANS

5. Dice the onion.

6. Trim the green beans.

7. Place onion and green beans in an airtight container. Store in the refrigerator for up to 1 week.

Feast Day

TIME: 1 hour

Tools: Medium roasting pan, measuring cups and spoons, small bowl, basting brush, aluminum foil, medium saucepan, knife, medium skillet

CORNISH GAME HENS

1. Preheat the oven to 350°F.

2. Place the hens in a medium roasting pan and surround with the garlic. Pour over the chicken broth. Cover with aluminum foil and roast for 25 minutes.

3. Raise the oven temperature to 450°F.

4. Uncover and roast for 35 minutes more, basting every 10 minutes. The hens are done when the skin is golden brown and their juices run clear. Transfer the hens to a serving platter and tent with foil to keep warm.

5. Pour the pan juices and garlic into a medium saucepan and set over high heat. Bring to a boil, whisking, and cook until the liquids have reduced to a sauce consistency, about 10 minutes.

6. When ready to serve, halve the hens lengthwise (optional) and plate. Spoon the sauce and garlic over the top.

SAUTÉED GREEN BEANS

7. In a large skillet, melt the ghee over medium heat.

8. Add the onions and green beans and sauté until tender, about 10 minutes. Serve with the hens and their sauce.

Pulled Pork Sliders

These sliders certainly don't feel like food from a diet book. The pork is tender and juicy with just enough spice, and the silver-dollar plantains make the perfect "bun." Stack three of these beauties on a plate, topped off with a super-simple creamy slaw, and you have a meal fit for the most ravenous appetite. The recipe uses half of the BBQ sauce, so there's plenty to save for dipping chicken or pouring over roasted ribs.

Serves: 4

PREP DAY TIME: 1 hour, 20 minutes

FEAST DAY TIME: 6 to 8 hours

Ingredients

WILD BBQ SAUCE
1 small sweet onion
6 garlic cloves
2 (16-ounce) cans tomato sauce
½ cup apple cider vinegar
½ cup pure maple syrup

1 tablespoon smoked paprika
1 teaspoon cayenne pepper
1 teaspoon freshly ground black
   pepper
1 to 2 teaspoons sea salt

CREAMY CHOPPED SLAW
2 cups finely chopped green cabbage
   (about ¼ head)
2 tablespoons minced red onion
2 tablespoons plain Greek yogurt or
   coconut cream (see Note, page 259)

2 teaspoons white vinegar
2 teaspoons raw honey, melted,
   or pure dried stevia leaf
Sea salt and cracked black pepper

PULLED PORK
2 pounds pork (pork roast, boneless chops, or tenderloin)
4 cups chicken broth or water

PLANTAIN "BUNS"
4 unripe (slightly green) medium plantains
4 large eggs
2 tablespoons grass-fed ghee

Prep Day

TIME: 1 hour 20 minutes

Tools: Blender, measuring spoons and cups, small pot, storage containers, knife, cutting board, garlic press

WILD BBQ SAUCE

1. Peel the onion, quarter it, and place it in a high-speed blender.
2. Peel the garlic cloves and add them to the blender.
3. Add the tomato sauce, vinegar, maple syrup, paprika, cayenne, and black pepper. Process until smooth. Season with salt, using more or less to taste.
4. Pour the sauce into a small heavy pot and set over very low heat. Gently simmer, stirring regularly, for about 1 hour. The sauce will darken and thicken.
5. Pour the sauce into a glass storage container with a tightly fitted lid and refrigerate for up to 10 days.

CREAMY CHOPPED SLAW

6. In a large bowl, combine the cabbage and red onion.
7. Mix in the yogurt, vinegar, honey, and salt and pepper to taste.
8. Store in an airtight container in the refrigerator for up to 4 days.

Feast Day

TIME: 6 to 8 hours, plus 20 minutes

Tools: Slow cooker, large griddle or frying pan, measuring spoons, blender, sharp paring knife, 2 forks, mixing spoon, spatula

PULLED PORK

1. Start the pulled pork in the morning before heading out for the day: Place the pork in the bottom of your slow cooker and cover with broth or water.

2. Cover and cook on low for 8 hours, or high for 6 hours. The time will vary according to the size and cut of meat. The pork is ready when it falls apart easily.

3. Pour off most of the broth or water, reserving a little bit in the bottom of the slow cooker for juicier sauce.

4. Using two forks, pull the pork apart into shreds (right in the slow cooker).

5. Pour in half of the Wild BBQ Sauce (or to taste) and mix to coat (the remaining BBQ sauce can be stored in the refrigerator for another use). Replace the lid and let this simmer while you make the plantain pancakes, up to 1 hour.

PLANTAIN PANCAKE "BUNS"

6. Using a sharp paring knife, cut away the peels from the plantains. You won't be able to peel them like a banana. If you can, they're too ripe.

7. Place the plantains in a blender. Crack in the eggs and blend until smooth.

8. Set a griddle over medium-high heat. Melt enough ghee on the griddle to coat.

9. Working in batches, spoon the plantain batter onto the hot griddle in ¼-cup increments. When the pancakes bubble in the middle and are browned on the edges, about 2 minutes, flip and cook the other side for about 1 minute. Transfer to a plate. Repeat until all the batter has been used.

10. Plate the "bottom" pancake buns. Scoop pulled pork onto half of the pancakes, top with slaw, and place a pancake "lid" on each. Enjoy!

11. Remaining pork can be refrigerated in an airtight container for up to 3 days or frozen for a few weeks. The pancakes can be frozen and reheated in the toaster oven.

Low-and-Slow Rubbed Ribs with Whipped Cauliflower

This is pork paradise with a side of whipped nirvana. The ribs are a little spicy, but you can turn down the heat by cutting back the cayenne and black pepper. Serve just as it is, or top with a dollop of Wild BBQ Sauce (page 159).

Serves: 4

PREP DAY TIME: 10 minutes

FEAST DAY TIME: 2½ hours

Ingredients

LOW-AND-SLOW RUBBED RIBS

1 teaspoon sea salt

1 teaspoon freshly ground black pepper

1 teaspoon cayenne pepper

1 teaspoon smoked paprika

1 (2-pound) slab baby back pork ribs

WHIPPED CAULIFLOWER

1 large head cauliflower

2 tablespoons grass-fed butter

Sea salt

Chopped fresh chives, for garnish

Prep Day

TIME: 10 minutes

Tools: Small bowl, aluminum foil, knife, measuring spoons, storage containers

LOW-AND-SLOW RUBBED RIBS

1. Make the dry rub by mixing together the salt, black pepper, cayenne, and paprika in a small bowl.
2. Lay out the slab of baby back ribs on a sheet of aluminum foil. Rub both sides with the dry rub. Pull up the sides of the foil and roll them at the top to create a pouch.
3. Store in the refrigerator for up to 2 days.

4. Wash the cauliflower and remove the stem and leaves.

5. Cut into florets and store in an airtight container in the refrigerator for up to 5 days.

Feast Day

TIME: 2½ hours

Tools: Large pot, blender or food processor, rimmed baking sheet, measuring tablespoon

LOW-AND-SLOW RUBBED RIBS

1. Preheat the oven to 250°F.

2. Place the ribs on a rimmed baking sheet, still in the foil packet, and bake for 1½ hours.

3. Crank up the heat to 375°F and continue baking for 1 hour more, or until the ribs are tender and slightly browned.

WHIPPED CAULIFLOWER

4. Place the cauliflower florets into a pot and add water to cover. Bring to a low boil over medium heat. Continue boiling until the cauliflower is very, very tender, about 15 minutes.

5. Drain the cauliflower and transfer to a blender or food processor.

6. Add the butter and salt to taste. Process until very light and fluffy.

7. Cut the ribs into sections and serve with a nice dollop of whipped cauliflower topped with chives.

Slow-Cooker Chicken with Roasted Broccoli and Mushrooms

Slow-cooking poultry is one of the best ways to keep it tender and juicy while retaining all of its vital nutrients. Put this chicken in the slow cooker before you go out for the day, and walk in the door to the incredible aroma of a home-cooked meal wafting through the house.

Serves: 4

PREP DAY TIME: 15 minutes

FEAST DAY TIME: 20 minutes, plus 5 to 6 hours in the slow cooker

Ingredients

SLOW-COOKER CHICKEN

2 teaspoons paprika

1 teaspoon cayenne pepper

1 teaspoon onion powder

1 teaspoon dried oregano

1 teaspoon garlic powder

½ teaspoon freshly ground black pepper

2 teaspoons sea salt

1 (3- to 4-pound) organic pastured whole chicken

1 large white or yellow onion

ROASTED BROCCOLI AND MUSHROOMS

½ pound white mushrooms

1 head broccoli

3 tablespoons grass-fed ghee

¼ cup coconut aminos

Prep Day

TIME: 15 minutes

Tools: Measuring spoons and cups, knife, cutting board, glass storage containers (or BPA-free plastic), paper towel

SLOW-COOKER CHICKEN

1. In a small bowl, combine the paprika, cayenne, onion powder, oregano, garlic powder, black pepper, and salt.
2. Clean the chicken and pat dry. Rub the spice mixture all over the chicken and under the skin.
3. Store in an airtight container in the refrigerator for up to 2 days, or freeze if making later in the week (allow a full day for thawing in the refrigerator).
4. Peel the onion, slice into thin rounds, and place in a storage container with a tight-fitting lid for up to 1 week.

ROASTED BROCCOLI AND MUSHROOMS

5. Rinse the mushrooms and trim the stems. Pat them *very* dry with a paper towel (otherwise they'll get slimy). Wrap in a dry paper towel and place in a storage container.
6. Rinse the broccoli and chop into florets. Pat dry and store in the container with the mushrooms in the refrigerator for up to 3 days.

Feast Day

TIME: 20 minutes, plus 5 to 6 hours in the slow cooker

Tools: slow cooker, measuring cups and spoons, baking sheet

SLOW-COOKER CHICKEN

1. Line the bottom of the slow cooker with the sliced onions.
2. Place the chicken, breast-side up, on top of the sliced onions. (No liquid is needed since the chicken will make its own juices.)
3. Cover and cook on low for 5 to 6 hours, until the meat is falling off the bone and the skin is a little bit crisp.

ROASTED BROCCOLI AND MUSHROOMS

4. Preheat the oven to 400°F.

5. Melt the ghee and toss it into the broccoli and mushrooms with the coconut aminos. Spread on a baking sheet and bake until the broccoli is tender and the mushrooms are dark and juicy, 15 to 20 minutes.

6. Plate the chicken and vegetables drizzled with the chicken drippings and topped with the slow-cooked onion slices.

Chipotle Steak and Veggie Fajitas with Fresh Guacamole

When you're in a hurry, whip up some fajitas. Whether you've prepped ahead or you're cutting it close, these fajitas come together fast . . . but no one would ever know it. You have a party on a plate without slaving all day, and everyone loves a fiesta!

Serves: 4

PREP DAY TIME: 20 minutes

FEAST DAY TIME: 20 minutes

Ingredients

CHIPOTLE STEAK

- 2 pounds grass-fed skirt or sirloin steak
- 4 garlic cloves
- 2 tablespoons organic extra-virgin olive oil
- Juice of 1 lime
- Juice of 1 lemon
- 2 teaspoons ground chipotle pepper
- 2 teaspoons ground cumin
- 1 teaspoon sea salt
- 1 teaspoon freshly ground black pepper

FAJITA VEGETABLES

- 4 mixed bell peppers (red, green, orange, yellow)
- 1 red onion
- 2 cups fresh mushrooms
- 1 teaspoon salt
- 1 teaspoon freshly ground black pepper
- 1 teaspoon ground chipotle pepper
- 1 tablespoon organic unrefined coconut oil

GUACAMOLE

1 garlic clove

½ white onion

½ teaspoon chopped fresh cilantro

Sea salt and freshly ground black pepper

Chili powder

2 avocados

Juice of 1 lime

1 Roma tomato

Prep Day

TIME: 20 minutes

Tools: Glass or BPA-free storage container with lid, medium mixing bowl, garlic press, wire whisk, paper towel

CHIPOTLE STEAK

1. Place the steaks in a storage container and set aside.
2. Peel and mince the garlic cloves.
3. In a medium bowl, combine the garlic, olive oil, lime juice, lemon juice, chipotle pepper, cumin, salt, and black pepper. Whisk thoroughly to create a marinade.
4. Pour the marinade over the steak and cover with a tight-fitting lid. Shake vigorously to completely coat the steaks. Cover and refrigerate for up to 2 days.

FAJITA VEGETABLES

5. Slice the bell peppers, discarding the seeds and stem. Place the slices in a storage container.
6. Thinly slice the onion and add it to the peppers.
7. Clean the mushrooms and pat them very dry with a paper towel. Slice and add to the container with the onions and peppers.
8. Sprinkle the salt, black pepper, and chipotle pepper over the vegetables and toss to coat. Cover and refrigerate for up to 2 days.

GUACAMOLE

9. Mince the garlic clove and finely chop the white onion. Season with cilantro, salt, pepper, and chili powder. Place together in an airtight container and refrigerate for up to 5 days.

Feast Day

TIME: 20 minutes

Tools: Medium ovenproof skillet, large skillet, tongs, sharp knife, cutting board

CHIPOTLE STEAK

1. Remove the steaks from the refrigerator and let rest until they are room temperature.
2. Preheat the oven to 500°F or to the broil setting. Adjust the oven shelf so the meat will be 2 to 3 inches from the flame. (Or use your oven's separate broiler rack.)
3. Grease a medium ovenproof skillet or baking dish and lay the steaks on the bottom. Broil for 4 to 5 minutes for a 2-inch-thick steak, or until the meat has browned on the top.
4. Remove from the oven, flip the steak with tongs, and broil for 4 to 5 minutes more. The steaks are done when they are browned on both sides and slightly pink in the center. (Or cook to the desired doneness.)
5. Transfer the steaks to a cutting board and slice into thin strips against the grain.

FAJITA VEGETABLES

6. Melt the coconut oil in a skillet over medium heat.
7. Add the onion-mushroom mixture and cook, stirring regularly, until the onions are translucent and the peppers are fork-tender, about 5 minutes.

GUACAMOLE

8. Using a sharp knife, halve the avocados, remove the pit, and scoop the flesh into a small bowl. Sprinkle with the lime juice and mash well.
9. Stir in the minced garlic and chopped onion until the guacamole has a soft, consistent texture.
10. Dice the tomato. Fold the tomato into the guacamole.
11. Plate the vegetables and top with the steak slices and guacamole. Serve immediately.

Bison Taco Salad with Avocado

Wild Community member and health coach Dawn Parker sent us this awesome recipe that deconstructs classic taco flavors to create a deliciously fresh salad. Utilize your prep day, or throw this one together at feast time. It's fast and filling, and truly a crowd-pleaser.

Serves: 2

PREP DAY TIME: 10 minutes

FEAST DAY TIME: 15 minutes

Ingredients

BISON

3 garlic cloves
1 large yellow onion
1 pound ground bison
1½ teaspoons ground cumin
1 tablespoon chili powder
½ teaspoon paprika

1 to 2 teaspoons salt
½ teaspoon freshly ground black pepper
½ teaspoon onion powder
¼ teaspoon red pepper flakes
¼ teaspoon dried oregano

TACO SALAD

1 yellow bell pepper
1 garden tomato
1 head green-leaf lettuce

1 large avocado
½ teaspoon freshly squeezed lemon juice

Prep Day

TIME: 10 minutes

Tools: Garlic press, knife, cutting board, small mixing bowl, measuring spoons, storage container

BISON

1. Peel and mince the garlic cloves and dice the onion. Set aside.

2. Place the bison in a large bowl and set aside.

3. In a small bowl, combine the cumin, chili powder, paprika, salt, black pepper, onion powder, red pepper flakes, and oregano. Stir until well combined.

4. Use your hands to evenly distribute the seasoning mixture, minced garlic, and chopped onion into the ground bison.

5. Transfer to an airtight container and refrigerate for up to 4 days, or freeze if making later in the week (thaw completely in the refrigerator before cooking).

TACO SALAD

6. Trim and chop the bell pepper and place in an airtight storage container.

7. Dice the tomato and place in a separate airtight storage container.

8. Wash, dry, and chop the lettuce and place in a produce bag.

9. Refrigerate all the prepared vegetables for up to 4 days.

Feast Day

TIME: 15 minutes

Tools: Large skillet, spoon

BISON

1. Heat a large skillet over medium heat. Add the bison mixture and cook, stirring frequently, until completely browned, 7 to 10 minutes. Add ¼ cup water and reduce the heat to maintain a simmer. Simmer the meat while you prepare the salad. This will create a nice, rich, saucy meat.

TACO SALAD

2. Halve the avocado lengthwise and remove the pit. Slip a metal spoon in between the flesh and skin and gently scoop out the flesh in one piece.

3. Slice the avocado flesh into wedges and drizzle with the lemon juice.

4. Divide the lettuce evenly among serving bowls or plates.

5. Spoon equal portions of the bison over the salad.

6. Top each salad evenly with avocado slices, tomato, and yellow bell pepper.

7. Serve immediately.

> **SWAP BOX**
>
> For a boost in antioxidants, lycopene, and anthocyanin, swap out the yellow onion for a red onion.
>
> Swap out the bison for grass-fed ground beef or pastured, organic ground turkey.

Ultimate Bacon Burger

This juicy burger has bacon on it . . . and in it! Laid on top of fresh lettuce and topped with the classic onion-and-tomato combo, you can be sure that burger night just got a little bit baconer—I mean, better.

Serves: 4

PREP DAY TIME: 15 minutes

FEAST DAY TIME: 20 minutes

Ingredients

1 (12-ounce) package nitrate-free bacon

1 pound grass-fed, organic ground beef

2 tablespoons coconut aminos (gluten-free soy sauce alternative)

1 small yellow onion

1 beefsteak or vine-ripened red tomato

4 leaves fresh broad-leafed lettuce

1 teaspoon organic extra-virgin olive oil (optional, if caramelizing the onion)

Sea salt and cracked black pepper

4 ounces grass-fed cheddar cheese (optional)

1 tablespoon grainy garlic mustard

Pickle spears, for serving (optional)

Prep Day

TIME: 15 minutes

Tools: Storage containers, sharp knife, cutting board, large bowl, measuring spoons

1. Divide the bacon slices into two portions, saving 4 to 8 slices to go on top of the burgers. Place the slices in a storage container in the refrigerator for up to 1 week. Mince the remaining slices as fine as possible and place in a large bowl.

2. Add the ground beef and coconut aminos to the minced bacon and use your hands to mix them together.

3. Divide the burger mixture into four equal portions, flattening each portion into a patty with the palms of your hands.

4. Place the burger patties in a single layer in an airtight storage container and refrigerate for up to 3 days, or freeze for up to 2 weeks (see Note, page 174).

5. Peel the onion and slice it into rings. Store in an airtight container in the refrigerator for up to 1 week.

6. Cut the tomato into thick slices and store in a separate storage container in the refrigerator for up to 3 days.

7. Rinse the lettuce and pat dry. Store in a produce bag in the refrigerator for up to 5 days.

Feast Day

TIME: 20 minutes

Tools: Grilling utensils, rimmed baking sheet, aluminum foil, small skillet, tongs or cooking spoon, gas grill or grill pan, paper towels

1. Preheat the oven to 400°F.

2. Line a rimmed baking sheet with aluminum foil, slightly crinkled.

3. Lay the reserved bacon in an even layer, ½ inch apart, on the foil-lined sheet.

4. Bake until the bacon is crisp, 12 to 15 minutes. Transfer to a paper towel–lined plate to drain excess fat.

5. While you can put those onions on fresh, a caramelized onion is so delicious. If desired, place the olive oil and onion rings in a small skillet over medium-low heat. Stir to coat the onions in the oil. Cook until the onions are just translucent, and then add ¼ cup water. Cook, stirring regularly, until the water has evaporated and the onions are beginning to brown, about 5 minutes. If the water has evaporated but the onions don't seem tender enough, add a few more tablespoons water and keep cooking until the desired consistency is reached. Remove from the heat and set aside until ready to serve.

6. Preheat a gas grill to medium, or set a grill pan over medium heat.

7. Season the burger patties with salt and pepper and place on the grill. Grill until the underside is browned, about 5 minutes. Flip the burgers and cook for 5 to 7 minutes more, until the meat is cooked through but the outside is *not charred*.

8. For each burger, lay a lettuce leaf on a plate and top with a burger, tomato, raw or caramelized onion, bacon, one slice of cheese (if desired), and garlic mustard. Serve with a fresh pickle on the side, if you'd like.

NOTES

Burgers can be grilled directly from the freezer. Increase cooking time by 3 to 5 minutes per side to ensure that the meat is cooked through.

Beef Brisket with Balsamic Mustard Greens

Thanks to the Foodie Alchemist Jaime Rothbard for submitting this family recipe. Put this brisket in the slow cooker before work, and you'll walk in to a hearty meal when you come home. Add some wilted mustard greens to round out your plate beautifully.

Serves: 6 to 8

PREP DAY TIME: 20 minutes

FEAST DAY TIME: 10 minutes, plus 6 to 8 hours in the slow cooker

Ingredients

BEEF BRISKET

1 tablespoon sea salt

1 tablespoon freshly ground black
   pepper

1 tablespoon ground chipotle pepper

1 (3-pound) beef brisket

1 tablespoon organic unrefined
   coconut oil

SAUCE

1 medium onion

6 garlic cloves

1 (2-inch) piece fresh ginger

½ habanero pepper

3 tablespoons tomato paste

1 teaspoon sea salt

1 teaspoon Chinese five-spice powder

1 teaspoon freshly ground black
   pepper

BALSAMIC MUSTARD GREENS

½ cup balsamic vinegar

2 tablespoons sliced raw almonds

1 large bunch mustard greens
   (about 6 cups)

½ teaspoon sea salt,
   or to taste

6 fresh strawberries

Prep Day

TIME: 20 minutes

Tools: Measuring spoons and cups, large heavy skillet, knife,
cutting board, food processor or blender, medium saucepan,
airtight containers, wooden spoon

BEEF BRISKET

1. In a small bowl, combine the salt, black pepper, and chipotle pepper. Rub the spice
   mixture all over the brisket until well seasoned.

2. Melt the coconut oil in a heavy skillet over medium heat. Add the brisket and sear
   on both sides.

3. Transfer to a heatproof glass storage container.

SAUCE

4. Coarsely chop the onion and transfer to a food processor or blender.

5. Peel the garlic and ginger and add to the onion in the food processor or blender.

6. Add the habanero pepper (seeds removed for less heat, if desired), tomato paste, salt, Chinese five-spice powder, and black pepper.

7. Add just enough water to facilitate blending and process until a smooth paste forms.

8. Spread the paste over the brisket. Wrap tightly or cover with a tight-fitting lid and refrigerate for up to 3 days, or freeze for up to 2 weeks (thaw completely in the refrigerator before cooking).

BALSAMIC MUSTARD GREENS

9. In a small saucepan, simmer the balsamic vinegar over low heat, stirring occasionally, until it reduces to half its original volume. Store the reduction in an airtight container at room temperature for up to 1 week.

10. Roast the almonds in a dry, hot skillet, stirring regularly, until browned, 3 to 5 minutes. Let cool completely. Store in an airtight container in the cupboard for up to 2 weeks.

Feast Day

TIME: 10 minutes, plus 6 to 8 hours in the slow cooker

Tools: Slow cooker, medium skillet, knife, cutting board

BEEF BRISKET

1. Place the brisket in the slow cooker before heading out for the day. Cook on low for 8 to 9 hours, or on high for 6 to 7 hours. The brisket is done when it shreds easily with a fork.

BALSAMIC MUSTARD GREENS

2. Rinse the mustard greens well to remove any sand. Do not dry.

3. Place the damp mustard greens in a large skillet and season with salt. Cook over medium heat, stirring occasionally, until just wilted, about 5 minutes.

4. Rinse and slice the strawberries.

5. Plate the brisket and arrange the greens alongside, topped with the balsamic reduction, toasted almonds, and strawberry slices.

SWAP BOX

Instead of cooking the brisket in the slow cooker, you can slow roast it in a Dutch oven at 215°F for 6 to 8 hours.

If mustard greens are too bitter for your palate, replace them with kale or spinach.

Wild Shepherd's Pie

Shepherd's pie is a true comfort food. Rich and hearty, topped with mashed potato, it's the kind of dinner you want to eat on a cold, rainy day or after an evening packed with activity—when you're ravenous.

Serves: 6

PREP DAY TIME: 30 minutes

FEAST DAY TIME: 30 minutes

Ingredients

4 medium white or Japanese sweet potatoes

4 tablespoons grass-fed butter

Sea salt and freshly ground black pepper

1 yellow onion

3 large carrots

1 garlic clove

1 pound grass-fed, organic ground beef, lamb, or bison

1 cup beef or vegetable broth

1 (5-ounce) package baby spinach or washed chopped spinach

1 teaspoon dried thyme

Paprika

Prep Day

TIME: 30 minutes

Tools: Peeler, cutting board, sharp kitchen knife, medium pot, handheld electric mixer, garlic press, large skillet, measuring cups and spoons, mixing spoon

1. Peel the sweet potatoes and cut into cubes.
2. Place the cubed potatoes in a pot and add water to cover. Bring the water to a boil and cook the potatoes until tender, 10 to 12 minutes.
3. Drain the potatoes and return them to the pot. Add the butter and using a handheld electric mixer, beat the potatoes and butter until a nice mash is formed. Set aside until ready to assemble.
4. Season with salt and pepper.
5. Peel and dice the yellow onion and set aside.
6. Scrub and dice the carrots.
7. Mince the garlic clove.
8. In a large skillet over medium heat, combine the onion, carrots, garlic, and ground meat. Cook, stirring regularly, until the meat is browned and the vegetables are tender, about 10 minutes.
9. Pour in the broth and simmer for about 7 minutes, until the broth has reduced slightly.
10. Stir in the spinach, thyme, and salt and pepper to taste. Stir and cook until the spinach has wilted, 2 to 3 minutes.
11. Pour the filling into a large casserole dish or pie pan.
12. Top with a layer of the mashed sweet potatoes. Cover with aluminum foil and refrigerate for up to a week, or freeze for up to 3 weeks.

Feast Day

TIME: 30 minutes

Tools: Oven

1. Preheat the oven to 350°F.
2. Uncover the shepherd's pie, sprinkle with paprika, and bake for about 30 minutes, or up to 1 hour if frozen. The pie is done when the filling is bubbling hot and the potatoes are heated through.
3. Scoop into shallow bowls or onto plates and serve piping hot.

Spicy Beef Chili with Mashed Sweet Potato

Everyone seems to have their own chili recipe. Some like it hot, some like it mild, some like tons of veggies, and others prefer more meat. With two different cuts of beef and whatever amount of spice pleases your palate, this meaty chili will win over even the pickiest chili lovers in your crowd.

Serves: 4

PREP DAY TIME: 35 minutes

FEAST DAY TIME: 7 to 8 hours in the slow cooker

Ingredients

SPICY BEEF CHILI

1 pound cubed grass-fed, organic beef stew meat

1 medium yellow onion

1 large carrot

1 medium zucchini

1 green bell pepper

1 red bell pepper

6 garlic cloves

1 pound grass-fed, organic ground
   beef
1 (28-ounce) can crushed tomatoes
1 cup beef broth or water

MASHED SWEET POTATO
1 large sweet potato
1 tablespoon grass-fed butter
Salt

3 tablespoons chili powder
1 teaspoon garlic powder
1 tablespoon ground cumin
Sea salt

Fresh chives, scallions, and/or
   crumbled bacon, for garnish

Prep Day

TIME: 35 minutes

Tools: Knife, cutting board, garlic press, large skillet, pot,
handheld electric mixer

SPICY BEEF CHILI

1. Cut the stew meat into small, bite-size pieces. Set aside.
2. Trim and coarsely chop the onion, carrot, zucchini, and bell peppers.
3. Peel and mince the garlic cloves.
4. In a large greased skillet over medium heat, combine the cubed stew meat, onion, and ground beef and cook until the onions are tender and the meat is browned.
5. Add the tomatoes, broth, zucchini, carrot, bell peppers, garlic, chili powder, garlic powder, cumin, and salt to taste. Stir well.
6. Transfer to an airtight container and refrigerate for up to 5 days.

MASHED SWEET POTATO

7. Place the unpeeled sweet potato in a pot and add water to cover. Bring to a boil over high heat and cook until the potato is soft, 30 to 40 minutes. Drain and set aside until cool enough to touch. Gently pull off the potato skin and discard.
8. Place the potato in a medium bowl. Add the butter and salt to taste.
9. Using a handheld electric mixer, beat the cooked potato until the mash has a creamy consistency. Alternately, blend or puree in a food processor.
10. Cover and refrigerate for up to 5 days.

Feast Day

TIME: 7 to 8 hours in the slow cooker

Tools: Slow cooker, small pot, mixing spoon

1. Pour the chili mixture into the slow cooker. Cover and cook on low until the tomato sauce thickens and the vegetables are soft, 7 to 8 hours.
2. When ready to serve, heat the sweet potato mash in a small pot set over low heat, stirring regularly, until warmed through.
3. Serve the chili in bowls topped with a dollop of mashed sweet potato and diced scallions or chives. A little crumbled bacon on top wouldn't hurt, either.
4. Freeze any remaining chili in an airtight container for up to 1 month. Simply reheat in a pot or slow cooker when ready to use.

Beef Tenderloin with Buttered Onions, Horseradish, and Arugula

Steak lovers, rejoice. Served with a simple arugula salad, you have a meal worthy of the finest restaurant in town. If you want to make it a bit heartier on the days that you've exerted extra energy, add a side of cauliflower mash or sweet potato.

Serves: 2

PREP DAY TIME: 10 minutes

FEAST DAY TIME: 45 minutes

Ingredients

BEEF TENDERLOIN
2 medium yellow onions
3 garlic cloves
2 tablespoons grass-fed butter
**2 (8-ounce) grass-fed, organic beef
   tenderloin steaks**

¼ cup coconut aminos
**2 tablespoons grated fresh
   horseradish**
1 tablespoon apple cider vinegar

ARUGULA SALAD
2 cups arugula
Organic extra-virgin olive oil

2 lemon wedges
Sea salt and cracked black pepper

Prep Day

TIME: 10 minutes

Tools: Knife, cutting board, garlic press, measuring cup, small
saucepan, storage container

BEEF TENDERLOIN

1. Peel and finely dice the onions. Mince the garlic. Set aside.
2. Melt the butter in a small saucepan over low heat and let it cool.
3. Place the steaks side by side in an airtight storage container, spoon the melted butter over the top, and sprinkle the onion, garlic, and coconut aminos over the steaks.
   Cover tightly and shake gently to coat.
4. Store in the refrigerator for up to 3 days.

Feast Day

TIME: 45 minutes

Tools: Grater, 9 x 9-inch baking dish, meat thermometer,
measuring cups and spoons

BEEF TENDERLOIN

1. Preheat the oven to 350°F.

2. Place the steaks in a 9 × 9-inch baking dish. Scoop all of the butter-and-onion mixture out of the storage container and completely smother the steak with it.

3. Bake for 10 minutes, then flip the steaks and continue to cook until the internal temperature of the steaks reaches 135°F, 20 to 35 minutes more.

4. Remove from the oven and set aside to rest.

5. Spoon the butter–coconut amino sauce from the baking dish into a separate bowl and mix with the horseradish and vinegar.

ARUGULA SALAD

6. Place the arugula in a medium bowl and drizzle with olive oil and a squeeze of lemon. Season with salt and pepper.

7. Plate the steaks and top with the onion-horseradish sauce. Serve immediately, with a side of arugula salad.

Chimichurri Steak and Roasted Brussels Sprouts

Chimichurri—Argentina's version of a barbecue sauce—is a tangy, pesto-like topping that will give any beef the Argentinean treatment. A perfect complement to steak, it's light and fresh and full of flavor . . . not to mention that fresh herbs are packed full of healing and detoxifying properties. I say, "Let them eat steak!"

Serves: 2

PREP DAY TIME: 10 minutes

FEAST DAY TIME: 30 minutes

Ingredients

ROASTED BRUSSELS SPROUTS
2 cups Brussels sprouts
3 tablespoons organic extra-virgin olive oil
Sea salt and freshly ground black pepper

CHIMICHURRI TOPPING
1 medium garlic clove
1 cup packed fresh parsley
½ cup packed fresh cilantro
⅓ cup organic extra-virgin olive oil

2 teaspoons freshly squeezed lemon juice
Sea salt and freshly ground black pepper

STEAK
1 tablespoon grass-fed ghee
2 (6-ounce) grass-fed, organic boneless top loin steaks
Sea salt and freshly ground black pepper

Prep Day

TIME: 10 minutes

Tools: Kitchen knife, storage container

ROASTED BRUSSELS SPROUTS

1. Wash and peel any yellow leaves from the sprouts. Cut the sprouts in half from tip to stem.
2. Place in a storage container and refrigerate for up to 3 days.

Feast Day

TIME: 30 minutes

Tools: Rimmed baking sheet or jelly-roll pan, medium skillet, food processor, measuring spoons

ROASTED BRUSSELS SPROUTS

1. Preheat the oven to 400°F.

2. Arrange the sprouts cut-side up on the rimmed baking sheet.

3. Drizzle olive oil all over the sprouts. Season with salt and pepper.

4. Bake for 15 minutes. Turn each sprout over and cook for 10 minutes more. The sprouts are done when the outside is slightly browned and the inside is tender.

CHIMICHURRI TOPPING

5. Peel the garlic clove and place it in a food processor with the parsley, cilantro, olive oil, lemon juice, and salt and black pepper to taste. Pulse a few times to combine. Set aside.

STEAK

6. While the Brussels sprouts are roasting, melt the ghee in a skillet over medium-high heat. Add the steaks and season with salt and pepper.

7. Cook until the steaks reach your desired doneness, 3 to 5 minutes on each side. Turn up the heat to high just before removing the steaks from the pan and lightly brown each side.

8. Transfer the steaks to a plate to rest.

9. Serve the steaks topped with chimichurri sauce with a side of roasted Brussels sprouts.

Ginger Lamb Chops with Roasted Vegetables

This recipe is actually a combo from our Community—the lamb recipe was sent to us by Erik Dyrr, and the recipe for the roasted vegetables was provided by Peggy Malone. Together, they make this astonishingly tasty dish.

Serves: 2

PREP DAY TIME: 25 minutes

FEAST DAY TIME: 1 hour

Ingredients

ROASTED VEGETABLES

1 large celery stalk
½ medium red onion
2 medium red or golden beets
1 medium sweet potato
1 garlic clove

1 tablespoon organic unrefined coconut oil, plus more as needed
Sea salt and freshly ground black pepper

GINGER LAMB CHOPS

1 (1-inch) piece fresh ginger
2 garlic cloves
Juice of 1 lemon
2 teaspoons Dijon mustard
2 tablespoons wheat-free tamari
2 tablespoons coconut palm sugar

2 teaspoons macadamia nut oil
⅛ teaspoon ground coriander
⅛ teaspoon red pepper flakes
Dash of sea salt and freshly ground black pepper
4 lamb chops

Prep Day

TIME: 25 minutes

Tools: Knife, cutting board, peeler, large bowl, grater, measuring spoons, storage containers, garlic press

ROASTED VEGETABLES

1. Trim the celery stalk and coarsely chop. Peel and dice the onion and beets. Peel, cube, and rinse the sweet potato. Peel and mince the garlic. Toss everything together and store in an airtight container in the refrigerator for up to 5 days.

GINGER LAMB CHOPS

2. Peel and grate the ginger into a large bowl.

3. Peel and mince the garlic and add to the bowl with the ginger.

4. Add the lemon juice, mustard, tamari, coconut palm sugar, macadamia nut oil, coriander, red pepper flakes, and salt and black pepper.

5. Using a fork, riddle the lamb chops with holes.

6. Place the chops in an airtight container and drench with the marinade.

7. Cover tightly and store in the refrigerator for up to 3 days.

Feast Day

TIME: 1 hour

Tools: 8 x 8-inch baking dish, knife, cutting board, grill and grilling utensils, measuring spoons

ROASTED VEGETABLES

1. Preheat the oven to 350°F. Grease a baking dish with the coconut oil.

2. Place the vegetable mixture in the greased baking dish.

3. Bake for 15 to 20 minutes, then stir the vegetables to completely coat with the oil. (Add more oil if needed.) Bake until the vegetables are tender on the inside and crisp on the outside, 25 to 40 minutes more.

GINGER LAMB CHOPS

4. Preheat a grill to medium-high. Grill the lamb for 3 to 4 minutes per side for medium-rare, or longer for your desired doneness. Do not char. Let the chops rest for 5 minutes before plating.

5. Serve with the roasted vegetables.

Sun-Dried Tomato Meatballs with Zucchini Noodles

love zucchini noodles, made from scratch in minutes using a spiralizer or julienne peeler. All the texture and pleasure of eating noodles without the carbs. While this recipe doesn't require a sauce, you could certainly add a little marinara if it calls to you.

Serves: 4

PREP DAY TIME: 20 minutes

FEAST DAY TIME: 20 minutes

Ingredients

SUN-DRIED TOMATO MEATBALLS
2 tablespoons chopped fresh chives
2 tablespoons chopped fresh basil
½ cup sun-dried tomatoes packed in olive oil
3 garlic cloves
1 pound grass-fed, organic ground beef
Sea salt and freshly ground black pepper
Cayenne pepper
2 tablespoons grass-fed butter

ZUCCHINI NOODLES
2 large zucchinis
2 teaspoons organic extra-virgin olive oil
Sea salt and cracked black pepper

Organic extra-virgin olive oil
Freshly grated Parmesan cheese (optional)

Prep Day

TIME: 20 minutes

Tools: Knife, cutting board, garlic press, food processor, measuring cups and spoons, storage containers, vegetable peeler or spiralizer, paper towels or kitchen towel

SUN-DRIED TOMATO MEATBALLS

1. Place the chives and basil in a large bowl.

2. Drain the oil from the sun-dried tomatoes and chop the tomatoes into very small bits. Add them to the bowl with the herbs.

3. Peel and mince the garlic cloves and add to the bowl with the herbs.

4. Add the ground beef, salt, pepper, and cayenne to taste and use clean hands to mix everything together.

5. Roll the mixture between your palms to form balls the size of golf balls. Repeat until all of the mixture has been used.

6. Place the meatballs in a single layer in a storage container with a tight-fitting lid and refrigerate for up to 2 days.

ZUCCHINI NOODLES

7. Rinse the zucchini and cut off the tips. Pass a vegetable peeler lengthwise over the zucchini to make long, thin ribbons, or use a spiralizer or a julienne peeler to make noodles.

8. Place the zucchini noodles in a paper-towel- or kitchen-towel-lined airtight storage container and refrigerate for up to 2 days.

Feast Day

TIME: 20 minutes

Tools: Measuring spoons, large skillet, baking sheet, aluminum foil, medium skillet, wooden spoon

SUN-DRIED TOMATO MEATBALLS

1. Preheat the oven to 375°F. Line a baking sheet with aluminum foil.
2. Melt the butter in an oven-safe skillet over medium to medium-high heat.
3. Add the meatballs in batches and cook until browned on all sides.
4. Transfer the meatballs to the prepared baking sheet.
5. Bake until the meat is cooked through, 10 to 12 minutes. The meatballs should be firm to the touch and lightly browned.

ZUCCHINI NOODLES

6. Heat the olive oil in a skillet over low heat.
7. Gently toss in the zucchini noodles and heat until just warmed. Season with salt and pepper.
8. Plate the zucchini noodles and top with the meatballs. Drizzle with a little extra olive oil and garnish with freshly grated Parmesan cheese, if you like.

Macadamia-Crusted Cod with Tender Greens

Cod, a favorite among my New England brethren, is a mild, flaky fish that stands up to any kind of cooking: It can be roasted, steamed, dropped into soup, or even chopped up to make fish balls. But this recipe utilizes the fish's blank canvas to create a macadamia-encrusted masterpiece.

Serves: 2 to 4

PREP DAY TIME: 15 minutes

FEAST DAY TIME: 20 minutes

Ingredients

MACADAMIA COD

1½ cups macadamia nuts

1 lemon

¼ cup fresh parsley leaves

¼ cup unsweetened shredded coconut

½ teaspoon salt

½ teaspoon freshly ground black pepper

2 large eggs

3 tablespoons unsweetened coconut milk

Organic unrefined coconut oil, for greasing

1 pound cod, cut into 4 fillets

TENDER GREENS

4 garlic cloves

1 large yellow onion

1 bunch fresh kale

1 tablespoon organic unrefined coconut oil

3 handfuls fresh spinach

2 tablespoons freshly squeezed lemon juice

2 tablespoons coconut aminos

1 teaspoon ground turmeric

Salt and freshly ground black pepper

Prep Day

TIME: 15 minutes

Tools: Food processor, zester/grater, 2 medium bowls, knife, cutting board, whisk, shallow baking dish, storage containers

MACADAMIA COD

1. Process the macadamia nuts in the food processor until coarsely chopped. Transfer to a medium bowl.
2. Zest the lemon and add to the bowl with the macadamias.
3. Coarsely chop the parsley and add to the bowl.
4. Add the shredded coconut, salt, and pepper.
5. In a separate bowl, whisk together the eggs and coconut milk until frothy.
6. Grease a shallow baking dish with coconut oil and set aside.
7. Dunk the cod fillets in the egg mixture, then dredge each one in the nut mixture, pressing the nuts into the fish firmly.
8. Lay the coated fillets in the prepared dish. Cover and refrigerate for up to 2 days, or freeze if making later in the week. This fish can go straight from the freezer to the oven.

TENDER GREENS

9. Peel and chop the garlic and onion. Store in an airtight container in the refrigerator for up to 1 week.
10. Wash, trim, and chop the kale. Remember to remove any thick stems, as they will be very fibrous and bitter. Store in a produce bag or salad spinner in the refrigerator for up to 3 days.

Feast Day

TIME: 20 minutes

Tools: Baking dish, skillet, metal spatula

MACADAMIA COD

1. Preheat the oven to 400°F.
2. Uncover the cod and bake until flaky, 13 to 18 minutes, or 36 to 40 minutes if frozen.

TENDER GREENS

3. Melt the coconut oil in a large skillet over medium heat.
4. Add the chopped garlic and onion and sauté until tender, 5 to 8 minutes.
5. Stir in the kale, spinach, lemon juice, coconut aminos, and turmeric.
6. Cook, stirring regularly, until the spinach has wilted and the kale is tender.
7. Season with salt and pepper.
8. Serve with the macadamia cod fillets.

Seared Ahi Tuna with Sesame-Ginger Asparagus

The delicate textures and flavors of this Asian-inspired dish are so exquisite that you'd never guess it takes just a few minutes to prepare. Fresh tuna is best when the center is rare, so sear this just long enough to warm the center.

Serves: 2

PREP DAY TIME: 10 minutes

FEAST DAY TIME: 15 minutes

Ingredients

SESAME-GINGER ASPARAGUS

16 to 20 asparagus spears
1 small knob peeled fresh ginger
   (about the size of a garlic clove)
1 garlic clove

1 tablespoon sesame oil
1 teaspoon black sesame seeds
Sea salt

SEARED AHI TUNA

2 (6- to 8-ounce) wild-caught ahi tuna
   steaks
1 teaspoon melted ghee or organic
   unrefined coconut oil
½ teaspoon finely ground black
   pepper

½ teaspoon mustard powder
½ teaspoon fine sea salt

Prep Day

TIME: 10 minutes

Tools: Knife, cutting board, garlic press, spoons, storage
containers

SESAME-GINGER ASPARAGUS

1. Rinse and trim the asparagus and place in a storage container.
2. Press the ginger and garlic clove through a garlic press, straight into the container
   with the asparagus. Cover and refrigerate for up to 3 days.

SEARED AHI TUNA

3. Rub the tuna steaks with the melted ghee or coconut oil.
4. Mix together the pepper, mustard powder, and salt in a small bowl and rub the spice
   mixture evenly into both sides of the tuna steaks.
5. Place the seasoned steaks in an airtight container, cover, and refrigerate for up to
   24 hours.

Feast Day

TIME: 15 minutes

Tools: 2 large heavy skillets, measuring spoons, metal spatula, tongs

SESAME-GINGER ASPARAGUS

1. Coat a pan with the sesame oil and heat over medium-high heat.
2. Add the asparagus with the garlic and ginger to the pan and toss to coat.
3. Cook, turning regularly, until the asparagus is crisp-tender, 5 to 8 minutes.
4. Pour in the sesame seeds and turn to coat. Season with salt.

SEARED AHI TUNA

5. Heat a skillet over high heat.
6. Place the tuna in the hot pan and sear for 2 to 3 minutes on each side. The center will be rare but warm.
7. Transfer to serving plates and pair with the sesame-ginger asparagus.

Parmesan Shrimp Lettuce Wraps with Avocado

These shrimp lettuce wraps are a regular in our house. They're also a great excuse to bust out the Frank's RedHot hot sauce. Handy in a pinch.

Serves: 4

PREP DAY TIME: 15 minutes

FEAST DAY TIME: 10 minutes

Ingredients

1 large yellow onion
1 pound raw medium shrimp
2 garlic cloves
1 teaspoon paprika
1 tablespoon ground cumin
½ teaspoon dried oregano
1 tablespoon chili powder
½ teaspoon red pepper flakes
1 teaspoon freshly ground black pepper

1 teaspoon sea salt
1 medium or large avocado
1 lemon wedge
½ bunch fresh cilantro
1 tablespoon grass-fed butter
1 head green- or red-leaf lettuce
Hot sauce or taco sauce
Shredded Parmesan cheese

Prep Day

TIME: 15 minutes

Tools: Knife, cutting board, strainer, mixing bowl, garlic press, measuring spoons, storage containers

1. Chop the onion and store in a small airtight container for up to 1 week.
2. Rinse, peel, and devein the shrimp. Place in a large airtight container and set aside.
3. Peel and mince the garlic cloves and place in a small bowl.
4. Add the paprika, cumin, oregano, chili powder, red pepper flakes, black pepper, and salt to the bowl with the garlic.
5. Toss the seasoning into the container with the shrimp. Close the lid securely and shake to coat. Refrigerate for up to 2 days.

Feast Day

TIME: 10 minutes

Tools: Measuring cups and spoons, knife, cutting board, pan, large skillet, storage container

1. Halve the avocado lengthwise, remove the pit, and use a large metal spoon to scoop out the flesh. Slice the flesh. Squeeze the juice from the lemon wedge over the avocado and set aside.

2. Coarsely chop the cilantro and set aside.

3. In a large skillet, melt the butter over medium-high heat.

4. Sauté the seasoned shrimp in the butter for 1 to 2 minutes, turn, and cook the other side until the shrimp has turned pink and the flesh is firm.

5. Plate the lettuce leaves and top each leaf with shrimp, onion, avocado, cilantro, hot sauce, and Parmesan. Serve immediately.

SWAP BOX

Don't have time to mince garlic? Replace it with a teaspoon of garlic powder in the seasoning. Make a double or triple batch to save a step next time.

Baked Pesto Salmon with Roasted Artichokes

Sure, salmon is healthy and delicious, yadda yadda yadda . . . Let's talk artichokes. Have you ever had a whole, fresh artichoke dunked in butter? Life-changing. If you don't have time for fresh artichokes or they're not in season, you can use frozen artichoke hearts and just eat them with a fork.

Serves: 4

PREP DAY TIME: 45 minutes
FEAST DAY TIME: 20 minutes

Ingredients

SUN-DRIED TOMATO PESTO

3 garlic cloves

½ cup sun-dried tomatoes packed in
olive oil

¾ cup organic extra-virgin
olive oil

½ cup raw pine nuts

2 cups fresh basil leaves

½ cup fresh flat-leaf parsley leaves

2 tablespoons chopped fresh
oregano

ROASTED ARTICHOKES

2 lemons

4 artichokes

1 garlic clove

¼ cup organic extra-virgin olive oil

Sea salt and freshly ground black
pepper

Grass-fed butter, for dipping

Chopped fresh flat-leaf parsley

SALMON

Melted ghee or organic unrefined coconut oil

2 pounds wild-caught salmon, cut into 4 fillets

Salt and freshly ground black pepper

Prep Day

TIME: 45 minutes

Tools: Measuring cups and spoons, food processor, knife,
cutting board, storage containers, large bowl or container,
ice, kitchen scissors, metal spoon

SUN-DRIED TOMATO PESTO

1. Peel the garlic cloves and place them in a food processor.

2. Drain the oil from the sun-dried tomatoes and add the tomatoes to the garlic.

3. Add the olive oil, pine nuts, basil, parsley, and oregano.

4. Process until the pesto has a grainy consistency but is not completely pureed.

5. Transfer to an airtight container and store in the refrigerator for up to 5 days. The color will gray a bit as the herbs lose their brilliance, but the flavor will be fine.

ROASTED ARTICHOKES

6. Fill a large lidded container with icy cold water. Squeeze in the juice of 2 lemons, and add their rinds to the water.

7. Working with one artichoke at a time, first remove the tough outer leaves by "shucking" them with a downward motion. You'll probably remove about 15 leaves.

8. Using kitchen scissors, snip the sharp ends off the remaining leaves (about one-third of the way down).

9. Cut the artichoke in half lengthwise and immediately immerse in the lemon water. Return it to the cutting board and scoop out the fuzzy choke and the small inner leaves (usually purple) with a small metal spoon. Immediately return the scooped artichoke, cut-side down, to the lemon water.

10. Repeat until all the artichokes are shucked, snipped, scooped, and submerged. Put a tightly fitted lid on the container and refrigerate for up to 2 days.

Feast Day

TIME: 20 minutes

Tools: Rimmed baking sheet, aluminum foil, measuring cups and spoons, garlic press, knife, cutting board, whisk, small bowl

SALMON

1. Preheat the oven to 400°F. Line a rimmed baking sheet with aluminum foil and grease the foil with ghee or coconut oil.

2. Remove any pin bones from the salmon.

3. Lay the salmon, skin-side down, on the foil and brush the tops with oil. Season with salt and pepper. Set aside.

4. Peel and mince the garlic clove and whisk it into the olive oil in a small bowl.

5. Place the artichokes, cut-side up, on a baking sheet. (This can be on the same sheet as the salmon, if there's room. A casserole dish will also work fine.)

6. Brush the artichokes with the garlic–olive oil to completely coat on all sides. Sprinkle with salt and pepper to taste.

7. Bake both the salmon and the artichokes until the salmon is cooked through and the artichokes are tender, 10 to 12 minutes.

8. Plate the salmon topped with the pesto, with the artichokes alongside. In a small bowl, stir together the melted butter and parsley and serve alongside the artichokes for dipping.

Bacon-Wrapped Scallops and Sweet Slaw

We enjoyed the delicate meat of scallops wrapped in crisp, savory bacon every Christmas Eve (sometimes drizzled with maple syrup—try it). If any of these little buggers actually make it out of the kitchen, they'll impress everyone at a party.

Serves: 4

PREP DAY TIME: 15 minutes
FEAST DAY TIME: 35 minutes

Ingredients

BACON-WRAPPED SCALLOPS

¼ teaspoon sea salt
¼ teaspoon freshly ground black pepper
⅛ teaspoon dried thyme
⅛ teaspoon onion powder

⅛ teaspoon garlic powder
⅛ teaspoon cayenne pepper
16 large scallops
8 slices thin-cut uncured bacon
Grass-fed butter, for greasing

SWEET SLAW

½ head purple cabbage
¼ cup white vinegar (or apple cider
 vinegar)
¼ cup organic extra-virgin olive oil

2 tablespoons raw honey or pure dried
 leaf stevia (to taste)
Sea salt and cracked black pepper
2 scallions

Prep Day

TIME: 15 minutes

Tools: Measuring cups and spoons, knife, cutting
board, mixing bowls, storage containers, toothpicks,
whisk

BACON-WRAPPED SCALLOPS

1. Place 16 toothpicks in a small bowl of water to soak.
2. In a separate small bowl, whisk together the salt, black pepper, thyme, onion powder, garlic powder, and cayenne.
3. Lay the scallops on a plate and sprinkle generously with the spice mixture.
4. Cut the bacon strips in half crosswise, turning each strip into two short pieces of bacon.
5. Wrap one half-strip around the outside of each scallop and secure in place with a soaked toothpick.
6. Place the bacon-wrapped scallops in an airtight storage container and store in the refrigerator for up to 2 days, or freeze for up to 2 weeks (thaw completely in the refrigerator before broiling).

SWEET SLAW

7. Slice the cabbage into thin strips and place in a large bowl.
8. In a small bowl, whisk together the vinegar, olive oil, honey, and salt and pepper to taste until it becomes a smooth dressing. Pour the dressing over the shredded cabbage.

9. Slice the scallions on an angle and add to the cabbage.

10. Using clean hands or a mixing spoon, turn the mixture until all of the cabbage is coated with the dressing and the scallions are incorporated.

11. Cover and refrigerate for up to 5 days.

Feast Day

TIME: 35 minutes

Tools: Rimmed baking sheet, aluminum foil

BACON-WRAPPED SCALLOPS

1. Preheat the oven to 500°F or set it to broil. Line a rimmed baking sheet with foil. Grease the foil with butter to prevent sticking.

2. Place the bacon-wrapped scallops at least ½ inch apart on the prepared baking sheet.

3. Broil about 5 inches from the heat for 3 minutes.

4. Remove from the oven, flip each scallop over, and broil for 3 minutes more, or until the scallops are firm to the touch and the bacon is crisp.

5. Serve with a side of sweet slaw.

Fish Tacos with Mango-Avocado Salsa

These mahimahi fillets are marinated in freshly squeezed lemon juice and topped with the sweet exotic punch of mango. This feast has a light, beachy feel but packs a serious protein punch . . . so you'll walk away totally satisfied.

Serves: 2

PREP DAY TIME: 15 minutes

FEAST DAY TIME: 30 minutes

Ingredients

MANGO-AVOCADO SALSA
1 medium ripe mango
1 medium or large avocado
1 medium Roma tomato
¼ cup chopped red onion

Juice of 1 lemon
¼ teaspoon cayenne pepper
Sea salt and freshly ground black
  pepper

FISH TACOS
¼ cup freshly squeezed lemon juice
Sea salt and freshly ground black
  pepper
2 (6-ounce) mahimahi fillets

Organic unrefined coconut oil or
  grass-fed butter, for brushing
  the grill
Large fresh lettuce leaves

Prep Day

TIME: 15 minutes

Tools: Measuring cups and spoons, knife, cutting board, medium bowl, small storage container, metal spoon

MANGO-AVOCADO SALSA

1. Using a sharp knife, peel the mango and cut the flesh away from the pit. Dice the mango flesh and place it in a small bowl.

2. Halve the avocado and remove the pit. Use a metal spoon to scoop out the flesh in one piece. Dice the avocado flesh and add it to the mango.

3. Dice the tomato and onion and add them to the bowl with the mango.

4. Squeeze in the lemon juice. Mix in the cayenne pepper and salt and black pepper to taste.

5. Stir to thoroughly combine.

6. Place the salsa in an airtight storage container and refrigerate for up to 3 days.

Feast Day

TIME: 30 minutes

Tools: Grill, measuring cup, airtight container with lid

FISH TACOS

1. Place the lemon juice, a pinch of salt and pepper, and the mahimahi in an airtight storage container. Toss to coat. Place in the refrigerator to marinate for 20 minutes.

2. Heat an electric or gas grill to medium-high. Brush the grill grates with coconut oil or butter to prevent sticking.

3. Place the fillets on the grill and grill for 3 to 4 minutes on each side, until just opaque inside and firm to the touch. Transfer to a plate to rest.

4. Serve each fillet on a bed of lettuce, topped with the salsa.

King Prawns and Seared Garlic Zucchini Spears

The garlic-infused goodness of these king prawns will please senses you didn't even know you had. Get your seafood as fresh as you can, and be careful not to over-cook it—low and slow, baby.

Serves: 2

PREP DAY TIME: 20 minutes

FEAST DAY TIME: 50 minutes

Ingredients

KING PRAWNS

5 garlic cloves
12 fresh or frozen king prawns (jumbo shrimp), thawed
¼ cup organic extra-virgin olive oil

SEARED GARLIC ZUCCHINI SPEARS

2 medium zucchinis

2 garlic cloves

Juice and zest of 1 lemon

Sea salt and cracked black pepper

Prep Day

TIME: 20 minutes

Tools: Measuring cups and spoons, knife, cutting board, paper towel, storage containers

KING PRAWNS

1. Peel and halve the garlic cloves.
2. Peel and devein the prawns, leaving the tails intact. Rinse each one under cold running water and pat dry with a clean paper towel.
3. Place the garlic and prawns in an airtight storage container and refrigerate for up to 2 days.

SEARED GARLIC ZUCCHINI SPEARS

4. Halve the zucchini lengthwise. Slice each half into 8 spears. Place in an airtight storage container.
5. Peel and mince the garlic cloves and place in a separate airtight storage container.
6. Refrigerate the zucchini and garlic for up to 2 days.

Feast Day

TIME: 50 minutes

Tools: Measuring cups and spoons, medium saucepan,
deep-fry or candy thermometer, skillet

KING PRAWNS

1. In a medium saucepan, heat the olive oil to about 160°F. Use a deep-fry or candy thermometer to test the temperature.

2. Remove the saucepan from the heat and add the garlic cloves. Let stand for 30 minutes to infuse.

3. Place the pan back on the heat and bring the temperature back to 160°F. Once it has reached the desired temperature, remove it again and place the prawns in the hot oil.

4. Allow the prawns to poach in the garlic-infused oil for about 10 minutes. Return the pan to the heat and bring the temperature back to 160°F. Remove from the heat. Turn the prawns to poach the other side for an additional 5 minutes. The prawns are done when they turn pinkish-white in color. Do not overcook.

5. Transfer the prawns to a clean towel or paper towel to drain well. Reserve the garlic-infused oil.

SEARED GARLIC ZUCCHINI SPEARS

6. Transfer 1 tablespoon of the garlic-infused oil from poaching the prawns to a heavy skillet and set over medium-high heat.

7. Add the zucchini spears to the skillet and squeeze a bit of lemon juice over the top. Sprinkle with the lemon zest. Cook until browned on all sides, about 5 minutes.

8. Transfer to a plate and season with salt and pepper. Serve alongside the prawns.

Lemon-Garlic Snapper

For Mexican-inspired fish that you can whip up in less than 20 minutes, this snapper can't be beat: jalapeños, fresh tomatoes, green olives, capers, onion, and the light flakiness of red snapper with a hint of lemon and garlic.

Serves: 2

PREP DAY TIME: 20 minutes

FEAST DAY TIME: 20 minutes

Ingredients

1 small Spanish onion or white onion

2 tablespoons organic extra-virgin olive oil

3 small garlic cloves

1 jalapeño pepper

¼ cup green olives, pitted

2 cups cherry tomatoes

¼ teaspoon ground coriander

1 teaspoon cayenne pepper

2 tablespoons capers

2 tablespoons chopped fresh oregano

Sea salt and cracked black pepper

2 (10-ounce) boneless skinless red snapper fillets

1 lemon

Chopped fresh chives, for garnish (optional)

Prep Day

TIME: 20 minutes

Tools: Measuring cups and spoons, knife, cutting board, large skillet, 2 individual ramekins/ceramic crocks (or a glass or metal baking dish)

1. Peel and finely dice the onion and set aside.
2. Pour the olive oil into a large skillet over medium heat. Add the onion and allow it to cook slightly while you're chopping the other vegetables, about 3 minutes.
3. Peel and mince the garlic cloves and transfer to a large bowl.
4. Slice the jalapeño and olives into thin rounds and add to the bowl with the garlic.

5. Cut the cherry tomatoes in half and add to the bowl.

6. Add the contents of the bowl to the skillet with the onion. Add the coriander, cayenne pepper, and capers and stir to combine.

7. Cook, stirring often, until the tomatoes soften and their skins wrinkle, 6 to 8 minutes.

8. Stir in the oregano and salt and pepper to taste.

9. Cut each snapper fillet in half, leaving you with four small fillets.

10. Grease the bottom of two ramekins or baking dishes with olive oil.

11. Scoop a small amount of the tomato mixture into each ramekin. Lay half of each fish fillet on top, season with salt and pepper to taste, and squeeze on some lemon juice.

12. Top with another scoop of the tomato mixture and the second half of the fish. Season each fillet with salt, pepper, and lemon juice and top with the remaining tomato mixture.

13. Cover tightly with aluminum foil and refrigerate for up to 3 days.

Feast Day

TIME: 20 minutes

Tools: Oven

1. Preheat the oven to 425°F.

2. Uncover the ramekins and bake for 15 to 20 minutes. When the fish is done, it will be light and flaky and the juices will run clear.

3. Serve hot, straight from the ramekins. Garnish with chives, if you'd like.

Swordfish with Spicy Peach Salsa

Fruit salsas are the perfect complement to spicy meat, poultry, and fish. They cool the palate, add texture, and are easy to whip up. This peach salsa has its own little kick, and I hope you enjoy it. Serve this over a bed of field greens for a complete, healthy, delicious meal.

Serves: 4

PREP DAY TIME: 20 minutes

FEAST DAY TIME: 15 minutes, plus 1 to 3 hours to marinate

Ingredients

SWORDFISH
2 tablespoons organic unrefined
    coconut oil, melted
2 tablespoons apple cider vinegar
2 teaspoons honey, melted

Juice of 1 lime
⅛ teaspoon cayenne pepper
4 swordfish fillets

SPICY PEACH SALSA
2 medium peaches
1 medium avocado
¼ large red onion
½ jalapeño pepper

½ cup fresh cilantro
Juice of 1 lemon
Sea salt and freshly ground black
    pepper

SERVING
Field greens

Prep Day

TIME: 20 minutes

Tools: Measuring spoons, mixing bowls, storage containers, knife, cutting board, whisk

SWORDFISH

1. In a bowl, whisk together the coconut oil, vinegar, honey, lime juice, and cayenne to create a marinade.

2. Place in an airtight storage container and refrigerate for up to 5 days.

SPICY PEACH SALSA

3. Halve and pit the peaches. Dice the flesh, leaving the skin on. Place in a large bowl and set aside.

4. Halve the avocado and remove the pit. Scoop out the flesh with a large metal spoon. Dice the avocado flesh and add it to the peaches.

5. Finely chop the red onion, jalapeño, and cilantro and add to the peach and avocado. Mix well.

6. Squeeze the juice of 1 lemon over the mixture, season with salt and pepper, and toss to coat. Place in an airtight storage container and refrigerate for up to 4 days.

Feast Day

TIME: 15 minutes, plus 1 to 3 hours to marinate

Tools: Grill and grill utensils

SWORDFISH

1. Dip each fillet in the marinade, coating both sides well. Lay the fillets in a storage container, cover, and refrigerate for at least 1 hour and up to 3 hours to marinate.

2. Heat a grill to medium.

3. Grill the fillets until the fish is firm to the touch and the juices run clear, 5 to 6 minutes per side. Do not char.

4. Serve each fillet on a bed of field greens topped with the spicy peach salsa.

Smoked Salmon and Kale Salad

This recipe, which was submitted by Kim Stace Thomas from our Community, is a delicious way to include salmon's vitamin-rich, omega-3 fatty acids in your diet. Smoked salmon requires no cooking, making this dish a quick, tasty protein when time is tight.

Serves: 4

PREP DAY TIME: 10 minutes

FEAST DAY TIME: 20 minutes

Ingredients

3 garlic cloves

1 tablespoon grass-fed butter

2 tablespoons organic extra-virgin olive oil

¼ teaspoon freshly ground black pepper

⅛ teaspoon red pepper flakes

Juice of 1 lemon

1 bunch fresh kale

1 large carrot

½ cup finely grated pecorino cheese

4 (6-ounce) smoked salmon fillets

Prep Day

TIME: 10 minutes

Tools: Measuring cups and spoons, knife, cutting board, large salad bowl, storage containers, whisk, garlic press, small saucepan

1. Peel and mince the garlic and place in a small saucepan. Add the butter and sauté over medium heat until the garlic is fragrant, about 2 minutes.

2. Pour the garlic-butter mixture into a small bowl and add the olive oil, black pepper, red pepper flakes, and lemon juice. Whisk thoroughly to form a salad dressing. Store in an airtight container in the refrigerator for up to 3 days.

3. Slice the kale into shreds, about ½ inch wide, and place in a storage container.

4. Grate the carrot into thin strands and toss with the kale.

5. Cover and refrigerate for up to 3 days.

Feast Day

TIME: 20 minutes

Tools: Small saucepan, measuring cups and spoons, small bowl, whisk

1. Warm the salad dressing in a small saucepan over low heat, stirring regularly.

2. Pour the warm salad dressing over the kale and carrots. Toss well until everything is coated. It's important to pour the dressing over the kale while the dressing is still warm. This will take some of the bitterness out of the kale and make it a bit more tender.

3. Add half of the pecorino and toss.

4. Divide the salad among four bowls, sprinkle with the remaining cheese, and top with equal portions of the salmon.

SWAP BOX

If you're not a kale fan, swap it out for another green, such as Swiss chard or red-leaf lettuce.

Green Monster Frittata with Bruschetta

Eggs aren't just for breakfast anymore. Chock-full of veggies and covered with your (new) favorite Italian bruschetta topping, this monster frittata will be sure to please even the pickiest eaters.

Serves: 4

PREP DAY TIME: 10 minutes

FEAST DAY TIME: 35 minutes

Ingredients

GREEN MONSTER FRITTATA

4 broccoli crowns (about 4 cups)

1 medium yellow onion

4 garlic cloves

4 tablespoons grass-fed butter

4 cups packed spinach

12 large eggs

¼ cup heavy cream (optional)

BRUSCHETTA TOPPING

1 large tomato, or 2 small tomatoes

½ cup packed fresh basil leaves

1 tablespoon organic extra-virgin olive oil

Sea salt and freshly ground black pepper

Prep Day

TIME: 10 minutes

Tools: Knife, cutting board, measuring cups, garlic press, storage container

GREEN MONSTER FRITTATA

1. With a sharp knife, cut the broccoli florets from the stems. Chop the florets into very small pieces and place in a large airtight container.
2. Slice the onion into thin rings, then cut the rings in half and add them to the broccoli.
3. Peel and mince the garlic cloves. Add them to the container with the broccoli and onion. Store in the refrigerator for up to 1 week.

BRUSCHETTA TOPPING

4. Quarter the tomato and remove the seeds. Dice the tomato and place it in an airtight container.
5. Chop the basil and add it to the tomato. Drizzle with the olive oil and turn to coat.
6. Season with salt and pepper. Cover and refrigerate for up to 3 days.

Feast Day

TIME: 35 minutes

Tools: Knife, cutting board, measuring cups and spoons, large ovenproof skillet, bowl, whisk, wooden spoon

1. Preheat the oven to 350°F.
2. Melt 2 tablespoons of the butter in a large ovenproof skillet over medium heat.
3. Add the broccoli, onion, and garlic and cook until tender, about 5 minutes.
4. Stir in the spinach and cook until wilted, about 2 minutes. Add the remaining butter and stir to melt.

5. Beat the eggs with the heavy cream (if using) until frothy. Slowly pour the eggs over the vegetables and cook until the edges begin to firm up and pull away from the sides of the pan, 5 to 7 minutes.

6. Place the pan in the oven on the top rack (as high as possible) and bake until the eggs are set and the top is golden brown, 15 to 20 minutes.

7. Slice the frittata into four triangles. Plate and top each slice with tomato bruschetta.

Field Green Salad with Apples and Buttered Pecans

This salad is light and fresh—the perfect combination of sweet and tart, topped off with the delicious crunch of pan-roasted buttery pecans.

Serves: 4

PREP DAY TIME: 15 minutes

FEAST DAY TIME: 5 minutes

Ingredients

FIELD GREEN SALAD
1 large Granny Smith apple
¼ lemon
1 tablespoon salted grass-fed butter
1 cup raw pecan halves

1 tablespoon pure maple syrup
¼ teaspoon ground cinnamon
¼ cup sweet red onion
5 to 6 ounces baby field greens

DRESSING
2 tablespoons balsamic vinegar
1 tablespoon macadamia nut oil
Juice of ½ orange

Prep Day

TIME: 15 minutes

Tools: Small heavy skillet, wooden spoon or rubber spatula,
measuring cups and spoons, sharp knife, cutting board,
storage containers, whisk, small bowl

FIELD GREEN SALAD

1. Core the apple and cut it into small pieces. Place the apple in an airtight container and squeeze the juice from the lemon quarter over the top; toss to coat. Cover and refrigerate for up to 2 days.

2. Melt the butter in a small skillet over low heat. Add the pecans, maple syrup, and cinnamon and stir to coat. Cook, stirring regularly, until the pecans darken and the coating is sticky, about 4 minutes.

3. Remove from the heat, stir, and let rest for a few minutes. The coating will harden as the pecans cool. (Try not to eat them all right out of the pan.)

4. When the pecans are completely cooled, store them in an airtight container in the cupboard for up to a few weeks.

5. Finely dice the onion and store it in an airtight container in the refrigerator for up to 1 week.

DRESSING

6. Place the balsamic vinegar, oil, and orange juice in a glass jar with a tight-fitting lid and shake to make the dressing. Store in the refrigerator for up to 1 week.

Feast Day

TIME: 5 minutes

Tools: Medium salad bowl, tongs

FIELD GREEN SALAD

1. Place the field greens in a large salad bowl. Give the dressing a shake and pour it over the greens.

2. Add the apple and chopped onion. Using tongs, turn to mix everything together and coat with dressing.

3. Plate the salad on four large dinner plates and top with the buttered pecans.

Creamy Roasted Vegetable Soup

This recipe was submitted by Wild Community member Lori Gemlin-Gingrich. If you've ever wondered if it's possible to create a creamy soup without dairy, we're about to make your day. This dairy-free soup is thick and rich, with a roasted flavor that adds a rustic touch to a creamy classic.

Serves: 4 to 6

PREP DAY TIME: 10 minutes

FEAST DAY TIME: 40 minutes

Ingredients

5 garlic cloves
1 large white sweet potato
3 large carrots
4 medium yellow onions
1 head cauliflower
2 medium heads broccoli
3 celery stalks
2 red bell peppers

⅓ cup organic extra-virgin olive oil
1 teaspoon dried rosemary
1 teaspoon dried oregano
1 teaspoon dried basil
About 4 cups vegetable, chicken, or bone broth (page 337)
Sea salt and cracked black pepper

Prep Day

TIME: 10 minutes

Tools: Peeler, knife, cutting board, large bowl, storage containers

1. Peel the garlic cloves and set aside.
2. Peel the sweet potato and cut it into small chunks.
3. Scrub, trim, and slice the carrots.
4. Peel and dice the onions.
5. Trim and chop the cauliflower, broccoli, celery, and red bell peppers into bite-size pieces.
6. Place all of the chopped vegetables and the garlic into a lidded storage container (a large roasting pan with a lid works well) and store in the refrigerator for up to 3 days.

Feast Day

TIME: 40 minutes

Tools: Measuring cup and spoons, 2 large rimmed baking sheets, food processor or high-powered blender, large soup pot, whisk

1. Preheat the oven to 375°F.
2. In a small bowl, whisk together the olive oil, rosemary, oregano, and basil.
3. Pour the olive oil mixture over the chopped vegetables and use your hands to completely coat the vegetables with the oil.
4. Arrange the vegetables in a single layer on two large rimmed baking sheets. Roast until the vegetables are fork-tender, 20 to 30 minutes. If they're getting too browned on top, turn them over with a spatula during roasting.
5. Reserve 1 cup of the roasted vegetables for garnish (and a little something to chew on). Working in batches, transfer the remaining vegetables to a food processor or blender. Puree until smooth, pouring each batch into a soup pot as you go.

6. Stir in the broth until you reach a desired soup consistency, about 4 cups. Heat over medium heat, stirring regularly, to heat through, about 5 minutes.

7. Pour into serving bowls or heavy mugs and top with the reserved roasted vegetables.

Cashew Cream Alfredo with Zucchini Noodles

If you crave pasta, try zucchini noodles. This dish is great for beginners—simple and ridiculously yummy. The cashew cream is packed with protein as well. Just remember that nuts are higher in carbs than meats, so try to limit this dish to "once in a while" if you're trying to burn fat.

Serves: 4

PREP DAY TIME: 20 minutes, plus 4 to 12 hours for soaking

FEAST DAY TIME: 10 minutes

Ingredients

2 cups raw cashews

1 cup filtered water, plus more as needed

½ cup plus 1 teaspoon organic extra-virgin olive oil

1 cup packed fresh basil leaves

6 garlic cloves

Juice of 2 lemons

½ teaspoon cayenne pepper

Sea salt and cracked black pepper

2 large carrots

4 small or medium zucchini

Prep Day

TIME: 20 minutes, plus 4 to 12 hours for soaking

Tools: Food processor or blender, julienne peeler or spiralizer, medium bowl, measuring cups and spoons, grater, storage containers

1. Place the cashews in a large bowl. Cover completely with filtered water and soak for 4 to 12 hours. Rinse and drain the cashews.
2. Place the soaked cashews, ½ cup of the olive oil, 1 cup filtered water, the basil, peeled garlic cloves, lemon juice, and cayenne pepper in a food processor or blender.
3. Blend until smooth and creamy, about 3 minutes. Add more water, if needed, to facilitate blending. Season with salt and pepper.
4. Scrub and shred the carrots.
5. Use a spiralizer or julienne peeler to turn the zucchini into noodles. Or use a peeler to peel the zucchini into long, thin ribbons.
6. Toss the zucchini noodles and shredded carrots together. Mix in as much cashew Alfredo sauce as needed to coat. Any remaining sauce can be frozen; just be sure to run it through the blender right after defrosting to eliminate any lumps.
7. Place the coated zucchini noodles in an airtight storage container and refrigerate for up to 4 days.

Feast Day

TIME: 10 minutes

Tools: Large skillet, mixing spoon

1. Grease a large skillet with the remaining 1 teaspoon of olive oil.
2. Add the zucchini noodles coated in the cashew Alfredo sauce and heat until warm, stirring regularly, 5 to 10 minutes. This dish can also be served cold.

Sweet Potato Hash

Packed with veggies and spices, this hash-and-egg dish comes together quickly in one pan. The color of the hash is bright and vibrant, worthy of even the most discerning social-media photographer.

Serves: 2

PREP DAY TIME: 20 minutes

FEAST DAY TIME: 20 minutes

Ingredients

1 small sweet potato

1 large leek

1 large garlic clove

3 red beets

2 tablespoons duck fat, lard, tallow, or organic extra-virgin olive oil

½ teaspoon dried thyme

½ teaspoon dried rosemary

Sea salt and cracked black pepper

4 large eggs

Fresh thyme, for garnish (if desired)

Prep Day

TIME: 20 minutes

Tools: Kitchen knife, cutting board, garlic press, peeler, storage containers

1. Peel and dice the sweet potato into very small pieces.
2. Dice the leek, discarding the leafy top.
3. Peel and mince the garlic clove.
4. Peel and dice the beets, discarding the stems and leaves.
5. Place everything in an airtight container and refrigerate for up to 3 days.

TIME: 20 minutes

Tools: Large heavy pan with a lid, spatula, measuring spoons

1. Melt the duck fat in a large skillet over medium-low heat. Swirl to coat the pan.
2. Add the chopped vegetables, thyme, rosemary, and salt and pepper to taste. Cover and cook for 5 minutes.
3. Uncover and cook, stirring regularly, until the vegetables are fork-tender and crisping at the edges, 10 to 12 minutes more.
4. Make four wells in the hash with a dinner spoon. Crack one egg into each well and cook, covered, until the eggs are soft-cooked with a runny yolk, 5 to 7 minutes.
5. Sprinkle with fresh thyme, if desired, and use a metal spatula to plate onto two dinner plates. Season with salt and pepper.

Immune-Boosting Veggie-Full Soup

Alyson made this "power soup" when I was under the weather last fall. It provides antioxidants, reduces inflammation, and helps stimulate the immune system.

Serves: 4

PREP TIME: 40 minutes

COOK TIME: 10 minutes

Ingredients

4 large garlic cloves
1 medium white or yellow
  onion

1 (3-inch) piece fresh ginger
1½ teaspoons organic unrefined
  coconut oil

3 broccoli crowns (about 3 cups), chopped

3 cups thinly sliced white mushrooms

4 small carrots, chopped

Sea salt and freshly ground black pepper

1 teaspoon garlic powder

1 teaspoon ground turmeric

1 tablespoon ground cumin

2 cups packed chopped kale

6 cups bone broth (page 337) or vegetable broth

3 large nori seaweed sheets

Prep Day

TIME: 40 minutes

Tools: Knife, cutting board, peeler, grater, measuring cups and spoons, large saucepan

1. Peel and mince the garlic cloves and set aside.

2. Peel and dice the onion and set aside.

3. Peel and grate the ginger.

4. Heat the coconut oil in a large stockpot over medium heat.

5. Add the minced garlic and onion and sauté, stirring regularly, until the onion is transparent, about 5 minutes.

6. Add the mushrooms, broccoli, and carrots, and season with salt and pepper. Stir and sauté for 2 minutes.

7. Stir in the grated ginger, garlic powder, turmeric, and cumin. Sauté until the vegetables are starting to darken in color, 2 minutes more.

8. Stir in the kale and broth.

9. Bring to a boil, then reduce the heat to low and simmer until the vegetables are tender, 15 to 20 minutes.

10. Cool, cover, and store in the refrigerator for up to 5 days, or freeze for up to several weeks.

Feast Day

TIME: 10 minutes

Tools: Large soup pot, scissors, soup ladle

1. In a large saucepan, bring the soup to a boil over medium heat. Remove from the heat.
2. Using sharp scissors, cut the nori into 1-inch strips.
3. Ladle the warm soup into bowls and top with seaweed strips.

Thai Carrot Curry Soup with Zucchini Chips

When ordering curry in Thailand, we noticed that the cook would run out the back door and come back with his arms full of vegetables and herbs harvested straight from his neighbor's garden—and he created the most vibrant food I've ever tasted. Use the best ingredients possible to get the full experience of fresh curry.

Serves: 2 to 4

PREP DAY TIME: 50 minutes

FEAST DAY TIME: 30 minutes

Ingredients

THAI CARROT CURRY SOUP

6 large carrots

1 large yellow onion

1 (2-inch) knob fresh ginger

1 tablespoon organic unrefined
   coconut oil

6 cups vegetable broth

⅓ cup full-fat unsweetened canned
   coconut milk

1 tablespoon dried basil, or
   2 tablespoons chopped fresh basil

1 teaspoon Thai red curry paste

Sea salt and freshly ground black
   pepper

ZUCCHINI CHIPS

1 medium or large zucchini

1 tablespoon coconut oil, melted, plus more for the baking sheet

Sea salt and cracked black pepper

Prep Day

TIME: 50 minutes

Tools: Kitchen knife, cutting board, peeler, measuring cups and spoons, storage containers, blender

THAI CARROT CURRY SOUP

1. Scrub and peel the carrots and cut them into thin slices. Set aside.

2. Peel and finely chop the onion.

3. Peel the ginger and cut it into thick slices.

4. Melt the coconut oil in a medium saucepan over medium-high heat. Add the carrots and ginger and turn to coat. Cook, stirring regularly, until the carrots begin to soften and the ginger is fragrant, about 8 minutes.

5. Add the onion and cook, stirring, until the onion begins to soften, about 2 minutes.

6. Add the broth, coconut milk, basil, and red curry paste. Stir and bring the mixture to a boil.

7. Reduce the heat to maintain a simmer and cook until the carrots are softened, about 20 minutes.

8. Working in batches, transfer the soup to a blender and puree until smooth and creamy. Season with salt and pepper.

9. Cool and store in an airtight container in the refrigerator for up to 4 days.

ZUCCHINI CHIPS

10. Cut the zucchini into ¼-inch-thick slices.

11. Place in an airtight storage container and refrigerate for up to 3 days.

Feast Day

TIME: 30 minutes

Tools: Basting brush, rimmed baking sheet, soup pot

THAI CARROT CURRY SOUP

1. In a soup pot, bring the soup to a boil over medium heat. Reduce the heat to maintain a simmer and cook for a few minutes to thoroughly warm.

ZUCCHINI CHIPS

2. Preheat the oven to 450°F. Grease a rimmed baking sheet with coconut oil.
3. Brush the zucchini slices with melted coconut oil and season with salt and pepper. Arrange the slices in one layer on the prepared baking sheet, at least ¼ inch apart.
4. Bake for 25 minutes, or until browned and crisp.
5. Serve the soup with a side of zucchini chips.

Roasted Red Pepper Mini Pizzas

Easier than kneading dough, these mini pizzas come in nature's own "crust"—jumbo portobello mushroom caps! The combination of roasted red peppers and creamy mozzarella go perfectly with the meatiness of this mushroom . . . and if you want to skip the cheese, substitute some of that yummy cashew Alfredo sauce (page 219) for a dairy-free vegan option.

Serves: 1

PREP DAY TIME: 15 minutes

FEAST DAY TIME: 15 minutes

Ingredients

2 large portobello mushroom caps

1 red bell pepper

1 tablespoon chopped fresh herbs, such as basil and parsley, or another combination

2 teaspoons organic extra-virgin olive oil

2 tablespoons marinara sauce or other tomato sauce

2 ounces fresh buffalo mozzarella, raw cheese, or goat cheese

Handful of microgreens

Drizzle of balsamic vinegar

Prep Day

TIME: 15 minutes

Tools: Kitchen knife, cutting board, rimmed baking sheet, tongs, brown paper bag, storage containers, paper towels

1. Preheat the broiler.

2. Clean and thoroughly dry the portobello mushrooms. Remove the stems and place the caps in an airtight container and refrigerate for up to 3 days.

3. Clean and dry the bell pepper. Place it on a rimmed baking sheet under the broiler until the skin begins to blister, about 2 minutes. Turn the pepper and repeat until all sides are blistered.

4. Using tongs or an oven mitt, transfer the roasted pepper to a paper bag. Roll the paper bag to close and let it sit on a plate for at least 15 minutes, until the pepper has softened.

5. Slice the pepper open from stem to base and remove the seeds and stem. If the skin is charred (black), remove the skin at this point. Slice the pepper into thin strips and store in an airtight container in the refrigerator for up to 3 days.

6. Place the herbs in an airtight container and refrigerate for up to 3 days.

Feast Day

TIME: 15 minutes

Tools: Baking sheet, knife, medium bowl, measuring spoons

1. Preheat the oven to 400°F.
2. Brush the mushroom caps on both sides with 1 teaspoon of the olive oil, then place the caps upside down on a baking sheet.
3. Spread 1 tablespoon of the marinara sauce over each mushroom cap.
4. Top with the herbs, cheese (one or two mozzarella balls, slices, or shreds), and roasted pepper strips.
5. Bake until the cheese is melted and bubbling, about 20 minutes.
6. While the pizzas bake, toss the microgreens with the remaining 1 teaspoon olive oil in a small bowl. Plate and drizzle with balsamic vinegar. Serve alongside the mini pizzas.

Hearty Pancake Breakfast

Thank you to Michael Tremba from our Community for this hearty pancake recipe. You die-hard pancake lovers won't believe that this is good for you.

Serves: 2

PREP DAY TIME: 10 minutes

FEAST DAY TIME: 20 minutes

Ingredients

2 large eggs
1 teaspoon pure vanilla extract

1¼ cups full-fat unsweetened canned coconut milk or heavy cream

¼ cup coconut flour
½ teaspoon baking soda
¼ teaspoon sea salt
6 slices bacon (optional)

Salted grass-fed butter, for frying and
 serving
2 tablespoons pure maple syrup
1 large grapefruit, halved, for serving

Prep Day

TIME: 10 minutes

Tools: Measuring cups and spoons, whisk, medium mixing
bowls, storage container

1. Place the eggs in a medium bowl and beat thoroughly. Add the vanilla and coconut milk and whisk a few times to mix.
2. In a separate bowl, whisk together the coconut flour, baking soda, and salt.
3. Stir the wet ingredients into the dry mixture until thoroughly combined.
4. Use immediately, or pour the pancake batter into an airtight storage container and store in the refrigerator for up to 2 days.

Feast Day

TIME: 20 minutes

Tools: Knife, cutting board, measuring spoons, large skillet or
electric griddle, rimmed baking sheet, aluminum foil

1. If you'd like to serve bacon on the side, preheat the oven to 400°F. Line a rimmed baking sheet with aluminum foil, slightly crinkled.
2. Lay the bacon slices in an even layer, ½ inch apart, on the foil-lined sheet.
3. Bake until the bacon is crisp, 12 to 15 minutes. Transfer to a paper towel–lined plate to drain.
4. Grease a skillet or electric griddle with butter and set over high heat.
5. Ladle desired amounts of pancake batter onto the skillet and cook until golden brown, 2 to 3 minutes per side. Do not flip until the pancake is cooked well on the bottom, or it will break.

6. Transfer the pancakes to serving plates and spread with butter, if desired, and drizzle with up to 1 tablespoon pure maple syrup or raw honey. Serve with a side of bacon and a grapefruit half.

Farmer's Omelets with Balsamic-Roasted Sweet Potatoes

A fluffy omelet packed with fresh veggies and with a side of roasted sweet potatoes? Believe it or not, this meal is so ludicrously good it doesn't even need bacon. Yeah, I said it.

Serves: 4 to 6

PREP DAY TIME: 20 minutes

FEAST DAY TIME: 35 minutes

Ingredients

FARMER'S OMELETS

2 medium red bell peppers
2 medium green bell peppers
10 white button mushrooms
½ large onion

6 tablespoons grass-fed ghee
12 large eggs
Sea salt and freshly ground black
   pepper

BALSAMIC-ROASTED SWEET POTATOES

2 large sweet potatoes
2 tablespoons organic unrefined coconut oil
1 tablespoon balsamic vinegar

Prep Day

TIME: 20 minutes

Tools: Knife, cutting board, measuring spoons, peeler, colander, storage containers

FARMER'S OMELETS

1. Trim the bell peppers and chop them into very small pieces. Place them in an airtight storage container.
2. Wash and dry the mushrooms and slice them into thin slices. Add them to the container with the peppers.
3. Peel and dice the onion and add it to the container. Cover and refrigerate for up to 3 days.

BALSAMIC-ROASTED SWEET POTATOES

4. Peel the sweet potatoes and cut into 1-inch cubes.
5. Rinse the potato cubes under cold water, drain, and store in an airtight container in the refrigerator for up to 3 days.

Feast Day

TIME: 35 minutes

Tools: Small saucepan, measuring spoons, rimmed baking sheet, large skillet, omelet pan, medium bowl, whisk, rubber spatula

BALSAMIC-ROASTED SWEET POTATOES

1. Preheat the oven to 400°F.
2. Melt the coconut oil in a small saucepan over low heat.
3. Toss the potato cubes with the melted coconut oil and spread in an even layer on a rimmed baking sheet. Bake until the potatoes darken in color and start to get tender, about 15 minutes.

4. Sprinkle with balsamic vinegar, turn to coat, and bake until tender and starting to caramelize, 5 to 10 minutes more.

FARMER'S OMELETS

5. While the potatoes are roasting, make the omelets: Melt 2 tablespoons of the ghee in a large skillet over medium heat. Place the bell peppers, mushrooms, and onions in the skillet and turn to coat with the ghee. Sauté until tender, about 5 minutes. Set aside.

6. In a large bowl, whisk the eggs until frothy.

7. In an individual (8- to 9-inch) omelet pan, melt 1 tablespoon of the ghee and swirl to coat the pan. Pour in one-quarter of the egg mixture and swirl to cover the entire pan.

8. Sprinkle one-quarter of the vegetable mixture into the egg.

9. Using a rubber spatula, push back the edges and tilt the pan to allow the uncooked egg to fill in the open spot so that everything cooks evenly. Do this a few times until the egg is cooked through but not overdone.

10. Fold the omelet in half and transfer to a dinner plate.

11. Repeat the process with remaining egg and vegetable mixture, making four omelets.

12. Season with salt and pepper. Serve with the sweet potatoes alongside.

GREEN SMOOTHIES

Green Smoothie Guidelines

If you want to burn fat, drink your green smoothie. It's super-easy, versatile, delicious, and a nutritional powerhouse.

The nutritional equivalent of eating a salad and then some, green smoothies are packed with vitamins and minerals, filling fiber, and raw food enzymes to aid digestion. Green smoothies are detoxifying and, best of all, alkalizing, which will encourage your body to burn off fat and restore health.

Store-bought "green smoothies" from the bottle are almost always devoid of fiber and packed with preservatives. Those that you buy from smoothie stores are more often than not well-marketed sugar bonanzas. They're more like Slurpees. They give smoothies a bad name and people the wrong idea. . . .

THIS IS HOW *NOT* TO MAKE A GREEN SMOOTHIE (I ACTUALLY FOUND THIS ON THE WEB RECENTLY):

- 2 cups reduced-fat vanilla ice cream
- 1 cup orange juice
- ⅔ cup spinach
- ¼ cup brown sugar
- 3 tablespoons fat-free frozen whipped topping

Brown sugar? Ice cream? Whipped cream?

Are you kidding me? This is a calorie-soaked, insulin-spiking devil's milk shake. And it will make you fat.

That's why it's essential that you make your own green smoothie at home. All you need is a blender, a drawer in your refrigerator with a few random vegetables, and a few minutes of your time.

So How Do You Make a Green Smoothie?

This is your Gateway Green Smoothie—opening the doors for many creative smoothies to come. Simply, you combine the following four categories of ingredients as you see fit:

- **Green (use one or more):** kale, spinach, bok choy, collard greens, cabbage, Swiss chard, beet greens, sprouts, cucumber, broccoli, celery, avocado, basil, mint, rosemary, cilantro, parsley
- **Liquid (use one):** water, tea, almond milk, coconut milk, coconut water, etc. Also add ice if you like your smoothie chilled.
- **Fruits/veggies (use one or more):** strawberries, blueberries, apples, cherries, coconut, carrots, beets (root), lemon, ginger, pumpkin, tomatoes, bell peppers, avocado.
- **Add-ins:** protein powder (with no added sugar), flax meal (for omega-3s), cinnamon (regulates blood sugar), stevia, spirulina, chlorella, hulled hemp seeds, chia seeds soaked in water, olive oil, powdered vitamin C

At first, it struck me as strange to slurp down a gelatinous green sludge in the morning. But once it hits your lips a few times, you'll be a convert. After a few weeks, I outright craved green smoothies in the morning. Now my days don't feel complete until I have one of these in my belly.

Give it a shot. Green smoothies rock.

Minted Melon Smoothie

Serves: 1 or 2

TOTAL TIME: 10 minutes

Tools: Blender, measuring cup and spoon

Ingredients

5 honeydew melon cubes, about 2
   inches each

3 to 5 large kale leaves

10 to 12 large fresh mint leaves

½ teaspoon pure vanilla extract

¼ cup hulled hemp seeds (optional)

Filtered ice and water

Dash of pure dried stevia leaf, or to
   taste

DIRECTIONS

1. Place the honeydew, kale, mint, vanilla, hemp seeds (if using), and a handful of ice in a blender. Add just enough water to facilitate blending.

2. Blend on high until smooth, about 1 minute.

3. Add the stevia and blend for about 15 seconds. Taste and adjust the sweetener as needed.

4. Drink immediately for maximum health benefit, or store in a jar in the refrigerator for up to 24 hours. Shake well before drinking.

Cucumber-Basil Smoothie

Serves: 1 or 2

TOTAL TIME: 10 minutes

Tools: Blender, measuring cup

Ingredients

1 small cucumber, cut into chunks

8 to 10 fresh basil leaves

1 large handful spinach leaves

½ cup fresh or frozen pineapple chunks

Filtered water and ice

Dash of pure dried stevia leaf, or to taste

DIRECTIONS

1. Place the cucumber, basil, spinach, and pineapple into a blender.

2. Add a handful of ice and enough water to facilitate blending.

3. Blend until smooth.

4. Add stevia to taste and blend to mix.

5. Drink immediately for maximum health benefits, or store in a jar in the refrigerator for up to 24 hours. Shake well before drinking.

Creamy Cilantro-Lime Smoothie

Serves: 1 or 2

TOTAL TIME: 10 minutes

Tools: Blender, measuring cups, metal spoon, knife, cutting board

Ingredients

1 medium ripe avocado

Juice of 1 lime

1 small celery stalk

¼ cup packed fresh cilantro leaves
and stems

½ cup cubed fresh or frozen pineapple
(about 10 chunks)

¼ cup coconut water

Large handful of watercress or other
mixed greens, plus more as
needed

Dash of pure dried stevia leaf,
or to taste

1 to 2 cups ice

OPTIONAL ADD-INs:

Ground flaxseeds

Raw hulled hemp seeds

Sea buckthorn juice powder

Noni powder

Royal jelly powder

DIRECTIONS

1. Halve the avocado and remove the pit. Slide a metal spoon between the skin and flesh and remove the flesh in one piece. Place the flesh in a blender and add the lime juice.

2. Scrub, trim, and coarsely chop the celery and add to the blender.

3. Add the cilantro, pineapple, coconut water, watercress, stevia, and ice.

4. Add any optional add-ins you'd like and blend until smooth.

5. If space frees up in the blender as you process, add more greens and blend until smooth.

6. Drink immediately for maximum health benefits, or store in a jar in the refrigerator for up to 24 hours. Shake well before drinking.

Rosemary-Raspberry Smoothie

Serves: 1 or 2

TOTAL TIME: 10 minutes

Tools: Blender, measuring cups and spoons, metal spoon

Ingredients

2 tablespoons chopped fresh rosemary

1 cup frozen or fresh raspberries

1 tablespoon chia seeds, soaked in filtered water for 5 to 60 minutes

Juice of 1 lemon

1 tablespoon avocado oil or organic extra-virgin olive oil

1 to 2 cups ice

Huge handful of baby kale, plus more as needed

Filtered water

Dash of pure dried stevia leaf, or to taste

DIRECTIONS

1. In a blender, combine the rosemary, raspberries, soaked chia seeds, lemon juice, avocado oil, and ice. Fill the rest of the blender with baby kale and just enough water to facilitate blending.

2. Blend until smooth, plunging down or stopping to mix with a spoon when necessary.

3. Add the stevia and blend to mix.

4. If space frees up in the blender, add more greens and blend until smooth.

5. Drink immediately for maximum health benefits, or store in a jar in the refrigerator for up to 24 hours. Shake well before drinking.

Strawberry "Milk Shake"

Serves: 1 or 2

TOTAL TIME: 10 minutes

Tools: Blender, measuring cups and spoons, peeler, knife, cutting board

Ingredients

8 large fresh or frozen strawberries

1 large handful beet greens

¼ cup diced peeled red beet

3 tablespoons coconut cream (see Note, page 259) or full-fat unsweetened canned coconut milk

1 teaspoon pure vanilla extract

1 to 2 cups ice

Filtered water

Dash of pure stevia leaf, or to taste

Coconut Whipped Cream (page 268), for garnish (optional)

DIRECTIONS

1. In a blender, combine the strawberries, beet greens, beet, coconut cream, vanilla, and ice.

2. Add just enough water to facilitate blending and blend until smooth.

3. Add the stevia and blend to incorporate.

4. Pour into a large glass and top with coconut whipped cream, if you'd like.

5. If not using immediately, store in a jar in the refrigerator for up to 24 hours. Shake well before drinking.

Spiced Blueberry Smoothie

Serves: 1 or 2

TOTAL TIME: 10 minutes

Tools: Blender, peeler, measuring cup and spoon

Ingredients

1 (1-inch) piece fresh ginger
1 cup fresh or frozen blueberries
1 small banana
1 tablespoon chia seeds, soaked in
    filtered water for 5 to 60 minutes
Large handful of baby spinach

¼ teaspoon ground cinnamon
Handful of ice
Filtered water
Dash of pure dried stevia leaf, or to
    taste

DIRECTIONS

1. Peel the ginger and place it in a blender.

2. Add the blueberries, banana, soaked chia seeds with their soaking water, baby spinach, cinnamon, ice, and just enough water to facilitate blending.

3. Blend until smooth. Add the stevia and blend to incorporate.

4. Drink immediately, or store in a jar in the refrigerator for up to 24 hours. Shake well before drinking.

Virgin Bloody Mary Smoothie

Serves: 2

TOTAL TIME: 12 minutes

Tools: Blender, peeler, grater, measuring spoons

Ingredients

1 garlic clove
1 medium ripe tomato
Thin slice peeled fresh ginger
1 teaspoon grated fresh or prepared
    horseradish
Juice of ½ lemon
Dash of hot sauce
Dash of Worcestershire sauce

4 small celery stalks
½ medium cucumber, peeled, if
    desired, for a redder smoothie
½ small yellow summer squash
1 tablespoon chopped fresh parsley
Filtered water
Salt and freshly ground black pepper
Ice (optional)

DIRECTIONS

1. Peel the garlic and set aside.

2. In a blender, combine the garlic, tomato, ginger, horseradish, lemon juice, hot sauce, Worcestershire sauce, 2 stalks of celery, cucumber, summer squash, and parsley.

3. If needed, add water to facilitate blending. Blend until smooth.

4. Season with salt and pepper, and blend to combine. Pour over ice and garnish with a whole celery stalk straight down the inside of the glass.

5. Drink immediately, or store in an airtight jar in the refrigerator for up to 24 hours. Shake well before drinking.

Chocolate-Cherry Smoothie

Serves: 1 or 2

TOTAL TIME: 12 minutes

Tools: Blender, peeler, measuring cups and spoons

Ingredients

½ cup fresh or frozen dark sweet
   cherries, pitted
1 large handful dandelion or other
   greens
1 tablespoon raw cacao powder

½ cup unsweetened almond milk
½ teaspoon pure vanilla extract
Handful of ice
Dash of dried pure stevia leaf, or to
   taste

DIRECTIONS

1. Place all the ingredients except the stevia in a blender and blend until smooth.

2. Add the stevia and blend to incorporate.

3. Drink immediately, or store in a jar in the refrigerator for up to 24 hours. Shake well before drinking.

Peaches 'n' Cream Smoothie

Serves: 1

TOTAL TIME: 12 minutes
Tools: Blender, measuring cup and spoon

Ingredients

1 pitted peach, or 1½ cups frozen
   peach chunks
1 small carrot, scrubbed and trimmed
Huge handful of fresh kale or other
   greens
½ cup full-fat unsweetened canned
   coconut milk

½ teaspoon pure vanilla extract
Dash of ground cinnamon
Dash of ground nutmeg
Handful of ice
Dash of pure dried stevia leaf, or to
   taste

DIRECTIONS

1. Place all the ingredients except the stevia in a blender and blend until smooth. (Add water to facilitate blending if neccessary.)

2. Add the stevia and blend to incorporate.

3. Drink immediately, or store in a jar in the refrigerator for up to 24 hours. Shake well before drinking.

DRINKS

Ginger-Lemongrass Tea

Serves: 1

TOTAL TIME: 12 minutes

Tools: Peeler, teakettle, fine sieve, measuring cup

Ingredients

1 (1-inch) piece fresh ginger

2 cups filtered water

2 stalks lemongrass

1 slice organic lemon

DIRECTIONS

1. Peel the ginger.

2. Bring the water to a boil in a teakettle. Remove from the heat.

3. Add the lemongrass, lemon, and ginger to the kettle. Steep for 5 to 10 minutes.

4. Set a fine sieve over a large mug and pour the tea through the strainer. Enjoy warm.

Ginger-Mint Tea

Serves: 1

TOTAL TIME: 12 minutes

Tools: Peeler, teakettle, fine sieve, measuring cup

Ingredients

1 (1-inch) piece fresh ginger
2 cups filtered water
1 sprig fresh mint (3 to 5 leaves)

DIRECTIONS

1. Peel the ginger.

2. Boil the water in a teakettle. Remove from the heat.

3. Place the mint and ginger in the kettle and steep for 5 to 10 minutes.

4. Set a fine sieve over a large mug and pour the tea through the strainer. Enjoy warm or chilled over ice.

Cucumber-Strawberry Spa Water

Serves: 8

TOTAL TIME: 10 minutes

Tools: Knife, pitcher

Ingredients

1 gallon filtered water
1 organic cucumber, sliced
5 organic strawberries, sliced

DIRECTIONS

1. Fill a pitcher with the water. Add the cucumber and strawberry slices.
2. If drinking immediately, add ice and serve. Otherwise, cover the pitcher and place in the refrigerator until ready to serve.
3. Enjoy chilled.

Citrus Spa Water

Serves: 8

TOTAL TIME: 10 minutes
Tools: Knife, cutting board, pitcher

Ingredients

1 organic orange
1 organic lemon
1 organic grapefruit

1 gallon filtered water
Leaves from 2 sprigs fresh mint

DIRECTIONS

1. Without peeling them, slice the orange, lemon, and grapefruit.
2. Fill a pitcher with the water and add citrus slices and the mint leaves.
3. If drinking immediately, add ice and serve. Otherwise, place the pitcher in the refrigerator until ready to serve.
4. Enjoy chilled.

Pear, Apple, and Rosemary Spa Water

Serves: 8

TOTAL TIME: 10 minutes

Tools: Knife, cutting board, pitcher

Ingredients

1 medium Anjou pear

1 medium Granny Smith apple

3 fresh rosemary sprigs

1 gallon filtered water

DIRECTIONS

1. Slice the pear and apple into thin rounds or wedges.

2. Place the pear and apple slices and the rosemary sprigs in a pitcher and pour in the water, leaving room for ice.

3. If drinking immediately, add ice and serve. Otherwise, cover the pitcher and place it in the refrigerator until ready to serve. It will keep for up to 2 days.

4. Enjoy chilled.

Lemon Water

Serves: 1

TOTAL TIME: 12 minutes

Tools: Knife, cutting board, measuring cup

Ingredients

½ large lemon

2 cups filtered water

DIRECTIONS

1. Slice the lemon into wedges and remove the seeds.
2. Place the water in a large glass. Squeeze the juice from the lemon into the water and add ice.
3. Wring the peel of the lemon over the water to release the oils, and place the lemon peel into the water.
4. Enjoy chilled.

Lime in the Coconut

Serves: 1

TOTAL TIME: 10 minutes

Tools: Muddler, measuring spoon, knife

Ingredients

1 young coconut
3 tablespoons fresh mint leaves
Juice of ½ lime
Ice

DIRECTIONS

1. Remove the top of the coconut.
2. Place the mint leaves in the bottom of a glass.
3. Pour about ½ cup coconut water from the coconut into the glass, along with the lime juice.
4. Place a muddler in the glass and press down gently, giving a few light twists.
5. Pour the lime juice–mint mixture back into the coconut.

6. Wring the rind of the lime over the young coconut to release the oils in the peel, and place it in the coconut.

7. Add ice and stir.

8. Enjoy chilled.

Green Juice Detox

Serves: 1

TOTAL TIME: 10 minutes

Tools: Blender, measuring cups

Ingredients

¼ cup aloe vera juice

2 cups packed baby spinach

2 medium celery stalks

1 small cucumber

Juice of 1 lime

Pure dried stevia leaf

   (optional)

Filtered water

DIRECTIONS

1. In a blender, combine the aloe vera juice, spinach, celery, cucumber, lime juice, stevia to taste (if using) and just enough water to facilitate blending.

2. Blend until smooth.

3. Drink chilled or over ice.

French-Pressed Fatty Coffee

Since coffee is one of the most-sprayed crops on earth, start with organic coffee to avoid exposure to pesticides. French-pressing coffee is a quick and dirty way to get full extraction from your coffee grounds. Get the freshest beans you can—most of coffee's flavors dissipate two weeks after roasting. I roast fair-trade, organic, green coffee beans at home on the stove to ensure I always have the best coffee possible. Get your beans whole and grind them immediately before brewing for best flavor. Great beans are worth it—you'll see.

Ingredients

2 cups hot French-pressed coffee
1 teaspoon heavy cream or organic grass-fed butter
1 teaspoon MCT oil (medium-chain triglyceride oil—found in most health food stores)

DIRECTIONS

1. Pour the hot coffee into a large bowl or pitcher. Add the butter and MCT oil.
2. Using a handheld milk frother, skim along the mixture just below the surface. The frother will whip air into the coffee mixture and a nice froth will begin to form on the top. Fully immerse the frother a couple of times just to mix everything up underneath.
3. Pour into a nice big mug and enjoy.

Peanut Butter Chocolate "Cheesecake" with Hazelnut Crust

Store these in the freezer and indulge in chocolaty peanut butter goodness when you get a craving for something sweet. Fun fact: I ate three of these the night before my photo shoot on the front of this book.

Serves: 20

PREP TIME: 20 minutes

COOK TIME: 10 minutes

Ingredients

CRUST

2 cups hazelnuts, processed into meal

1 teaspoon pure vanilla extract

¼ cup organic unrefined coconut oil, melted

¼ teaspoon salt

3 tablespoons pure maple syrup

FILLING

3 cups raw cashews, soaked in filtered water to cover overnight (or at least 4 hours) and drained

Juice of 4 large lemons

1 cup organic unrefined coconut oil, melted

1 cup full-fat unsweetened canned coconut milk (just use the cream on top)

1 cup unsweetened cocoa powder

½ cup unsweetened smooth peanut butter

½ cup raw honey or maple syrup

¼ to ½ teaspoon pure dried stevia leaf

½ teaspoon sea salt

½ cup dark chocolate chips or chocolate shavings

Directions

CRUST

1. Preheat the oven to 350°F. Line two standard muffin pans with paper liners.
2. In a large bowl, combine all the crust ingredients and stir until they form a coarse meal.
3. Press the crust into the muffin liners, covering the bottom in a layer about ¼ inch thick.
4. Bake for 10 minutes, or until the crusts are set and golden.

FILLING

5. In a blender, combine all the filling ingredients except the chocolate chips and blend until smooth. Add more coconut milk or water, if needed, to facilitate blending.
6. Pour the filling over the crusts and sprinkle the tops with a few chocolate chips.
7. Freeze until the cheesecakes are firm, 30 minutes to 1 hour.
8. Peel the muffin liners from the individual cheesecakes and wrap each in aluminum foil.
9. Store in airtight storage containers in the freezer until ready to serve. Remove from the freezer, lay on a plate, and let the cheesecakes thaw for about 10 minutes before serving for cheesecake consistency, or serve frozen for ice cream consistency.

Choco-nut Cookies

A snap to make, these chewy coconut cookies with crisp brown edges make a monthly appearance in our house. These are best warm from the oven, and great from the freezer, too.

Serves: 12

PREP TIME: 10 minutes

COOK TIME: 15 minutes

Ingredients

2½ cups shredded unsweetened coconut

¼ cup coconut palm sugar, plus more to taste

¼ teaspoon sea salt

½ cup organic unrefined coconut oil, at room temperature

1 tablespoon pure vanilla extract

2 large eggs

½ cup dark chocolate chips

½ cup walnut pieces

Directions

1. Preheat the oven to 350°F. Line a baking sheet with parchment paper.
2. In a large bowl, mix together the shredded coconut, coconut palm sugar, and salt until well incorporated.
3. Stir in the coconut oil, vanilla, and eggs. Work everything together with your clean hands.
4. Stir in the chocolate chips and walnut pieces.
5. Scoop tablespoons of the batter onto the prepared baking sheet and flatten each ball into fat patties.
6. Bake until the edges are golden brown and the cookies are soft-set, 15 to 20 minutes.
7. Store in an airtight container in the freezer. Eat these cookies at room temperature or right out of the icebox.

Peanut Butter Chocolate Chunk Cookies

Serves: 12

PREP TIME: 10 minutes

COOK TIME: 15 minutes

Ingredients

1 duck egg or large chicken egg
½ teaspoon baking soda
½ cup coconut palm sugar
½ teaspoon pure vanilla extract
1 cup organic no-sugar-added chunky
    peanut butter

¼ teaspoon sea salt
½ cup organic dark chocolate
    chunks

Directions

1. Preheat the oven to 350°F. Line a baking sheet with parchment paper.
2. In the bowl of a stand mixer fitted with the paddle attachment, beat together the egg and baking soda until frothy.
3. Add the coconut palm sugar and vanilla and beat until mixed. Add the peanut butter and salt and beat on low until a thick dough forms.
4. Stir in the chocolate chunks by hand until evenly distributed.
5. Drop tablespoons of the dough at least 2 inches apart onto the prepared baking sheet.
6. Bake until lightly browned and soft in the middle, 10 to 12 minutes.
7. Let cool on the baking sheet before transferring to a wire rack to cool completely. Store the cooled cookies in an airtight container at room temperature for up to 1 week.

Pumpkin Pie

Serves: 8

PREP TIME: 20 minutes

COOK TIME: 1 hour

Ingredients

CRUST

½ cup coconut flour

½ cup almond flour

3 tablespoons flaxseed meal

½ teaspoon sea salt

3 tablespoons organic unrefined coconut oil, melted

½ cup full-fat unsweetened canned coconut milk

1 tablespoon pure maple syrup

FILLING

1 (15-ounce) can 100% pumpkin puree (or 1¾ cups fresh pumpkin puree)

6 dates, pits removed

¼ teaspoon pure dried stevia leaf

2 cups evaporated goat milk (or full-fat unsweetened coconut cream—see Note, page 259)

4 tablespoons (½ stick) unsalted butter, melted, or organic unrefined coconut oil

½ teaspoon ground cinnamon

¼ teaspoon ground ginger

¼ teaspoon ground cloves

¼ teaspoon ground nutmeg

¼ teaspoon sea salt

1 duck or large chicken egg

2 duck or large chicken egg yolks

Directions

CRUST

1. Preheat the oven to 425°F. Grease a pie pan with butter or coconut oil.

2. In a large bowl, whisk together the coconut flour, almond flour, flaxseed meal, and salt.

3. Add the melted coconut oil, coconut milk, and maple syrup. Mix until well combined.

4. Press the dough into the greased pie pan. Freeze the pie shell while you make the filling.

FILLING

5. In a blender, blend the pumpkin puree, dates, stevia, evaporated goat milk, butter, cinnamon, ginger, cloves, nutmeg, and salt until the dates are broken up and well-incorporated. Taste and add more spices, if desired.

6. Add the egg and egg yolks and blend until combined.

7. Pour the filling into the pie shell. Bake for 15 minutes.

8. Reduce the oven temperature to 350°F. Bake until a knife inserted near the center comes out clean, 40 to 50 minutes.

9. Remove from the oven and cool for 2 hours. Serve immediately, or cover and refrigerate until ready to serve.

Apple Cider Donuts

These gluten-free goodies are so tasty, you won't even want to dunk them in your coffee. . . .

Serves: 6

PREP TIME: 15 minutes

COOK TIME: 12 minutes

Ingredients

2 tablespoons organic unrefined coconut oil, melted, plus more for the pan

½ cup coconut flour

½ cup fine blanched almond flour

½ teaspoon baking powder

¼ cup arrowroot flour

½ teaspoon ground nutmeg

½ teaspoon ground cinnamon, plus more for sprinkling

¼ teaspoon sea salt

½ cup coconut palm sugar

2 tablespoons molasses

½ cup apple cider

1 large egg

2 tablespoons grass-fed butter or lard, melted

Shredded unsweetened coconut or coconut palm sugar, for rolling

Directions

1. Preheat the oven to 350°F. Grease a mini donut pan with coconut oil.

2. In a large bowl, mix together the coconut flour, almond flour, baking powder, arrowroot flour, nutmeg, cinnamon, salt, and coconut palm sugar.

3. In a separate bowl, combine the molasses, apple cider, egg, and melted coconut oil. Mix well with a wire whisk or handheld electric mixer.

4. Add the dry ingredients to the wet ingredients and stir well.

5. Spoon the dough into the greased donut pan, filling each space just slightly above the top. Bake until golden brown, 10 to 12 minutes.

6. Let cool in the pan or on a wire rack until cool enough to touch.

7. Remove the donuts from the pan. Dip each donut in the melted butter, roll in the shredded coconut, and sprinkle with cinnamon.

8. Serve warm.

Alyson's Coffee Cake

This coffee cake is the reason I wake up on Saturdays.

Serves: 1 or 2

PREP TIME: 10 minutes

COOK TIME: 30 minutes

Ingredients

COFFEE CAKE

1 tablespoon organic unrefined coconut oil, plus more for greasing

¼ cup coconut palm sugar

1 large egg

¼ cup unsweetened applesauce

¼ teaspoon pure vanilla extract

½ cup almond flour

¼ teaspoon baking soda

¼ teaspoon baking powder

Dash of sea salt

1 tablespoon coconut palm sugar

¼ teaspoon ground cinnamon

2 tablespoons chopped walnuts

Directions

COFFEE CAKE

1. Preheat the oven to 350°F. Grease a 6-ounce ramekin with coconut oil.
2. In a bowl using a handheld electric mixer, cream together the coconut oil and coconut palm sugar. Add the egg, applesauce, and vanilla and beat to combine.
3. In a separate bowl, whisk together the almond flour, baking soda, baking powder, and salt.
4. Add the dry mixture to the wet mixture and stir until well combined.
5. Pour the batter into the prepared ramekin.

TOPPING

6. In a small bowl, stir together the coconut palm sugar, cinnamon, and walnuts. Sprinkle the mixture over the top of the coffee cake batter.
7. Bake until a toothpick inserted into the center comes out clean, 15 to 20 minutes.
8. Serve warm, with a steaming cup of coffee.

Carrot Cake

Carrot cake topped with whipped coconut cream frosting and pecans. . . . Mmm, there's just nothing like it.

Serves: 12

PREP TIME: 20 minutes

COOK TIME: 35 minutes

Ingredients

CARROT CAKE

Grass-fed butter, for the pan

1½ cups almond flour

½ cup coconut flour

1 teaspoon baking soda

1 teaspoon baking powder

2 teaspoons ground cinnamon

½ cup coconut palm sugar

½ cup unsweetened applesauce

2 cups shredded carrots

3 large eggs, beaten

1 cup organic unrefined coconut oil, melted

1 cup unsweetened shredded coconut

1 cup canned unsweetened crushed pineapple with juice

1 cup chopped pecans, plus more for topping

FROSTING

½ cup grass-fed butter, softened

½ cup unsweetened coconut cream (see Note, page 259)

½ teaspoon pure vanilla extract

½ cup coconut palm sugar

1 teaspoon arrowroot flour

¾ cup unsweetened shredded coconut

Directions

CARROT CAKE

1. Preheat the oven to 350°F. Grease a 9-inch springform pan with butter.

2. In a large bowl, whisk together the almond flour, coconut flour, baking soda, baking powder, cinnamon, and coconut palm sugar.

3. In a separate large bowl, mix together the applesauce, carrots, eggs, melted coconut oil, shredded coconut, and pineapple.

4. Stir the dry mixture into the wet mixture. Mix well with a wooden spoon.

5. Stir in the pecans.

6. Pour the batter into the prepared pan and bake until a toothpick inserted into the center comes out clean, 30 to 35 minutes. Let cool completely in the pan.

FROSTING

7. In the bowl of a stand mixer fitted with the paddle attachment, beat together the butter and coconut cream.

8. Add the vanilla, coconut palm sugar, arrowroot flour, and shredded coconut. Beat until creamy.

9. After the cake has cooled, remove the ring of the springform pan and first frost the sides of the cake with the coconut frosting. Place a dollop of frosting in the middle of the top of the cake (if desired). Press pecan pieces all over the frosted sides and sprinkle over the dollop in the center.

10. Slice and serve. Store any leftover cake covered in the refrigerator for up to 5 days.

NOTES

To get the coconut cream from a can of full-fat coconut milk, place the unopened can upside down in the refrigerator overnight. When ready to use, carefully invert the can and open it. Scoop out the thick, white cream from the top, reserving the clear liquid in the can for another use.

Birthday Cake with Whipped Chocolate Topping

Do you have a Wild birthday to celebrate? Bust out the candles and slice up the fun! Serve this moist, delicious cake with a scoop of Mint Chip Ice Cream (page 261).

Serves: 8

PREP TIME: 15 minutes

BAKE AND COOL TIME: 45 minutes

Ingredients

CAKE

½ cup organic unrefined coconut oil, melted, plus more for the pan

1 cup almond flour

¼ cup coconut flour

1 teaspoon baking soda

½ teaspoon baking powder

½ teaspoon sea salt

¼ teaspoon pure dried stevia leaf

¼ cup unsweetened coconut cream

3 Medjool dates, pitted

½ cup unsweetened applesauce

1 teaspoon pure vanilla extract

4 large eggs

TOPPING

1 cup coconut cream (see Note, page 259) or organic dairy heavy cream

2 tablespoons raw cacao powder

2 tablespoons pure maple syrup

½ teaspoon pure vanilla extract

Directions

CAKE

1. Preheat the oven to 350°F. Grease an 8-inch springform pan with coconut oil.

2. In a large bowl, whisk together the almond flour, coconut flour, baking soda, baking powder, salt, and stevia. Set aside.

3. Place the coconut cream in a blender. Add the dates, applesauce, and melted coconut oil. Blend on high until the dates are well incorporated and there are no longer any chunks.

4. Add the vanilla and eggs and pulse until both are fully incorporated.

5. Pour the wet mixture into the dry mixture and stir until well combined.

6. Pour the batter into the prepared pan. Bake until a toothpick inserted into the center comes out clean, about 35 minutes.

7. Let cool in the pan before topping.

TOPPING

8. In the bowl of a stand mixer fitted with the whisk attachment, beat the coconut cream on medium speed until fluffy.

9. Add the cacao powder, maple syrup, and vanilla. Continue to whip until thick like whipped cream.

10. Spread the topping over the cake just before serving.

Mint Chip Ice Cream

Cool and creamy, with just enough dark chocolate to soothe the savage beast, mint chip ice cream is truly a dessert for all occasions, all ages, and every sweet craving. Garnish with a bit of fresh mint and a dash of cacao powder. Simple perfection.

Serves: 4 to 6

PREP TIME: 30 minutes

TOTAL TIME: 5 minutes

Ingredients

2 (16-ounce) cans full-fat unsweetened coconut milk (see Note, page 262)

4 Medjool dates, pitted

1 teaspoon peppermint extract

1 teaspoon pure vanilla extract

¼ teaspoon pure dried stevia leaf

½ teaspoon salt

Raw honey (optional)

½ cup Enjoy Life mini dark chocolate chips

½ cup macadamia nuts

Directions

1. Place the coconut milk and dates in a blender. Blend on high until the dates are well incorporated and the mixture is smooth.

2. Add the peppermint extract, vanilla, stevia, and salt. Blend to combine.

3. Taste the mixture and add a small amount of raw honey, if desired.

4. Add half of the chocolate chips and all of the macadamia nuts to the blender and blend until the chips and nuts are broken into small pieces.

5. Add the remaining chocolate chips and stir.

6. Transfer the mixture to your ice cream maker and churn according to the manufacturer's instructions.

7. Serve immediately or freeze in an airtight container for up to 10 days.

If possible, buy organic full-fat canned coconut milk (not "lite"). If guar gum is not included in the ingredients, dissolve ½ teaspoon unflavored powdered gelatin in 2 tablespoons boiling water and add it to the blender as you blend.

For other ice cream flavors: Omit the peppermint extract, chocolate chips, and macadamia nuts. Add whatever ingredients you love best in ice cream. Cherries, nuts, and chunks of chocolate, or cocoa powder and roasted coffee beans—the sky is the limit!

Old-Fashioned Apple Pie

This pie, like many of our treats, is a collaborative effort between generations of Bascoms, Bridges, and more to create an old-fashioned apple pie for the twenty-first century in all of its gluten-free glory.

Serves: 6

PREP TIME: 30 minutes

COOK TIME: 45 minutes

Ingredients

CRUST

1 cup grass-fed butter, cut into chunks and chilled, plus more for the pan

2 cups brown rice flour

½ cup quinoa flour

⅓ cup arrowroot flour

½ teaspoon sea salt

1 teaspoon xanthan gum

1 teaspoon ground cinnamon

2 tablespoons filtered water

1 tablespoon freshly squeezed lemon juice

1 tablespoon pure maple syrup

FILLING

5 large Granny Smith apples, peeled,
    cored, and sliced

Juice of ½ lemon

½ cup unsalted grass-fed butter

3 tablespoons almond flour

2 tablespoons filtered water

¾ cup coconut palm sugar

1 teaspoon ground cinnamon

½ teaspoon ground nutmeg

1 tablespoon pure vanilla extract

1 large egg, lightly beaten

Directions

CRUST

1. Preheat the oven to 350°F. Grease a pie pan with butter.

2. In a large bowl, whisk together the brown rice flour, quinoa flour, arrowroot flour, salt, xanthan gum, and cinnamon.

3. Cut the chilled butter into chunks. Using clean hands, work the butter into the flour mixture until a dough begins to form.

4. Sprinkle the water over the dough. Drizzle in the lemon juice and maple syrup and continue to mix with your fingers until incorporated.

5. Cut the dough in half. Press half of the dough into the bottom and up the sides of the prepared pie pan. Set the other half of the dough aside.

FILLING

6. Place the apple slices in a large bowl and toss with the lemon juice.

7. Melt the butter in a small saucepan over low heat.

8. Stir in the almond flour, water, coconut palm sugar, cinnamon, nutmeg, and vanilla. Bring to a simmer.

9. Reserve 3 tablespoons of the sauce mixture to pour over the crust right before baking. Mix the remaining portion of the sauce with the apple slices to completely coat. Pour the apple mixture into the prepared crust, mounding the filling slightly in the center.

10. Flatten out the second half of the dough on a lightly floured surface or waxed paper until it is about ¼ inch thick. Cut the crust into six strips. Make a lattice pattern

over the filling. (Alternatively, make one round top crust and cut slices in it for ventilation while baking.)

11. Brush the egg over the top crust.

12. If the reserved sauce has thickened, heat it on the stove top for a minute or two until liquid. Gently pour the sauce over the top crust.

13. Bake until the crust is golden brown and the filling is hot and bubbling, 40 to 50 minutes. Let cool on a wire rack until just warm. Enjoy with whipped cream or a cup of coffee. Alternatively, cover and refrigerate overnight or for up to 5 days.

Nan's Blueberry Salad

This is our take on a treat my grandmother Nan made for us every summer from the bountiful blueberry bushes in front of her house. No baking is required.

Serves: 24

PREP TIME: 30 minutes

COOK TIME: 5 minutes

CHILL TIME: 4 hours to overnight

Ingredients

GELATIN FILLING

3 cups boiling water

¼ cup unflavored organic powdered gelatin

½ cup coconut palm sugar

1 (16-ounce) can unsweetened crushed pineapple, well drained (see Note, page 265)

2 cups fresh blueberries

FROSTING

1 (8-ounce) package full-fat organic cream cheese, at room temperature

½ cup coconut palm sugar

1 cup full-fat organic sour cream

½ teaspoon pure vanilla extract

TOPPING

1 tablespoon organic unrefined
coconut oil, plus more for the pan

1 cup chopped raw pecans

½ teaspoon salt

2 tablespoons pure maple syrup

½ teaspoon pure vanilla extract

Directions

GELATIN FILLING

1. Place the boiling water in a large bowl. Dissolve the gelatin and coconut palm sugar into the boiling water, stirring to break up any chunks.

2. Stir in the pineapple and blueberries.

3. Pour the mixture into a 7 x 13-inch glass dish and chill for 4 hours or overnight, until firm to the touch.

FROSTING

4. In a large bowl using a handheld electric mixer, blend together the softened cream cheese, coconut palm sugar, sour cream, and vanilla.

5. Spread the cream cheese mixture over the chilled gelatin layer.

TOPPING

6. Preheat the oven to 350°F. Grease a baking sheet with coconut oil.

7. In a small bowl, mix together the pecans, coconut oil, salt, maple syrup, and vanilla.

8. Spread the pecans evenly over the prepared baking sheet and toast in the oven until they become aromatic, about 5 minutes. Watch them carefully, as the pecans can burn quickly.

9. Let the pecans cool in the pan for at least 5 minutes.

10. Sprinkle the pecan mixture over the cream cheese frosting. Cover and chill until ready to serve.

> **NOTES**
>
> Do not use fresh pineapple in this recipe. Enzymes found in fresh pineapple will break down the gelatin and your dessert will not set. The canning process neutralizes these enzymes.

Butter Pecan Ice Cream

Two minutes after Alyson invented this ice cream, it was gone. All of it. And since she doesn't do well with dairy, this masterpiece is made with coconut milk.

Serves: 6 to 8

PREP TIME: 15 minutes

TOTAL TIME: 1 hour

Ingredients

3 tablespoons grass-fed butter

3 cups pecans

3 (16-ounce) cans full-fat unsweetened canned coconut milk (see Note, page 262)

9 Medjool dates, pitted

½ teaspoon ground cinnamon

½ teaspoon sea salt, plus more as needed

1 tablespoon pure vanilla extract

¼ cup coconut palm sugar

Directions

1. In a skillet, melt the butter over medium-low heat. Add the pecans and toast, stirring frequently, until lightly browned and fragrant. Be careful not to burn the pecans. Remove from the heat and set aside.

2. In a blender, combine 2 cans of the coconut milk and the dates and blend well, until the dates are well incorporated and there are no longer any chunks.

3. Add the remaining can of coconut milk along with the cinnamon, salt, and vanilla. Blend well.

4. Add half of the toasted pecans and blend well.

5. Taste and add the coconut palm sugar and more salt to taste.

6. Add the remaining toasted pecans and pulse a couple of times to break them up into chunks.

7. Transfer the mixture to an ice cream maker and churn according to the manufacturer's instructions.

8. Enjoy cold.

Pumpkin Bread

This pumpkin bread has all the wonderful earthy cinnamon-spice flavors of fall, with just enough sweetness to make you feel like you're indulging in dessert.

Serves: 8

PREP TIME: 15 minutes

COOK TIME: 45 minutes

Ingredients

PUMPKIN BREAD

¼ cup organic unrefined coconut oil, melted, plus more for the pan

1½ cups almond flour

¼ cup coconut flour

¼ flaxseed meal

½ teaspoon sea salt

1 teaspoon baking soda

2 tablespoons ground cinnamon

2 teaspoons ground nutmeg

1 teaspoon ground cloves

½ teaspoon ground ginger

¾ teaspoon pure dried stevia leaf

1 cup organic pumpkin puree

1 teaspoon pure vanilla extract

3 Medjool dates, pitted

6 large eggs

1 teaspoon freshly squeezed lemon juice

TOPPING

2 tablespoons grass-fed salted butter, plus more for serving

1 tablespoon coconut palm sugar

½ teaspoon ground cinnamon

Directions

PUMPKIN BREAD

1. Preheat the oven to 350°F. Grease a loaf pan with coconut oil.

2. In a large bowl, whisk together the almond flour, coconut flour, flaxseed meal, salt, baking soda, cinnamon, nutmeg, cloves, ginger, and stevia. Set aside.

3. In a blender, combine the pumpkin puree, vanilla, dates, 3 of the eggs, the melted

coconut oil, and the lemon juice. Blend until the dates are broken up and well incorporated.

4. Add the remaining 3 eggs and blend until smooth.

5. Add the pumpkin mixture to the flour mixture and stir until well combined.

6. Pour the batter into the prepared loaf pan and bake until a toothpick inserted into the center comes out clean, 35 to 45 minutes.

TOPPING

7. While the pumpkin bread is in the oven, melt the butter in a small saucepan over low heat. Stir in the coconut palm sugar and cinnamon. Spoon the mixture over the pumpkin bread during the last 15 minutes in the oven.

8. Slice and serve with grass-fed salted butter for spreading.

Coconut Whipped Cream

Coconut whipped cream looks like that tub of white stuff you get in the grocer's freezer, but the two actually taste nothing alike. Coconut whipped cream is made from one ingredient: coconut milk. That tub of white stuff is made up of . . . a whole bunch of stuff that I'd rather not mention. So we put this white stuff, or pure organic dairy whipped cream from pasture-grazed cows, on our coffee drinks instead.

Serves: 4

PREP TIME: Overnight, plus 5 minutes

Ingredients

1 (15-ounce) can full-fat unsweetened coconut milk
1 teaspoon pure vanilla extract (optional)

Directions

1. Flip the can of coconut milk upside down and leave it in the refrigerator overnight. Carefully invert the can and open it. The cream will all be on the top. Scoop it into the bowl of a stand mixer fitted with the whisk attachment. Add the vanilla. Whisk until light and fluffy.

2. Store any unused coconut whipped cream in an airtight container in the refrigerator for up to 5 days.

How to Soak and Dehydrate Nuts and Seeds

Almonds

Soak 2 cups of raw organic almonds in warm filtered water with 1½ teaspoons sea salt for 7 to 24 hours. Drain and rinse. Dehydrate at 105°F to 150°F until dry and crisp, 7 to 24 hours. Store in an airtight container in the freezer.

Cashews

Soak 2 cups of cashews in warm filtered water with 1½ teaspoons sea salt for 2 to 6 hours. Drain and rinse. Dehydrate at 105°F to 150°F until dry and crisp, 12 to 24 hours. Store in an airtight container in the freezer.

Hazelnuts

Soak 2 cups of raw hazelnuts in warm filtered water with 1½ teaspoons sea salt for 7 to 12 hours. Drain and rinse. Dehydrate at 105°F to 150°F until dry and crisp, 12 to 24 hours. Store in an airtight container in the freezer.

Peanuts

Soak 2 cups of raw organic peanuts in warm filtered water with 1½ teaspoons sea salt for 7 to 24 hours. Drain and rinse. Dehydrate at 105°F to 150°F until dry and crisp, 12 to 24 hours. Store in an airtight container in the freezer.

Pecans

Soak 2 cups of raw pecans in warm filtered water with 1 teaspoon sea salt for 7 to 24 hours. Drain and rinse. Dehydrate at 105°F to 150°F until dry and crisp, 12 to 24 hours. Store in an airtight container in the freezer.

Pine Nuts

Soak 2 cups of raw pine nuts in warm filtered water with 1½ teaspoons sea salt for 6 to 8 hours. Drain and rinse. Dehydrate at 105°F to 150°F until dry and crisp, 12 to 24 hours. Store in an airtight container in the freezer.

Pumpkin Seeds

Soak 2 cups of raw pumpkin seeds in warm filtered water with 1½ teaspoons sea salt for 6 to 8 hours. Drain and rinse. Dehydrate at 105°F to 150°F until dry and crisp, 12 to 24 hours. Store in an airtight container in the freezer.

Sunflower Seeds

Soak 2 cups of raw sunflower seeds in warm filtered water with 1 teaspoon sea salt for 6 to 8 hours. Drain and rinse. Dehydrate at 105°F to 150°F until dry and crisp, 12 to 24 hours. Store in an airtight container in the freezer.

Walnuts

Soak 2 cups of raw walnuts in warm filtered water with 1 teaspoon sea salt for 7 to 24 hours. Drain and rinse. Dehydrate at 105°F to 150°F until dry and crisp, 12 to 24 hours. Store in an airtight container in the freezer.

How to Soak Beans and Legumes

Soaking and boiling your own beans and legumes is a far healthier way to eat them than to buy them in a can at the grocery store. You cut down on additives and sodium, ensure quality, and keep it cheap (bonus!). Prepare a large batch of beans and freeze a portion for later. Remember, legumes and other carbs can be inflammatory and worsen autoimmune conditions, so eat them with intention.

Serves: 8

PREP/SOAK TIME: 12 to 24 hours

COOK TIME: 4 hours

Ingredients

2 cups dried beans or legumes
2 tablespoons apple cider vinegar, freshly squeezed lemon juice, or grass-fed whey
Filtered water

Directions

1. Pour the beans into a strainer and rinse thoroughly under cold water, removing any stones or other debris. Pour the beans into a large heavy pot, add the vinegar, and cover with filtered water.

2. Cover the pot and let soak at room temperature for 12 to 24 hours.

3. Drain and thoroughly rinse the beans.

4. Fill the pot with fresh filtered water to at least three-quarters full (enough to cover the beans) and bring to a boil over medium-high heat. Return the beans to the pot and reduce the heat to maintain a simmer.

5. Simmer until the beans are soft, about 1 to 4 hours. Check the tenderness of the bean by removing one with a spoon and pressing it with the side of a butter knife. The bean is done when it mashes easily.

How to Make Sprouted Flours

If you're going to eat grains—which you might, if you're working out or require more carbohydrates, as some women do—it's far healthier to eat sprouted grains. So go ahead, sprout your own! It's not that difficult, and kind of fun. Make it a culinary science experiment for your kids (or yourself)!

Serves: 6 to 10

PREP TIME: About 3 days soaking
COOK TIME: 12 to 18 hours in dehydrator

Ingredients

2 cups organic grain (amaranth, buckwheat, millet, or quinoa)
Warm filtered water
1 tablespoon apple cider vinegar, freshly squeezed lemon juice, grass-fed whey, grass-fed buttermilk, or kefir

Directions

1. Rinse the grains well.

2. Place the grain in a glass bowl or jar and pour over just enough warm filtered water to cover by 2 inches. Add vinegar.

3. Tightly cover the bowl and let soak at room temperature for 18 to 24 hours. If it's chilly in the house, place the container in the oven with the pilot light on or next to a warm slow cooker to keep it warm.

4. Drain and rinse the grains.

5. Return the grains to the bowl with warm filtered water to cover, and continue rinsing and stirring twice a day for 2 to 3 days, until a tiny sprout starts to emerge from the end of the grains.

6. Drain the grains and transfer to dehydrator trays. Dehydrate until firm and dry, 12 to 18 hours.

7. Process the grains in a grain grinder to a fine flour and store in an airtight container in the freezer until ready to use.

Grandma's Oatmeal

Believe it or not, real oatmeal doesn't come in little packets coated in powdery sugar substances to be microwaved until thick and gooey. No, real oatmeal is hearty and chewy with a deep earthy flavor that pairs perfectly with a bit of butter and cinnamon—or even with savory meats and vegetables. It sticks to your ribs and warms your soul.

Serves: 2

PREP TIME: 7 to 24 hours soaking

COOK TIME: 5 minutes

Ingredients

1 cup gluten-free rolled oats (not
   quick-cooking oats)
2 cups warm filtered water, plus 1 cup
   boiling filtered water
2 tablespoons apple cider vinegar or
   freshly squeezed lemon juice

1 teaspoon sea salt
Grass-fed butter
Raw local honey
Ground cinnamon (optional)

Directions

1. In a small bowl, stir together the oats, 2 cups warm filtered water, the vinegar, and ½ teaspoon of the salt.
2. Cover and let soak at room temperature for 7 to 24 hours.
3. In a medium saucepan, dissolve the remaining ½ teaspoon salt in boiling filtered water.
4. Add the soaked oats and simmer for about 5 minutes.
5. Serve warm, with grass-fed butter and honey—and maybe a dash of cinnamon.

Brown Rice

Brown rice is a good carb choice to add after a particularly tough workout or to keep up your energy on high-output days. Always choose an organic brown rice and prepare it according to these directions for optimal nutritional value and minimal impact on digestion.

Serves: 2

PREP TIME: 8 to 24 hours soaking
COOK TIME: 30 to 40 minutes

Ingredients

1 cup dry organic whole-grain brown rice

Hot filtered water

1 tablespoon apple cider vinegar, freshly squeezed lemon juice, grass-fed whey, grass-fed buttermilk, or kefir

Grass-fed butter

Sea salt

Directions

1. Pour the rice into a 1-quart mason jar and add enough hot filtered water to cover.

2. Add the vinegar and tightly close the jar lid.

3. Let soak at room temperature for 8 to 24 hours. If it's chilly in the house, place the jar in the oven with the pilot light on or next to a warm slow cooker to keep it warm.

4. Drain the rice in a fine-mesh sieve set over a bowl; reserve the soaking liquid for the next time you make brown rice (it will keep in an airtight container in the refrigerator for 6 months or longer). Gently rinse the rice.

5. Bring 1¾ cups filtered water to a boil in a medium saucepan.

6. Add the rice, reduce the heat to maintain a simmer, and cook until the water has been absorbed and the rice is tender, 30 to 40 minutes.

7. Add a chunk of butter and salt to taste.

Simple Sauerkraut

Fermented foods are excellent for restoring gut health . . . and sauerkraut might just be the simplest to make. Eat it alone or pair it with a nice piece of roast beef or fresh organic sausage.

Serves: 8

PREP TIME: 20 minutes

TOTAL TIME: 3 to 10 days

Ingredients

1 organic head green cabbage (2 to 3 pounds)

1 to 2 tablespoons sea salt

1 large organic carrot, shredded (optional)

1 teaspoon caraway seeds (optional)

Directions

1. Thoroughly clean a wide-mouth mason jar, chopping knife, cutting board, large bowl, and your hands.

2. Rinse the cabbage and carefully peel off the two outer layers. Lay these two cabbage leaves on top of your jar like a "lid." Use a knife or clean scissors to cut the cabbage leaves about an inch wider than the jar all around. You'll use these cabbage leaf rounds to hold the sauerkraut below the brining liquid in a later step.

3. Quarter the head of cabbage and chop out the thick core from each quarter. Slice each cabbage quarter lengthwise into thin ribbons.

4. Put each handful of cabbage you cut into a large bowl and sprinkle it with salt. Add salt as you go to help keep the cabbage crisp. In the end, you want to have added between 1 and 2 tablespoons of salt.

5. Use your hands to massage the cabbage with the salt until it becomes watery and limp, 5 to 10 minutes.

6. Add the shredded carrot and caraway seeds to the cabbage and mix with your hands to combine.

7. Take handfuls of the cabbage mixture and press them into the bottom of the mason jar, packing them tight with each handful so the liquid (created by salting and massaging in step 5) rises to the top over the cabbage.

8. Take the cabbage rounds you cut in step 2 and press them into the jar so they hold the cabbage under the liquid.

9. Wipe the jar mouth clean and cover it with a cloth, cheesecloth, or paper towel and secure in place with a rubber band or twine. This allows air into the jar but prevents insects from getting in.

10. Over the next 24 hours, press down on the cabbage leaves to keep the cabbage packed under the liquid as it ferments and rises. If needed, you can add more brining liquid by mixing filtered water with a bit of salt (1 teaspoon salt dissolved in 1 cup filtered water).

11. Allow the sauerkraut to ferment at room temperature out of direct sunlight for 3 to 10 days, checking daily to make sure the cabbage is not floating above the liquid. Taste every few days until the desired taste is achieved.

12. The sauerkraut will keep in the sealed jar in the refrigerator for at least 2 months.

Roasted Bone Marrow

Bone marrow is an often-discarded part of the animal that deserves to be eaten! It's high in nutritive properties, helps rebuild tissue and cells, and works to remineralize teeth and bones.

Serves: 4

PREP TIME: 5 minutes

COOK TIME: 15 minutes

Ingredients

4 grass-fed beef marrow bones
Fleur de sel or sea salt
Chopped fresh flat-leaf parsley

Directions

1. Preheat the oven to 450°F. Line a rimmed baking sheet with aluminum foil.
2. Stand the marrow bones upright on the baking sheet and roast for 15 minutes.
3. Scoop the marrow onto four small serving plates and sprinkle with fleur de sel and chopped parsley.

Hard-Boiled Eggs

Hard-boiled eggs are an excellent protein snack, so I keep them in the fridge all the time. Add them to salads, eat them plain, or whip up some delicious deviled eggs!

Serves: 4

PREP TIME: 2 minutes

COOK TIME: 10 minutes

Ingredients

8 large free-range eggs

Directions

1. Fill a 2-quart pot three-quarters full of water and bring to a boil. Fill a bowl with ice and water and set aside.
2. Use a slotted spoon to gently place the eggs into the boiling water.
3. Let boil for 10 minutes exactly.
4. Using the slotted spoon, remove the eggs from the boiling water and plunge directly into the bowl of ice water. Chill for a few minutes, until cool to the touch.
5. Peel immediately.
6. Store in an airtight container in the refrigerator for up to 5 days.

Hot-as-the-Devil Eggs

Deviled eggs with pickled jalapeño and hot sauce, topped with crumbled bacon and scallions, are far more fiery than your typical devil.

Serves: 6

PREP TIME: 8 minutes

COOK TIME: 10 minutes

Ingredients

1 recipe Hard-Boiled Eggs (page 279)

2 slices bacon

2 teaspoons prepared yellow mustard

½ teaspoon freshly squeezed lemon juice

½ teaspoon paprika, plus more for sprinkling

5 pickled jalapeño slices, finely diced

1 tablespoon pickled jalapeño juice, or to taste

Dash of hot sauce, or to taste

½ teaspoon garlic powder

Sea salt and freshly ground black pepper

1 tablespoon organic extra-virgin olive oil, plus more as needed

3 scallions, chopped

Directions

1. Cut the boiled eggs in half lengthwise, removing the egg yolks as you go and placing them in a medium bowl.

2. Arrange the egg whites on a serving plate.

3. In a skillet, cook the bacon over medium heat, flipping halfway through cooking to sear the bacon evenly, about 5 minutes. Set the bacon aside and pour the rendered bacon fat from the skillet into the bowl with the egg yolks. Mash with a fork and mix to combine.

4. Add the mustard, lemon juice, paprika, jalapeños, jalapeño juice, hot sauce, and garlic powder. Mix thoroughly.

5. Season with salt and pepper.

6. Add the olive oil to the egg yolk mixture and mash with a fork until everything is well incorporated. Add more olive oil to reach the desired consistency.

7. Taste and add more salt, hot sauce, or jalapeño juice as desired.

8. Scoop the egg yolk mixture into the egg white halves, evenly distributing the yolk mixture. Sprinkle with the scallions. Crumble the bacon over the top and sprinkle with paprika.

9. Serve immediately, or cover and store in the fridge for up to 3 days.

PART VI

The Wild Diet Challenge

> **The magic is inside you. There ain't no crystal ball.**
>
> —*Dolly Parton*

YOUR FIRST TASK

Pick a day to start and go 100 percent. Once you start, stick to it for at least forty days. Your rapid progress will motivate you. With a strong commitment to the Wild lifestyle, your results will be dramatic. Before you begin, take "before" pictures from the front and side. These images will be very useful in the weeks ahead as you measure your progress.

Remember that although the Wild Diet Challenge gives you the tools to get results as quickly as possible, this is not meant to be a crash diet. It's a way of eating for the rest of your life. You don't need to "watch what you eat" if you simply refuse to settle for low-quality food. Stick to the good stuff and your body will reward you with boundless energy and a lean, sculpted frame. And once you try this food, there's no looking back.

Sure, you'll avoid some food that you are accustomed to eating, but the Wild Diet also gives you implicit permission to indulge in foods you probably once thought were fattening. Bacon is back on the menu. So push the stale bread aside, lick your chops, and sink your teeth into that juicy, grass-fed porterhouse knowing that it is good for you and will help you burn fat.

And when you find something in front of you that doesn't align with your goals, don't say to yourself, "I *can't* eat that." Say instead, "I *don't* eat that." See how much more empowering that feels? Let your good decisions motivate you.

It might take a few weeks for your body to adjust after years of eating low-quality food. If you've been running on carbs, it will take a few days or even a week for your body to produce the fat-burning enzymes needed to kick-start fat metabolism.

Most people who go Wild find that their enjoyment of food *increases* over time. Your tastes will change as your palate adapts to a new normal. The less sugar you eat, the sweeter all food tastes. As your palate becomes more sensitive and your body more finely attuned to the effects of your meals, you will find yourself craving foods you never thought you liked—like kale chips or cauliflower rice. For what might be the first time in your life, you'll be able to taste all the nuances in the vast spectrum of flavors in real food.

HOW TO TRACK YOUR PROGRESS

Don't trust your scale. Trust your clothes. Once a week, take your tightest pair of pants and put them on first thing in the morning. If they feel loose, it's working. If they don't, scale back on starches, dairy, nuts, fruit, sweets, and/or alcohol in favor of lean protein and non-starchy vegetables.

Assuming you make progress on the Wild Diet, you will lose fat and gain muscle. Since muscle weighs more than fat, it's possible that you'll see a temporary uptick in the numbers on the scale. If you're eating plenty of protein and building muscle, then your muscle will increase your metabolism and help you burn more fat in the weeks ahead. You may notice your waist size shrinks very quickly—6 pounds of fat take up almost a gallon of volume on your frame!

Many men and some women lose upward of 5 pounds in the first week. However, 1 pound a week of fat loss is a much more realistic goal for most. But again, how you look and feel is far more important than anything the scale will tell you. As you get the hang of living Wild, your body will begin to look and feel so amazing that you won't be able to imagine how you used to eat any other way.

Losing 20 pounds in 40 days is quite possible, but not if you don't have 20 pounds to lose. You may lose less or more, but keep it up, and you'll see that the benefits to your lifestyle go well beyond just losing pounds. Keep in mind that you can gain or lose weight for many reasons that have precious little to do with whether your eating is in balance. Be good to your body and it'll be good to you.

Before we begin, I want to get something off my chest. I despise rules, and I've spent the majority of my life ignoring them. So before I give you a bit of dogmatism to help you lose fat as quickly as possible in the next forty days, let me say this:

Don't do what the rules tell you. Do what works.

Remember: This is about you—your needs, your tastes, your preferences, and your pleasures. Experiment and have fun!

Step 1: Toss the Low-Quality Food

Purge your pantry and fridge of all foods not found on the Wild Diet Staples or Secondary food lists. Don't leave any tempting foods in the house—they'll only add to cravings and wear down on your precious willpower. Grab the bread, rice, pasta, cookies, crackers, pudding, ice cream, waffles, juice, sodas, cereals, sugar, flour, artificial sweeteners, canned soups, noodles . . . every single refined, packaged junk food you can find. Bag it all up and give it away. It might take a few weeks for your body to adapt to burning fat instead of sugar. You may crave junk foods temporarily. If there's no junk in your house to tempt you, you'll find it much easier to stay on task.

Step 2: Shop for Great Food

Go shopping and stock up on Wild Diet Staple foods (see page 132). You don't need to buy any special or branded foods to follow the Wild Diet—in fact, it's better if you don't. Nearly everything you need can probably be found where you shop for food already. Here's a quick tip: Stick to the perimeter of the grocery store, because the center aisles are typically filled with processed junk. Remember: Real food is perishable, so shop for fresh foods at least once a week or buy flash-frozen produce in bulk.

Buy the highest-quality foods you can find and afford. When you buy packaged food, look for the following labels:

☐ Organic	☐ Cold pressed
☐ Local	☐ Raw
☐ Grass fed	☐ Unpasteurized
☐ Pasture raised	☐ Non-GMO verified
☐ Wild caught	☐ BPA-free
☐ Extra virgin	

Do yourself a favor and grab some real dark chocolate (more than 70% cocoa content) to keep on hand for "chocolate emergencies." My favorite chocolate is single origin, stone ground, and raw. Just promise me you won't polish off the bar in one sitting. Get the good stuff and savor it one square at a time as a treat.

Step 3: Feast

Eat liberally from the Wild Diet Staples list. Limit Wild Diet Secondary Foods to two servings a day.

- Eat at least two to three times as much green and colorful veggies as meats, fats, and oils. Eat all the green and non-starchy vegetables you can. Heaping veggies will boost your nutrient intake and get your digestive system in order.
- Don't let yourself go hungry—always keep Wild Diet food on hand. Fill yourself up in this priority:
  - Green and non-starchy vegetables
  - Protein
  - Fat
  - Everything else
- Enjoy all of the eggs, seafood, poultry, and red meat as you want, but there's no need to overdo it—your body will tell you when you've had enough. Protein will boost your metabolism and replace some of the calories you previously sourced from carbohydrates.
- Make 30 minutes the minimum for each meal to avoid spikes in blood sugar.
- Eat your greens and veggies first—a salad, a vegetable, or a piece of lower-

sugar fruit—to start every meal. Fruits and vegetables are low in calorie density and high in bulk and water. Those who consume soup or salad before a meal eat an average of 30 percent fewer calories than those who go straight to the entrée.

- Drink as much unsweetened coffee, tea, and seltzer as you like, but avoid caffeine after noon.
- Drink at least eight 8-ounce glasses of clean water a day. Add trace minerals to improve taste and nutrition.

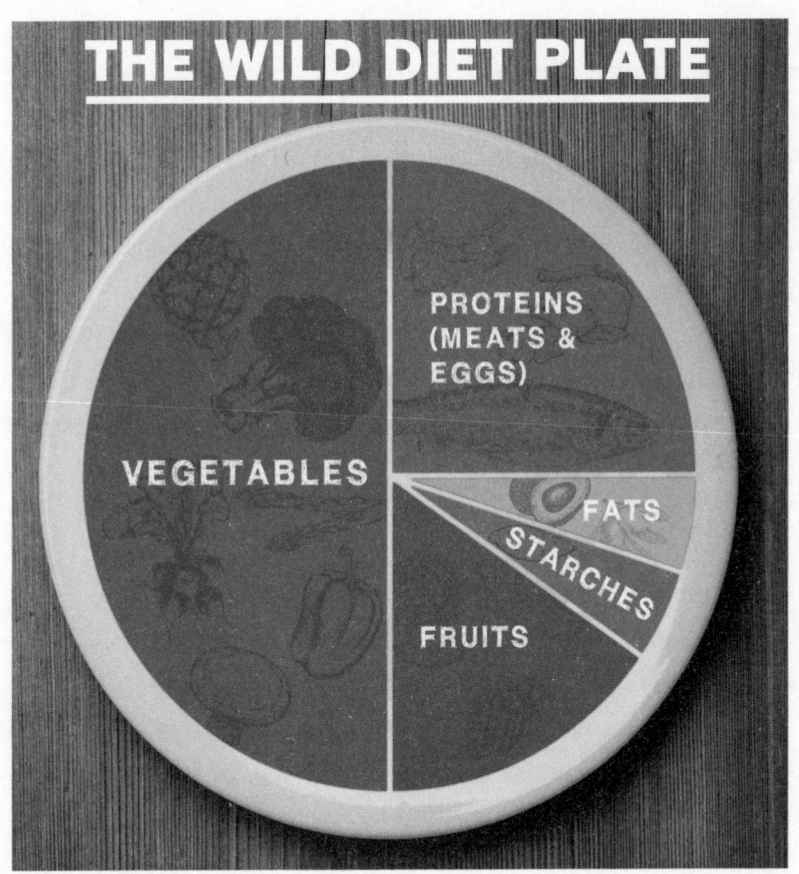

1. Most of your plate should be covered with fresh leafy vegetables such as kale, spinach, arugula, collards, or other greens. Raw is best, but steamed or lightly cooked veggies count, too. Fresh organic veggies are preferable, but flash-frozen works well in a pinch. When eating out, ask for extra greens or other colorful veggies instead of a starch.

2. Proteins such as grass-fed beef, chicken, turkey, pork, eggs, or seafood should make up about a quarter of your plate. A generous serving of protein is the size of the palm of your hand. If you're still hungry, feel free to eat protein and green veggies until you're satisfied.

3. Eat whole fruit as a snack or use to sweeten other foods. Limit to one to two servings of whole fruit a day to maximize fat loss.

4. Add energy to your meals with nutrient-dense fat. Fat should come from grass-fed meat, butter, coconut oil, avocado oil, olive oil, or unsalted nuts such as almonds, pecans, macadamias, or walnuts. Avoid processed oils.

5. If you are particularly active, have a high metabolism, or are less tolerant of fat or protein, consider a side of starch such as boiled sweet potato or whole-grain rice with lunch or dinner. If you find that carbs slow your fat loss, skip the starch and eat extra protein, veggies, or fat instead.

Step 4: Avoid These Foods

- No white carbohydrates, including: bread, rice, cereal, potatoes, pasta, and fried food with breading.

    Why? White carbohydrates are typically processed and high glycemic, which raises insulin levels, increases hunger, and leads to fat storing.

- No processed foods or "carbage."

    Why? Processed foods are packed with chemicals and do not ultimately satiate your hunger because they contain a high amount of calories with very little nutrition.

- No wheat, corn, or other modern grains.

  Why? Domesticated, GMO, and processed grains spike blood sugar, increase insulin levels, and cause fat storage. Heirloom, heritage, and ancient varieties are always better.

- No liquid calories: fruit juice, sports drinks, soda, or fat-free milk.

  Why? Pure high-glycemic carbs, such as fruit juice and sports drinks, cause a rapid rise in blood sugar resulting in high insulin levels that stop fat burning in its tracks.

TIPS TO MAXIMIZE FAT LOSS AND HEALTH

- Focus on native plant and animal foods, local sources, and traditional food preparation, preservation, and cooking techniques.
- Use small utensils or chopsticks to eat your meals. Taking many small bites is more satisfying and less likely to result in overeating than chomping on larger bites with giant silverware.
- Eat from small plates and bowls, preferably blue or white plates. Avoid the color red in your eating environment—the color red is often used by fast food and chain restaurants to increase arousal and get you to eat more.
- Eat animals nose to tail (or eat complete foods like oysters and eggs) to ensure that you get a full spectrum of nutrients.
- Cook meats, veggies, and starches low and slow to minimize impact on blood sugar. Add vinegar, citrus, and fermented foods to meals to aid in digestion and reduce the glycemic load of your meals.
- Be vigilant: It's your responsibility to judge the quality of food before you choose to consume it. You have 100 percent free agency over what you eat. Before you eat, ask yourself, "Would this look like fresh food to my ancestors?"

Step 5: Exercise

1. Break a sweat every day doing something you love. Walk often, preferably outdoors in the sun.

2. For faster results, complete one Wild Workout and at least one strength training workout per week. Schedule workouts in your calendar and stick to them as if you've booked a flight.

WHAT TO LOOK FORWARD TO

The Bad

- A heightened awareness of what food does to your body and how it makes you feel. Low-quality foods that you used to eat all the time might make you feel ill, and rightly so.
- Increased elimination, mostly resulting from an increase in intake of natural fiber in plant foods. Sure, this may mean more frequent trips to the restroom at first, but this is good—your body is eliminating toxins that have built up in your system from years of abuse.
- Temporary sugar cravings, lack of energy, and brain fog as your body adjusts to burning fat instead of relying on carbohydrates for energy. Your carb hangover might last about a week, but the cravings should subside as your body heals and you transform from a sugar burner to a fat burner.

GARBAGE IN, GARBAGE OUT

You'll notice that your digestive machinery becomes much more "productive" than it might have been on your previous diet. This is great, actually—fiber from fresh greens, fruit, nuts, and seeds detoxifies and cleanses the digestive tract on its way out.

The state of what comes out is a good indicator of how well you're doing with your diet and digestive health. Have you ever seen the little pile of poo left by a bear in the wilderness? Yours should look kind of like that—full of seeds, shells, and fiber. That means you're eating your fruits and veggies like you're supposed to.

The Good

As long as you eat real, fresh, clean foods and move your body every day, you will look and feel better. I promise. Most people experience rapid weight loss for the first few days (often as much as 5 pounds in the first week). This initial weight loss is the result of your body flushing retained water and toxins; more sustainable fat loss will stabilize after about a week. Let your rapid results *become* the motivation for further progress. In the first few days and weeks of this program, you might notice the following:

- ☐ Rapid fat loss
- ☐ Clearer skin and decreased acne
- ☐ Healthy color in skin and even tone
- ☐ Less water retention and puffiness
- ☐ Reduced allergies
- ☐ Reduced inflammation
- ☐ Improved sleep
- ☐ Increased lean muscle
- ☐ Increased energy level
- ☐ Improved strength, speed, and athletic performance
- ☐ Decreased recovery time

- ☐ Increased sex drive and sexual performance
- ☐ Heightened sensitivity in taste and smell
- ☐ Decreased blood pressure
- ☐ Reduced inflammation
- ☐ Improved digestion
- ☐ Little to zero gas
- ☐ Decreased dandruff
- ☐ Decreased acid reflux
- ☐ Decreased migraines
- ☐ Reduced body odor

Keep in mind that when you experience these improvements to your health and vitality, this is the way your body was meant to function—disease- and symptom-free.

7-DAY SAMPLE MEAL PLAN

SUNDAY—DAY 1

Breakfast: Eggs, bacon, and tomato with a half grapefruit

Lunch: Giant salad with avocado, cucumber, and feta over mixed greens drizzled with olive oil and balsamic

Snack: Plain yogurt with cinnamon and berries

Dinner: Beef Tenderloin with Buttered Onions, Horseradish, and Arugula (page 181)

Dessert: Strawberries and real grass-fed whipped cream

MONDAY—DAY 2

Breakfast: Gateway Green Smoothie (page 234)

Lunch: Bison Taco Salad with Avocado (page 170)

Snack: Broccoli florets and cucumber slices with hummus

Dinner: Mustard-Roasted Chicken Legs with Peach Salad (page 146)

Dessert: Chocolate, cheese, and fruit

TUESDAY—DAY 3

Breakfast: French-Pressed Fatty Coffee (page 249)

Lunch: Smoked Salmon and Kale Salad (page 211)

Snack: Bone Broth (page 337)

Dinner: Chicken Parmesan with Mixed Greens (page 143)

Dessert: 1 Peanut Butter Chocolate Chunk Cookie (page 253) and herbal tea

WEDNESDAY—DAY 4

Breakfast: Strawberry "Milk Shake" (page 239)

Lunch: Mom's Homemade Chicken Soup (page 150)

Snack: Avocado with tomato, basil, and balsamic vinegar

Dinner: Macadamia-Crusted Cod with Tender Greens (page 191)

Dessert: Blackberries with Coconut Whipped Cream (page 268) and Ginger-Lemongrass Tea (page 243)

THURSDAY—DAY 5

Breakfast: French-Pressed Fatty Coffee (page 249)

Lunch: Arugula salad with chopped apple, walnuts, and feta drizzled with olive oil and balsamic

Snack: Carrots and guacamole

Dinner: Ultimate Bacon Burger (page 172) with "the works"

Dessert: Alyson's Coffee Cake (page 256) with decaf coffee

FRIDAY—DAY 6

Breakfast: Green Monster Frittata with Bruschetta (page 213)

Lunch: Cucumber-Basil Smoothie (page 236)

Snack: Flax crackers with raw cheese

Dinner: Slow-Cooker Chicken with Roasted Broccoli and Mushrooms (page 164)

Dessert: Prunes, Brie cheese, and toasted hazelnuts

SATURDAY—DAY 7

Breakfast: French-Pressed Fatty Coffee (page 249)

Lunch: Cashew Cream Alfredo with Zucchini Noodles (page 219)

Snack: Hot-as-the-Devil Eggs (page 280)

Dinner: Chipotle Steak and Veggie Fajitas with Fresh Guacamole (page 167)

Dessert: Carrot Cake (page 257)

WHAT TO DO AFTER YOU REACH
YOUR GOAL WEIGHT

Here's some good news: *Maintaining* a lean and healthy body is much easier than creating one. Once you reach your ideal body composition, experiment with eating more starches, fruit, ancient grains, or anything else you like. If you love fruit, starchy vegetables, or dairy, enjoy them more often and see how your body responds. If you suddenly gain weight, you know the culprit. If your weight begins to drift and you can't isolate it to one food in particular, boost your protein and scale back your fat and carbs.

When your body is in perfect balance, you feel so mentally sharp, physically strong, and energetic that you may no longer take great pleasure in the low-quality foods you once craved. If you don't feel the need to schedule indulgences, there's no need to force it. Relaxing your standards on a whim throughout the week may work better for you. As long as you stick to the Wild Diet 80 to 90 percent of the time, the results will come, perhaps even more quickly than you think.

PART VII

The Wild Diet
Survival Guide

> **Expect problems and eat them for breakfast.**
>
> —*Alfred A. Montapert*

As an undergraduate, I led wilderness trips for the Dartmouth Outdoors Club where I'd teach incoming freshmen how to live in the woods. Despite the fact that these freshmen were the cream of the Ivy League crop—valedictorians, football stars, child prodigies, and more—most had never built a fire, cooked, treated a wound, identified wild berries, built a shelter, pooped outside, or spent more than an hour away from their phones. But after a week in the wilderness, these kids always walked out of the woods transformed—self-reliant, confident, and ready for whatever the world throws at them.

If you got through this whole book, there's a good chance that you'll be making a transformation, too. So, before I send you on your way, I'd like to make sure you have all the tools you need to kick some butt. As anyone who loves the outdoors will tell you, the best way to prevent disaster is by planning ahead. This section will help you stay one step ahead of the challenges waiting for you in the weeks ahead.

HOW TO GET THE MOST OUT OF YOUR FOOD DOLLAR

When it comes to food, you usually get what you pay for. That said, local foods from mom-and-pop shops or small farms generally give you the best bang for your buck. While popcorn and soda are often marked up more than 1,000 percent, grass-fed beef and organic eggs are usually sold close to cost. While some food from small farms may seem expensive, trust me—most farmers aren't doing it for the money. Small-scale organic farmers like my brother Mark are doing well if they break even every year. Make sure your food dollar goes to the farmer and the next harvest, not the Big Food marketing exec with the Maserati. Buy the food, not the package.

Processed food is impossibly cheap because it's not really food, but a combination of inexpensive fat, sugar, flour, and salt with little to no nutritional benefit. When you go to the grocery store, you will find that the cheapest calories are the ones that are going to make you the fattest and sickest. Will you be spending more money on certain foods? Sometimes. But since real foods are nutrient dense and filling, you'll find that you won't need to eat as much to feel satisfied. It's important to make a shift when thinking about food value: Measure your food by how much it satisfies you, not the size package it comes in or the bulk on your plate.

When I started buying RAW (Recently Alive and Well) food like local meats, farm fresh eggs, and seasonal fruits and vegetables, I actually saved money on my monthly food expenses. Why? Because I was eating less (but feeling full), buying in-season produce, and leaving out the branded processed junk. Real food has more bounce to the ounce.

Here are some tips to get the most out of your food dollar.

- ☐ Buy in bulk and cook large meals ahead of time.
- ☐ Shop at a food co-op. Pay a small fee to become a member and you'll even get a discount.
- ☐ Join a Community Supported Agriculture (CSA) farm, where you can purchase "shares" of fresh seasonal produce in bulk, straight from a local farm. It feels good to know where your food comes from.
- ☐ Shop at farmers' markets. Often you will find high-quality food and wares for far less than you'd pay in the grocery store.
- ☐ Look into volunteering at local farms. Many farms allow you to work for a day or even a few hours in exchange for a basket full of their fresh food. It's a great deal if you're on a budget.
- ☐ Join a local Meetup group. In most major cities, you can find groups that

sponsor feasts based upon farm-to-table, Paleo, Primal, Wild, and Slow Food principles and more.

☐ Grow your own groceries. Plucking food from your garden is as fresh as it gets.

☐ Eat your weeds. Whenever we go home to New Hampshire, we have plates full of milkweed, purslane, dandelion, and other plants that grow wild for free in most backyards.

☐ Learn how to forage for wild berries, plants, and mushrooms.

☐ If you like to fish or hunt, catch your own dinner. Nothing like fresh trout sautéed in real butter.

☐ Save the drippings from fatty meats like bacon, beef, duck, and pork and use them instead of buying cooking fats.

☐ Buy offcuts and organ meats instead of steaks like tenderloin, prime rib, T-bone, and sirloin, which are expensive not because they're better for you but because they're in high demand.

☐ Buy fat-heavy, nutrient-dense foods. Grass-fed butter, full-cream yogurt, cheese, avocado, nuts and nut butter, eggs, meats, coconut, beans, and sardines will fill you up more than their low-fat counterparts.

SAVE A BUCK WITH THE DIRTY DOZEN AND CLEAN FIFTEEN

My friends at the Environmental Working Group developed a list of the most and least polluted produce in America. Sometimes organic is too expensive, isn't available, or isn't in season. No problem. Here's a list of the most contaminated conventional fruits and vegetables that you should always buy organic (the Dirty Dozen) and the ones that are safer if you go for the non-organic variety (the Clean Fifteen).

Buy Organic—The Dirty Dozen. When conventionally grown on industrial farms, these fruits and veggies tested for at least forty-seven different chemicals, toxins, and pesticides—and some had as many as sixty-seven!

- Apples
- Strawberries
- Grapes
- Celery
- Peaches
- Spinach

- Sweet bell peppers
- Imported nectarines
- Cucumbers
- Cherry tomatoes
- Imported snap peas
- Potatoes

Save a Buck with the Clean Fifteen. These fruits and vegetables bear little or no traces of chemicals, and are safe to buy conventionally grown (preferably still local) if your budget is tight.

- Onions
- Avocados
- Pineapples
- Mango
- Sweet peas
- Asparagus
- Kiwi fruit
- Cabbage

- Eggplant
- Cantaloupe
- Papaya
- Grapefruit
- Sweet potatoes
- Sweet onions
- Sweet corn (but this is genetically modified unless organic)

HOW TO ORDER AT A RESTAURANT

Eating out without a plan can make it really difficult to shed fat. Most restaurants will accommodate your eating preferences, but you may need to take initiative and order with a keener eye and thicker hide than you have in the past.

Here are a few tips for eating out:

- Choose the restaurant yourself—always favor farm-to-table over fast-food and chain restaurants. If you can find a restaurant that uses locally sourced produce and meats—even better!

- Ask your waiter if they have a "gluten-free" menu. If not, ask which dishes are gluten-free. The waiter is your friend—let them know that you do not eat MSG, gluten, or added sugar. If you have to, tell them that these foods make you ill. If you're at a nice restaurant, often the chef will visit the table to speak with you and create a special meal.
- Order a salad, soup, or lean protein appetizer. Make green veggies the first thing that hit your belly.
- Ignore the bread, chips, or other cheap carbs—these cheap, high-glycemic foods are meant to stimulate your appetite to encourage you to order more.
- Ask for sauces and dressings on the side.
- Always choose raw, boiled, steamed, poached, or grilled over baked or fried.
- Order a lean protein and vegetable dish for your entrée.
- Ask for extra vegetables instead of the starch.
- You don't need to clean your plate—ask for a doggie bag.
- Eat slowly and push the plate away when you are 80 percent full.
- If you want dessert, order chocolate, fruit, or cheese and split with a companion. Never eat dessert alone.

Remember, *you* are putting the food into *your* body, and most of the time, *you* are paying for the meal. You don't have to be abrasive, but always order what you want, how you want it. Talking through the order to get food exactly as you prefer pays huge dividends for your health and happiness.

HOW TO SAVOR YOUR MEAL

Have you ever eaten dinner in Italy? It lasts all night! The night's feast means gathering around the table with family and friends and enjoying meals for hours, laughing, relaxing, and carrying on in merriment. That's what dinner should be—the best time of the day. In the face of relentless media messaging designed to convince us that eating is a chore, resist the temptation to settle for mediocre meals. There's not much joy in the act of choking down a greasy burger or burrito in the front seat of the car. Weight loss has just as much to do with how you think about food as what you actually put in your mouth.

As you experience your meal, remember that most of your perception of taste comes from your sense of smell. Make it a game with your little ones—smell each bite and see how many ingredients your nose and palate can perceive. You'll find fresh food tastes much better when you really learn how to increase the sensitivity of your palate and savor each morsel.

Cut into that fresh grapefruit and smell it before you take a piece. Twist the rind to extract its oil and sense how it differs from the flesh in taste, smell, and touch. Crush a bit of cilantro or mint between your fingers and let the smell of it settle into your nostrils. There is so much pleasure that comes from the olfactory senses, and we're missing out on it because we have never been taught how to experience our food. But we can learn.

As I advanced in studying jazz, an interesting thing happened to how I perceive music. While many people hear a song as a complete sound in and of itself, students of music learn to focus their attention to listen to each instrument, voice, string, and note individually. With careful practice, you can develop the same ability for the foods you eat to taste your food like a true connoisseur. Dogs also are born with this ability in their incredible sense of smell; while a human may smell "tomato sauce," the dog can sense canned tomatoes, burnt butter, rancid oil, high-fructose corn syrup, and other constituent parts. You can learn to do this, too.

Taste your food as you cook, adjusting it to your palate. Pretend you're a toddler again, trying new foods as if you are diving into an exciting new experience. Relax and enjoy your meals, the company of your family and friends, and remember to express gratitude for the food that nourishes your body.

Make mealtime an occasion to be enjoyed. Don't slop food on your plate like the dog's dinner. Sit down, break out your auntie's best china, and feast like royalty. Look forward to what you eat and seize the opportunity to make incredible food one of the great joys of your life.

A FEW TIPS

- You can eat only so much food every day. Make it delicious and never settle for boring meals. No need to eat whatever is put in front of you if it doesn't align with your goals.
- Taste food like a wine connoisseur would enjoy a select vintage on his or her night off. Smell, savor, and experience the delight of every sensation.
- Offer a few words of gratitude before your meal.
- Take deep breaths as you smell, taste, and savor your food.
- See how many ingredients you can identify through smell and taste.
- Serve yourself just enough food to fill up 80 percent of the way. The Japanese call this *hara hachi bu*.
- Eat your green veggies and fiber first to decrease the glycemic load of the meal.
- Smell each bite and wait to take the next bite until you finish the first. Don't be afraid to make "mmm" and "yummm" sounds in between, like Alyson does.
- If you choose to eat dessert, always share it with a friend.

HOW TO SNACK ON THE WILD DIET

Eat protein, fat, fibrous vegetables, or fruit as snacks. If you're a snacker, keep a protein snack (like jerky, yogurt, or salmon) handy at all times. Keep snacks on hand for hunger pangs, travel, and emergencies. As long as you eat Wild throughout the day and avoid bingeing, the exact number of meals you choose to eat is immaterial.

Fasting and Feasting, the cycle of eating light foods or fasting during the day and luxurious feasts at night, is a powerful fat-loss tool. As you learned in Part II, I find that eating my first meal, often a green smoothie or eggs with fruit and veggies, between noon and three p.m. gives me great energy and balance. This amounts to sixteen to eighteen hours of "fasting" or undereating each day and six to eight hours of meals and snacking.

During my "feasting" phase, I always have snacks on hand. Here are a few of my favorites.

- Leftovers
  - Lean proteins (e.g., hard-boiled eggs, turkey breast, canned fish, homemade jerky, leftover chicken)
  - Green smoothie
  - Soup or broth
  - Nuts and seeds
  - Raw vegetables
  - Dehydrated vegetable snacks
  - Seaweed
  - Plain yogurt or cottage cheese with nuts and berries
  - Homemade protein snacks

Growing up in a house full of brothers, there never seemed to be enough food around. I picked up the habit of hunting for fresh fruits, vegetables, and fungi wherever I could find it. I could scrounge up something to eat almost year-round in the backyard gardens or woods—tart apples from the tree behind the house, blueberries from the bushes by the fishing spot, or even a hardy stalk of kale peeking up through the snow. There are more than 10,000 edible wild plants in Europe alone—take a class and snack for free on your hikes!

When traveling, I almost always bring a few raw cucumbers as a snack, chomping on them like Bugs Bunny would a carrot. Sure, people look at you funny for eating a vegetable in public (you should have seen the way the Brazilians pointed at my cucumber), but once you get over the shame of it all, you realize that raw veggies are the ultimate snack. Like an apple, the tough skin that surrounds the cucumber protects it during transport, and its bulk and size usually allows the vegetable to remain cool on a hot day. Since fresh veggies are mostly water, you're actually hydrating while you eat—the fluid in cucumbers alone has probably saved my life on a few extended adventures through the desert. Raw veggies like leafy greens, cucumbers, squash, zucchini, carrots, and celery provide slow-burning fiber, and numerous phytonutrients to keep you properly fueled, as well. In addition to raw veggies, fill your pack with energy-dense foods like nuts, berries, and fresh fruits that give you steady energy and nourishment for your adventures during the day.

HOW TO HYDRATE

It is impossible to overemphasize the importance of hydrating properly. As the most abundant and essential nutrient in your body, water makes up 90 percent of your blood, 85 percent of your gray matter, 78 percent of your brain, 70 percent of your muscles, and even 20 percent of your bones. Even mild dehydration of 3 percent of your body weight can decrease muscle contractile strength by 10 percent; when 5 percent of your total weight is lost in water, muscular and aerobic endurance can decrease by 20 to 30 percent. Go without water for a few days and you flat-out *die*.

But let's get to the point—drinking plenty of water helps you burn fat.

Drinking pure water encourages fat metabolism by enabling the liver, the primary fat-burning organ in the body, to function optimally. Your body is assaulted daily with thousands of harmful substances such as smog, secondhand smoke, food additives, fluoride, chlorine, drugs, alcohol, heavy metals, pharmaceuticals, and other chemicals. Your liver works tirelessly to disassemble these harmful substances into molecules that can be dissolved in water so they can be easily eliminated. Due to all of the toxins we are exposed to in our environment or consume directly in our food, most people's livers are overtaxed. From a survival standpoint, burning fat is low in the pecking order. It's more important for your liver to filter toxins and keep you alive than to burn fat and give you a perfect beach body.

In addition to enabling your liver to burn fat, drinking plenty of water also:

- Regulates and suppresses appetite
- Increases metabolism
- Boosts energy levels
- Releases toxins from the body
- Reduces water retention
- Alleviates headaches
- Reduces blood pressure
- Eases joint pain

- Reduces risk of kidney stones
- Improves skin

HOW TO DRINK MORE WATER

- Carry a water bottle everywhere (most healthy people do this).
- Drink unsweetened teas and tonics throughout the day.
- Drink spa water with fresh fruits, herbs, cucumber, mint, etc.
- Drink green smoothies.
- Eat more whole veggies and fruits, which are mostly water.
- Drink water with lemon.
- Drink a vinegar tonic: Morning/refreshing tonic: Combine 2 tablespoons of apple cider vinegar, a slice of lemon, a dash of cinnamon, and stevia to taste in a glass of ice water and enjoy.
- Drink one glass of fresh water with each alcoholic drink.
- Drink a glass of water 20 minutes before your meal.

Generally speaking, you don't feel thirsty until *after you're already dehydrated*. In fact, since food and water are such related and interconnected needs, you often feel hungry when you're actually thirsty.

Consume water on a regular basis and before you are thirsty. While drinking water with every meal is beneficial, limit yourself to one glass. Too much water consumed with or directly before meals will dilute the stomach juices and prevent effective digestion. Most tea aids hydration, while coffee and other stimulants, diuretics, and prescription drugs borrow against it.

Do your best to drink clean water—this may take some effort on your part. Tap water is often treated with chlorine, which can damage your digestive system and gut flora. Fluoride is added to many water systems despite the fact that studies have shown that it is linked to problems with the thyroid, kidneys, central nervous system, and skeletal systems.

HOW TO DROP 25 POUNDS IN A MONTH

In 2003, a friend on the Dartmouth crew team was faced with a seemingly impossible challenge. After a few too many keg stands in the off-season, his coach came back to him with an ultimatum: "Lose twenty pounds in less than thirty days or you're off the team."

Now, it should be said that many bodybuilders, wrestlers, and even fitness models can drop an insane amount of weight by using performance-enhancing drugs, diuretics, or severe water restriction. It "works," but it's not particularly good for you, fair, or sustainable.

So my friend dug deep into old wives' tales and legends of the crew team and beyond to find a fix. After all, rowers had faced the same problem for decades. He finally found a long-retired crew coach who claimed to have the answer to his prayers. The coach said that his trick:

- Does not involve any drugs/herbs/or magic potions
- Requires no special foods
- Is very simple
- Requires little deprivation but considerable self-control

So how do you shave off 20 pounds in a month in a way that's fair, healthy, and legal?

Drink water. Only water. No fruit juice, soda, diet soda, coffee, beer, sports drinks, energy drinks, or anything else. Nothing but fresh water for a month.

My friend was dubious, but he decided to grit his teeth and give it a shot. He started drinking a glass of cool, fresh water every morning and continued to drink plenty throughout the day. He still made appearances at parties and get-togethers, where he politely and confidently sipped from his water bottle, staying delightfully clear-headed while everyone else transformed into slobbering idiots.

Did it work?

Yep, he lost 25 pounds in a month, dropping 5 pounds more than he planned. His body transformed from chubby to chiseled. He ate exactly the same foods, ignored all of the mysterious-colored liquids on the convenience-store shelves, and drank more water instead. He also noticed that he wasn't any hungrier, since liquid calories are rarely satisfying or filling.

Our ancestors survived for thousands of years on clean water wherever they could find it. There were no Slurpees, caramel macchiatos, or double-chocolate stouts. In a sense, we are built to drink water and little else. It's incredible how easy it is to take in hundreds of extra, unneeded, empty, and unfulfilling calories in the many drinks you consume over the course of the day. Don't make the mistake of watching your food and ignoring the liquid calories.

Here are the worst offenders that you should cut out first:

- Milk shakes
- Sugary alcoholic drinks (e.g., margaritas, rum and Coke, etc.)
- Fruit juice (even 100% juice)
- Meal-replacement drinks
- Soda
- Energy drinks
- Beer
- Diet soda (artificial sweeteners alter insulin response and leave you craving more sugar)
- Flavored milk
- Sugary drive-thru drinks (the famed caramel cappuccino)
- Sugar in coffee or tea
- Powdered drink mixes
- Sports drinks

When you want to spice up your water, throw in some citrus or mint. Cheers!

THE WILD DIET FOR ATHLETES

If you're physically active, you're going to need more fuel, usually in the form of carbs, to aid in recovery and replenish your frequently depleted muscle and liver glycogen stores. But remember that our hunter-gathering ancestors could run a hundred miles in a day with little more than an ostrich egg filled with water for subsistence. They certainly weren't suckling on sugar goo and sports drinks mile after mile.

When you're training, go ahead and fuel up with extra carbs from starchy vegetables, fruits, legumes, and gluten-free whole grains. A bit of fruit can help some people before workouts or a big adventure. Fruit is fine on an empty stomach as long as it's eaten whole, but stay away from fruit juices. As always, use your hunger as a guide. If you feel low on energy and you're not gaining fat, don't be afraid of eating more low-glycemic carbs like boiled sweet potatoes, whole-grain rice, gluten-free oatmeal, carrots, beets, legumes, and fruit. The best time to fuel up with carbs is directly following physical activity or with your evening meal to induce the "carb coma" that helps you sleep.

If you want to cut fat to improve speed, try cycling carbs during training. High-fat, low-carb ketogenic diets are intermittently used by elite athletes, movie stars, bodybuilders, and physique competitors to drop fat rapidly. For beginners, eating fewer than 20 grams of carbs a day throughout the week and refeeding with more than 150 to 300 grams of natural carbs one or two days a week can accelerate fat loss and encourage fat adaptation without sacrificing performance.

Occasional fasting can cut fat, optimize health, and improve performance for athletes. Understand, however, that if you're accustomed to eating small meals throughout the day, then you might need to eat more than usual during your post-workout feast to properly refuel. Remember, everyone has a unique body composition—so there's no one-size-fits-all guideline. Listen to your body and eat whole, Wild food until you're not hungry anymore. If you're an athlete and crave carbs, go for starchy veggies like boiled sweet potatoes, whole-grain rice, ancient grains, or fruit.

Resist the temptation to eat high-sugar products like drinks, bars, and shakes that are specifically marketed to athletes. While you might be able to get away with eating more sweets than your less active peers without gaining as much fat, know that excess sugar depresses your immune system, taxes your pancreas and liver, encourages brain fog and lethargy, disturbs sleep, and worse. Like our ancestors did for thousands of years, you can get all the carbs and nutrition you need from real food and water with natural electrolytes.

THE WILD DIET FOR VEGETARIANS AND VEGANS

If you avoid meat for health reasons, know that eating nutrient-dense foods from healthy animals will improve your health, not sacrifice it. But if you choose not to eat animal foods because of ethical reasons, I get it. In my teens and part of my twenties, I considered myself an ethical vegetarian, avoiding meat on and off for nearly a decade. I made many mistakes as a vegetarian, though, and missed out on the critical nutrients that are difficult or impossible to source without animal foods.

Since the Wild Diet isn't a dogmatic program that tells you exactly what you can and can't eat, there is plenty of space to experiment with a plant-based or even raw version of this diet (and we have on many occasions). In practice, Alyson and I joke that we're 80 percent vegetarian and 20 percent Paleo, since the vast majority of our food comes from plants, not animals. In fact, most of the store-bought snacks in our pantry are 100 percent plant-based—we find many healthy treats, often dehydrated veggies, nuts, and fruits, in the Raw / Vegan / Vegetarian aisles of the health food store. They're not cheap, but they're tasty. On a budget, dehydrated plant-based snacks—crackers, cereals, and treats—can also be made easily at home.

A crucial part of the Wild Diet is eating foods that were RAW, plants and animals alike. We fight against conventional feedlots and mistreated animals as fervently as many vegans—we often meet our animals in person to make sure they live in great health and happiness on the farm in the way nature intended.

If you avoid meat for ethical reasons, know that you don't *need* to eat the meat of animals to achieve great health. If you choose to avoid animal foods completely, I suggest that you work with a plant-based nutritionist to spackle the gaps in your nutrient profile. An experienced professional can tailor your meals to make sure you get access to nutrients that are difficult to source without eating animal foods, like choline, B_{12}, iron, K_2, collagen, and more.

Alternatively, consider consuming the eggs or dairy from healthy animals on pasture, which provide critical nutrients for health without harming the animal. Seafood like oysters, clams, and mussels can also be powerful additions to a plant-based diet. Oysters are especially rich in iron, zinc, B_{12}, selenium, copper, and vitamin A. These sea creatures, called bivalves, lack a central nervous system and are not considered sentient by most criteria.

Of course, eliminating meat, eggs, and dairy from this diet will change the plan tremendously—but if you follow the guidelines here for eating local and organic as much as possible, soaking and cooking/roasting your own nuts, seeds, and legumes, and steering clear of wheat and processed grains, you can find incredible success incorporating Wild principles into a plant-based diet.

Substitutions: Here are a few basic substitutions for animal products when cooking or baking Wild Diet recipes. Remember that these substitutes won't replicate the recipe exactly, so have some fun and tweak them on your own with plant-based ingredients that please your palate.

- Grass-fed butter: coconut oil (or other oil)
- Cream or milk: coconut milk, coconut cream, unsweetened almond milk
- Cheese (sauce): Cashew Cream Alfredo (page 219)
- Eggs (baking): 1 tablespoon flax meal mixed with 3 tablespoons filtered water, per egg
- Chicken (cubed or sliced): tempeh (fermented soy is better for your gut)
- Ground beef or bison: black beans (whole or mashed)

Remember, just because food is labeled "vegan," "plant-based," "vegetarian," "gluten-free," "raw," or anything else doesn't mean that it's good for you. Processed imitation meat dishes marketed to vegans and vegetarians are often more artificial than a Big Mac, containing GMOs, modern gluten, artificial flavors, and other nasties. Regardless of whether or not you eat animal foods, always get the least processed, highest-quality foods you can find and afford.

THE WILD DIET FOR KIDS

The kids' menu at most restaurants is a far cry from what children should be eating—battered fish sticks, cheese pizza, chicken nuggets, and French fries to name a few familiar options. But if anyone should be eating nutrient-dense, high-quality, fresh food, it's kids.

Here are a few tips to feed your kids Wild:

- Kids like what's around them, so keep plenty of chopped veggies and other healthy snacks in the refrigerator. If your child can get into the fridge, keep these healthy foods in their sight and reach and get rid of or hide any sugar-filled snacks.
- It can take time for kids to adjust to eating new foods. You may need to introduce a new food up to a dozen times before your kids will like it. Try again—you call the shots!
- Make comments on how much you enjoy a food. Describe the taste, texture, and smell to help pique their interest.
- Start a garden and help your kids see where their food comes from.
- Make food fun by dropping interesting facts about what they're eating. For example:
  - Beets are cool because they turn your pee red!
  - Your garlic breath keeps vampires away.
  - That headcheese is made out of brains!
  - Eating carrots gives you better night vision.
  - Apples float in water because they're 25 percent air.

SIMPLE WILD RECIPES AND SNACKS THAT KIDS LOVE

- Sweet potato chips cooked with coconut oil and sprinkled with cinnamon and salt
- Kale wrapped around dates and avocados, drizzled with olive oil
- A yogurt "sundae" with nuts and berries
- Deviled eggs

- Zucchini noodles with tomato sauce and meatballs
- Spaghetti squash with olive oil, basil, tomato, olives, feta, and salt
- Canned tuna or salmon mixed with fresh parsley, mustard, diced red onion, lemon juice, and pepper, lightly cooked and spread on celery sticks
- Taco-seasoned ground beef cooked and served in butter lettuce with shredded cheese, diced tomato, grilled onions, and guacamole
- Turkey rolled around spinach, tomato, and cheese
- Carrot and cucumber slices with hummus
- Green smoothie with kale, avocado, and strawberries
- Homemade trail mix with macadamia nuts, shredded coconut, pumpkin seeds, sunflower seeds, cinnamon, coconut oil, and dark chocolate chips
- Apple slices with almond butter
- Cauliflower rice with chopped sautéed onion, butter, and salt
- Salad with mixed greens, sprouts, pine nuts, strawberries, and feta cheese

TOMATOES MAKE KIDS SMART

While living in Washington, D.C., I volunteered to teach troubled teens how to cook. I was surprised to see how quickly even the "cool kids" took to the kitchen. They loved the smells, sounds, flavors, and choose-your-own-adventure mentality of cooking—it's like they came alive. One afternoon, one particularly feisty teen pointed a batter-covered finger toward the tomato on my cutting board. She scrunched her nose and asked, "What is that thing?"

"It's a tomato. . . . You've never seen one before?"

"Nope!"

As she took a slice and tasted the juicy, purplish beefsteak tomato I snatched from the farmers' market a few blocks away, her face lit up. "I never liked vegetables. But I like this."

I think our kids need to see more fresh tomatoes. Many kids don't like vegetables because all they've tasted is the flavorless glop that comes out of cans. Even you may think that you don't like vegetables, but find a fresh one straight off the vine and you'll be coming back for more. If we want the next generation to grow up to be health nuts, we need to make sure they get some dirt under their fingernails and learn how to feed themselves fresh food.

When I worked on a best-practices consulting project with the Department of Education, I visited some of the top high schools for troubled youth in America. Several of these schools were known for finding homeless children who had dropped out of school and convincing them to come back to school and get their diplomas. One student was found homeless sleeping in an abandoned truck just outside of Wasilla, Alaska (Sarah Palin's stomping grounds—you can see Russia from there). Now he's a straight-A student just a month away from graduation, and I asked him: "So if you dropped out of every other school, why did you keep coming back to this one?"

"For the food. The teachers always help us find good food."

Many of these remarkable schools had gardens that not only taught students how to grow their own food but also fed them throughout the day. Study after study has shown that when you improve the source of food in schools, behavior problems vanish, test scores skyrocket, and children truly thrive. And that was the secret to getting high school dropouts back to school to finish their diplomas: Feed them well.

THE WILD DIET FOR PETS

A few years ago, I had a problem. Three days after Christmas in 2012, Alyson and I adventured to a ranch in West Texas to pick up our new puppy, Bailey. As the fluffy little creature snuggled a wet nose into Alyson's neck, the breeder thrust a bag of dry food into my chest.

"There are thirty chickens in every bag," he declared. "I only feed my pups the best."

Sounds like good marketing, I thought. But since it's best to keep a young pup's diet consistent for the first few days, we gave her a few bowls as we began to introduce her to raw meat, the natural diet for dogs in the wild. We hopped down to the farmers' market and picked up a few raw, meaty bones. It was the best day of her little puppy life.

A few days later, as Alyson set the last bowl of the breeder's dry food on the floor, a surprising thing happened. Bailey barked, jumped up, and snatched the food bowl in her mouth. She shook the bowl as hard as she could, spewing brown pebbles across the kitchen floor. She wouldn't touch kibble after that. Sounds like my dog, right?

It made me wonder—what's *in* kibble, anyway? Dogs have been eating certain types of foods for thousands of years, and it has only been in the last few generations that we've started feeding them "dog food." Today's supermarket has aisles for "dog food" and "human food," but isn't it all just food?

Before the invention of pet foods, most dogs and cats lived off of meats, table scraps, and homemade food from their owners. After World War I, canned horsemeat was introduced in the United States under the Ken-L Ration brand as a means to dispose of deceased horses. It's gone downhill ever since. If you think the standards of quality for processed human food are low, you'll be stunned by the ingredients passed off as dog "food."

Here's a quick look at what these terms really mean on the label of pet food:

- *Meat by-products* can actually mean slaughterhouse fecal waste, poultry feather meal, connective tissue, leather meal, and horse and cattle hair. By-products can actually be toxic products from spoiled foodstuffs, non-nutritive fillers, heavy metal contaminants, sugar, pesticides and herbicides, drug residues, artificial colors, flavors, and preservatives, bacteria and fungi contaminants.
- *Chicken and chicken by-products* are often diseased and damaged, declared unfit for human consumption by the USDA.
- *Corn gluten* is usually a GMO substance used as a filler, with no nutritional value.
- *Dried beet pulp/beet sugar* is a GMO sugar with no nutritional value.
- *Corn syrup* (usually derived from GMO corn) is an empty source of calories that stresses the pancreas and adrenals.
- *Natural flavors* may or may not contain the anal secretions of beavers (see page 32).
- *Fiber* can come from peanut hulls, hair, or even newspaper. Often, these types of ingredients can be disguised as a vague ingredient label, or not listed at all.

- *Water/water sufficient for processing*, if listed as the first ingredient, means there is more water than any other ingredient.

If processed food for humans didn't scare you off, with its mutant grains, hunger-hijacking chemicals, and toxic pesticides, I hope this section encourages you to feed your pets real food as often as you can. As with humans, fresh foods from healthy plants and animals create healthy bodies for your pets, too.

DNA testing indicates that a split occurred between dogs and wolves about 100,000 years ago. But even after all that time, dogs have nearly identical genes to their wolf ancestors. While your cuddly mutt may seem almost human at times, her DNA expects her to be running with the wolves and thriving on a wild diet of ruminants and rodents.

While regular DNA derives equally from both parents, giving you all shapes and sizes of dog breeds, there is another kind of DNA that doesn't rapidly change from generation to generation: mitochondrial DNA (small cells within the cells of animals that convert stored food into energy). This type of DNA changes at a very slow pace, at around 1 or 2 percent every 100,000 years. From a nutritional point of view, dogs aren't all that different from wolves.

Wolves don't use ovens. As we learned from Pottenger's cats on page 109, it's important to feed your animals as they would have eaten in the wild. If you have a dog, think raw meaty bones, organ meats, offal, and perhaps a small amount of cooked vegetables, fruit, or grain to simulate the contents of the stomach of canine prey. Our death-defying cat, Nugs, survived eighteen years in the backwoods of New Hampshire, eating birds, squirrels, bats, weasels, rabbits, chipmunks, and anything else she could catch.

What to Feed Fido

The common idea that your dog shouldn't eat table scraps because "it will make them fat and sick" is ridiculous (but gives some insight into the state of *our* food). The environmentalist and cheapskate in me loves having a dog and feeding her Wild. If I'm the human compost, devouring everything in the fridge that's about to go bad, Bailey is the vacuum cleaner—the second line of defense from waste and excess spending. Bailey polishes off everything I don't get around to. Any table scraps, battered cooking bowls, odd-smelling leftovers, expired dairy, or other food that would otherwise be thrown away goes straight into the dog bowl. Even better, all of that food that might have been garbage comes right out of our "dog food" budget, since we need to buy less to feed her.

Although she does get a fair amount of our table scraps and leftovers, the bulk of our dog's diet comes from raw meat and bones. While overachieving canines like sledding and racing dogs have long eaten a native diet, feeding your dog this way might be new to you.

Contrary to what you might have heard, variations in your dog's diet is one of the best ways to make sure they get the spectrum of nutrients their bodies require.

Let's look at the diet of our dog's ancestors that lived in the wild. Muscle, bone, and organs made up 65 to 80 percent of their diet by volume, with 10 to 25 percent coming from carbohydrates found in the intestines of small prey.

What happens to the domesticated canine gone Wild?

- Shinier coats
- Fewer stomach issues
- Cleaner teeth
- Increased energy
- Healthier skin
- Less poop
- Stronger immune system

There are a few risks to feeding your dog raw meat and bones, however, including bacterial contamination to both you and your dog. Get the best meat you can and know where it comes from. If you don't have access to high-quality, farm-raised meats, buy lean meats in your local grocery store. Since conventional meats often harbor harmful bacteria such as E. coli and salmonella, lightly cook the meat before feeding it to your dog. To add calories and bulk at low cost, simmer the meat low and slow with vegetables and starches like sweet potatoes or whole grains such as oats or rice. Add fats and oils from your kitchen before serving to provide more energy for larger and more active dogs.

These days, you can also order raw dog food online or at most pet stores, although it's not always cheap. If you're not up for raw feeding, just "throw your dog a bone" once in a while—a real, raw beef bone with meat still on it. These bones provide great nutrition and exercise for your furry friend. Keep it outside if you want to spare your carpet from stains, but Fido probably ruined that already.

So, what's on your dog's menu?

- Bones with muscle meat attached
- Raw bones either left whole or ground
- Organ meats (liver, gizzards, heart)
- Bone marrow
- Raw eggs
- Vegetables (broccoli, celery, carrot, spinach, etc.)
- Fruits (tart apples, bananas, strawberries, etc.)

To make your dog's meal more Wild without changing their current food, mix canned or dry food with nutrient-dense eggs, heavy cream, fish oil, butter, sweet potato, pumpkin, or squash. Leftovers that are a little past their prime also go great in the dog dish as long as they're not too spicy for the canine constitution, if you catch my drift.

It's not uncommon to feel a little overwhelmed when first preparing your dog's meals. Don't fret! You can start by working one or two raw meals into your dog's eating schedule each week, and gradually increasing over a few months. Or start by feeding raw in the morning and regular food in the evenings.

Fasting for Pets

In addition to feeding our pets real food, you won't be surprised to learn that we "fast" our pup, too. Every Sunday, Bailey skips breakfast, going twenty-four hours—from dinner to dinner—without a meal. Eating nutrient-dense real food and fasting once a week, our pets thrive with strong teeth, shiny coats, and lean physiques.

One of the first indications that our dog has a bug is that she loses her appetite. This is an instinctive strategy to spare the body the burden of digestion and starve bacterial and viral cells of their main fuel source, glucose. Taking a page out of Fido's book, I started listening to my body whenever I felt ill—when it feels right, fasting might be just what the doctor ordered.

Note: A guideline for feeding your dog is about 1 cup of food per 20 pounds of body weight. So, a 10-pound dog might eat only ½ cup of food per day, plus a small treat or two. However, a 60-pound dog might eat 3 cups of food, plus healthy treats.

Beef Supreme

TOTAL TIME: 10 minutes

Ingredients

2 pounds raw grass-fed ground beef
1 cup plain yogurt
1 cup pumpkin puree
1 cup broccoli, steamed and chopped
2 tablespoons ground kelp

5 large eggs
2 tablespoon fish oil
1 teaspoon Eggshell Calcium
   Supplement (page 325)

DIRECTIONS

1. In a bowl, mix together all the ingredients until well incorporated.

2. Divide the mixture into individual servings in resealable bags.

3. Refrigerate 2 days' worth of food and freeze the remaining portions.

4. Remove from freezer to thaw as needed.

Half Chicken

TOTAL TIME: 5 minutes

Ingredients

½ raw chicken

DIRECTIONS

1. Depending on the size of your dog, cut the chicken into a sizable portion.
2. Give the raw chicken to your dog.

> **NOTES**
>
> Your dog is likely to consume the meat and bones—never give your dog cooked bones, which can splinter and damage the stomach. Check with your vet to see which bone types are suitable for your dog's breed and size.
>
> Turkey, duck, and other foul can replace the chicken in this recipe.

Raw Meaty Bones

Raw meaty bones can make up to half of your dog's diet.

TOTAL TIME: 1 minute

Ingredients

Raw meaty bones

DIRECTIONS

1. Go in the yard and give your dog the meaty bone.

2. Store raw bones in the refrigerator for up to 2 days, or freeze for later.

NOTES

> Instead of beef bones, you can also feed your dog raw chicken necks, legs, quarters, backs, etc.

Dried Beef Liver Treats

TOTAL TIME: 2 to 4 hours

Ingredients

1 pound grass-fed beef liver

DIRECTIONS

1. Preheat the oven to 250°F. Line a baking sheet with aluminum foil.

2. Cut the liver into bite-size pieces and spread them on the prepared baking sheet.

3. Bake until the liver is dry to the touch, 2 to 4 hours.

4. Store in an airtight container in the refrigerator or freezer for up to 2 months.

NOTES

> Alternatively, you can feed the liver to your dog raw.
>
> While liver offers many benefits, feeding too much to your dog can result in an overdose of vitamin A and can be harmful.

Eggshell Calcium Supplement

TOTAL TIME: 20 minutes

Ingredients

Eggshells

DIRECTIONS

1. Gather the empty eggshells from your breakfast and put them outside to dry in the sun.
2. Use a coffee grinder or mortar and pestle to grind the shells into a fine powder.
3. Add the eggshell powder to your dog's food—start slow and work up to ½ teaspoon powder to each pound of food.
4. Store in an airtight container in the refrigerator.

Steak and Eggs

TOTAL TIME: 2 minutes

1 raw grass-fed steak or other hunk of beef appropriate for the size of your dog
1 to 3 large free-range eggs

Directions

1. Place the raw steak in your dog's food dish.
2. Crack 1 to 3 raw eggs over the meat.
3. Bring your dog outside to enjoy the meal.

Fast Sunday

TOTAL TIME: Zero

Ingredients

Nope.

DIRECTIONS

1. Tell Fido that he's skipping breakfast once a week.

Avoid Feeding These Foods to Dogs

While for the most part canines can eat almost everything a human can, some foods that are perfectly safe for humans are toxic for dogs. Never feed your dog cooked bones, which can splinter and cause internal bleeding. Even if your dog "begs" for these foods, don't give in. Avoid feeding your dog:

- Alcohol
- Avocado
- Baking items, such as spices, baking soda, baking powder
- Caffeine
- Chocolate
- Cooked bones
- Garlic (small amounts are fine)
- Grapes and raisins
- Hops
- Macadamia nuts
- Moldy or spoiled foods
- Onions (small amounts are fine)
- Pits from persimmons, peaches, and plums
- Salty foods
- Sugary foods
- Xylitol
- Yeast dough

LIVE LIKE YOU CAMP

Take a second and listen to what's around you. What do you hear? A TV? Traffic? Construction? That insufferable vent fan that never shuts off?

Our serene soundscape of soft ruffling leaves and babbling brooks has been drowned out by clanking construction, blaring sirens, and booming jets. We carry phones that make our pockets buzz and blurp every single time someone else wants our attention. We even use alarms designed to sound like a bomb drill to start our day. It's no wonder we're all stressed out of our minds.

Once you silence all of those noisy machines, you get your brain back. We think that we can't live without the strange contraptions and the web that connect, liberate, and shackle us, but once you unplug, you learn that you must. And it's only then that most people feel truly alive. My lawyer loves to tell me that I can't ignore e-mail and my phone, but my family and friends know that when something important is happening, I'll be there.

Growing up in the frosty backwoods of New Hampshire, thunderstorms, ice storms, and blizzards often knocked us straight back into the Stone Age; we sometimes went without electricity and phone for more than a week at a time. And something remarkable happened. The lack of TV, phones, and other distractions *forced* us to change our behavior. Instead of watching the evening news, we curled up with books. After long days spent sledding, snowshoeing, and cross-country skiing, we warmed our toes and chatted in the gentle warmth of the wood stove. With no computers or gadgets, our nights were filled instead with epic family battles of Risk, Clue, and Monopoly by candlelight. . . . It certainly wasn't my sentiment at the time, but accidentally living off-the-grid produced some of the happiest moments of my childhood. That's why, these days, we live like we camp (see page 342).

One of life's greatest pleasures is also the simplest—the opportunity to reconnect with nature. This has been known for thousands of years. When indigenous shamans hadn't seen enough healing someone with plants, they would send them out in the woods for several days to be healed by nature. I think we get a small taste of what they were after when we spend a night under the stars, dive into the ocean, or trot barefoot in the grass.

Science once again confirms common sense. In a study in the 1970s in Ann Arbor, Roger S. Ulrich used an EEG to measure alpha wave activity in the brains of his subjects. When looking at natural scenes, people showed reduced anger, aggression, and anxiety. Japan has a national movement called *shinrin-yoku*, which translates to "basking or bathing in the forest," to reduce stress and accelerate healing. Spending the day barefoot is a wonderful thing, with recent science showing that "grounding" with your bare feet on grass, stone, or earth has incredible health benefits—reversing disease, reducing inflammation, and improving recovery. You can even make your home more Wild through styles of living such as Zen and feng shui, which are designed to learn from and live harmoniously with nature.

SITTING IS FOR SUCKERS

While sitting all day is just about the worst thing you can do to your body, standing up works wonders for your body and your mind. Many great thinkers experienced moments of clarity and genius while they were standing up. Ben Franklin, Thomas Edison, Ernest Hemingway, and many others knew this well, spending most of their days and nights scurrying about, notebook in hand, cranking out earth-shattering ideas. Most of my employees work standing up, often fasted. But the simple act of standing at work isn't for philosophers, authors, and barefooted app developers anymore—everybody is standing these days.

In fact, as I wrote this book my editors at Penguin Random House, Megan and Gigi, said that they swear by using a standing desk, and they've recently even convinced three other editors to stand as well. While ridiculous standing desks will set you back more than five thousand dollars, you can build your own at home with a few parts from IKEA or your local hardware store for less than twenty bucks.

Ask your higher-up for permission to use a standing desk at work, and they may even splurge on your behalf since they know you'll be happier and more productive for it. Your hunched shoulders and achy back will thank you.

In a world where nearly every machine in the house bleeps and bloops at you all day, it's more important than ever to escape them and go on an adventure. Hiking, camping, walking, running, playing sports, riding a horse, it doesn't matter—just find something you and your family love and do it as often as you can.

Don't get me wrong—I love technology as much as the next nerd, but I find it's impossible to relax or get real work done when devices are screaming at me all day. These days, I spend most of my time unplugged, checking my e-mail and phone a few times a week but often going days without them.

Since most of our jobs and personal lives require time in the house, school, or office, make excuses to enjoy more time in nature, preferably every day. And if you must be in front of a screen, see if you can use a tablet or a laptop and work outside, perhaps while enjoying a refreshing drink.

ABEL'S ENVIRONMENTAL HACKS TO MAKE HEALTHY HABITS AUTOMATIC

We are what we repeatedly do. Excellence, then, is not an act, but a habit.

—*Aristotle*

- **Light:** Get fifteen minutes of sunlight shortly after sunrise and at least a few minutes midday or in the afternoon. Avoid artificial light after sundown, or use blue-blocking glasses to filter out blue light from screens, which disrupts the natural release of melatonin, a hormone that regulates the circadian rhythm.
- **Sight:** Cultivate a living and working space conducive to production, clear thinking, and exercising good habits. Keep junk food, alcohol, TV, computers, clutter, and other distractions out of sight. Instead, keep notebooks, sketchpads, musical instruments, books, and fresh produce in view. Make some places dedicated to work and others to play. Work outside or next to a window as often as possible to help regulate circadian rhythm, boost energy, and improve mood. Set up your

work environment so you can take breaks often, every twenty to thirty minutes or whenever necessary.

- **Sound:** Listen to nature sounds, chimes, music, or binaural beats during the day. Turn off notifications on computers and devices as much as possible. In noisy places, use a fan or air purifier to provide white noise to cover ambient sounds. As a last resort, wear earplugs. Play your favorite music often.
- **Smell:** Avoid areas of pollution and/or run an air purifier while sleeping. Use natural incense, essential oils, or old-fashioned home cookin' to lighten the mood and cover unwanted smells to create a comfortable environment. Hand-roasting green coffee beans once a week does the trick.
- **Skin:** Have you ever stopped to consider the sheer number of chemicals in the personal products we use every day: soap, shampoo, antiperspirant, toothpaste, and so on? Don't put anything on your skin that you wouldn't eat. The skin is your body's largest organ and absorbs substances into the body within seconds. Avoid products made with chemicals such as sodium lauryl sulfate, triclosan, petrolatum, and more that disrupt hormone function and cause weight gain and disease. Avoid petrochemicals and instead use plant-based or earth-based products like food-grade oil, aloe vera, clay, salt, and other natural products to cleanse, moisturize, and condition the skin.
- **Grounding and the Outdoors:** Spend at least ten minutes a day with bare feet or body in contact with the ground, especially after travel to ease jet lag, speed recovery, and improve sleep. In terms of temperature, our bodies are meant to respond and adapt to changing seasons. Let your body feel the change in the weather—sweating and shivering are biological mechanisms that are meant to be exercised and experienced. Don't be afraid to get cold in the winter and hot in the summer; your body is meant to adapt.
- **Air:** Do your best to breathe clean air from the natural environment as often as possible by visiting or living in the wilderness. We spend most of the year breathing thin mountain air since it's less polluted, and adapting to high elevations can improve lung capacity. Close your eyes and focus on breath every morning

and throughout the day to de-stress, clear the head, and focus thoughts. Breathe before you need to.

- **Water:** Drink clean water free of toxins, chlorine, fluoride, heavy metals, BPA, and other contaminants. Consume mineral water or supplement with magnesium, salt, and other electrolytes when drinking filtered water. Drink water before you're thirsty and always have it handy. Add trace minerals to your drinking source to improve taste and nutrition.

HOW TO USE LAZINESS TO YOUR ADVANTAGE

As we all know, changing your habits isn't easy. But if you want to change the way you eat, then you'll need to ditch some bad habits and trade them for good ones. We all want to believe that if we force ourselves to make the "right" decisions, our willpower will make it happen. But willpower is weak, and that's why 92 percent of New Year's resolutions fail.

One of the best ways to make good behavior automatic is to intentionally engineer your environment to make good decisions convenient and bad decisions inconvenient. I call this "environmental design," the act of setting up your surroundings to drive good behavior and discourage bad.

For instance, your brain craves what it knows is around you, so make the act of procuring fat-storing foods like ice cream a *chore*. It's easy to build the habit of taking a bite of Ben and Jerry's every time you have a bad day when it's in the freezer, but not if you need to find your wallet, put on your shoes, drive to the store, pick some up, and drive back before you dig in. You know that bowl of candy that's always on the counter at the doctor's office? Do the opposite of that. Hide the candy and put cookies in the freezer to save them for your feast. Out of sight, out of mind.

If you want to exercise every morning, a positive habit, set out your gym clothes and shoes the night before so you're ready to hit the gym and pump some iron as soon as you wake up. Workouts take effort, so make it easy on yourself. I keep kettlebells handy and a pull-up bar on one of my doors so I can get my blood pumping anytime I walk by.

This concept doesn't just apply to health and fitness, however. If you want to learn how to play guitar, for example, set it on a stand that you can see so it's easy to pick it up and play for a few minutes. Most of us have far too much stuff—eliminate clutter to clear your head. Set up your home and workplace to remind you of good habits so the bad ones never even cross your mind.

30-SECOND VISUALIZATION EXERCISE

Experimental and clinical psychologists have proved beyond a shadow of a doubt that the human nervous system cannot tell the difference between an "actual" experience and an experience *imagined vividly and in detail.*

—Dr. Maxwell Maltz, author of *Psycho-Cybernetics*

Visualization is a spectacularly powerful tool for transforming your body and life. Because your brain often thinks in images, creating a clear mental picture of what you want to achieve will focus your progress.

Below is an exercise I learned from a professional drug-free bodybuilder. He said that a lot of other people obsess over their calories and macros, but his secret to getting down to 3 percent body fat whenever he wants is mental, not physical. When he wants to lose fat or build muscle in the weeks before a contest, he does this 30-second exercise every day:

Find a comfortable place to sit. Take a deep breath.

Close your eyes, relax, and imagine your body at its absolute best. You can see and feel your flat stomach, toned muscles, and athletic figure fitting perfectly into your favorite clothes. You feel comfortable in your own skin. Feel the strength build in the muscles in your arms, back, trunk, and legs, ready to burst into action at any moment. You are confident and feel a tremendous sense of accomplishment.

Hold the image of yourself at your best in your mind for a few moments, as long as you'd like. Then take a deep breath and open your eyes.

Feel good? Use visualization as a tool to focus your progress and keep yourself on track. If you find yourself in a tempting situation, stop, relax, and take 30 seconds to visualize your body at its best. The temptation will fade. If you are dreading exercise but you know you are overdue, visualize yourself having already finished your workout—sweating, energized, and pumping endorphins through your veins. Let that great after-workout glow you know is coming motivate you to crank through the rest of your workout.

Make it a goal to take 30 seconds to do this exercise every day until you reach your goal. The more you focus the image of your body at its best in your mind, the more your subconscious will strive to achieve that state of being. Train your mind to expect impossible things and it will make them happen.

HOW TO USE AN INJURY TO YOUR ADVANTAGE

It was a typical Friday. I hit the 4 p.m. lull and knew I needed a bit of adrenaline to get me into the rhythm of what promised to be an excellent night playing a gig out on the town. Time to squeeze in a quick session of Krav Maga. Krav Maga is an Israeli form of self-defense designed to be bone-crushingly efficient in survival scenarios—blows are punishing and there are no rules. The dirtier the better. So instead of practicing Katas and talking theoretically about what moves could possibly work in a self-defense situation, you spend most of your time getting kicked in the groin or returning the favor.

After the first 30 minutes of warming us up and tiring us out, we got to the combo. A reverse hammerfist, followed by two others and an elbow, an advancing front kick to the groin, two roundhouses and a flying scissor kick to close it out.

I executed the first few times around. But I was almost out of juice. So on the last combo, my reverse hammerfist didn't work out too well.

As soon as the meaty part of my fist hit the pad, I knew I screwed up. You know that piercing, burning, tweaking feeling like your joint is being electrocuted from the inside out? Sorry about that, shoulder.

I went to the chiropractor and asked for her professional opinion. What's my next move, doc?

"Don't use your shoulder for a few days, Abel. Just take it easy. Rest."

Ugh. I knew she'd say something like that.

If you're a serious athlete or competitor, you know that the torn ligament, busted thumb, or ripped cartilage is a very small part of your pain. The real sting is completely psychological. In life, I always want to be moving forward at 110 percent, so setbacks like these can be tough.

When I broke my foot earlier this year doing something stupid while scrambling down a canyon, I was bummed out—nearly all of my workouts became impossible. Dead-lifts don't work as well with a broken foot. Instead of wallowing in shame and feeling sorry for myself, I did my best to use it as an opportunity to cross-train. I abandoned dead lifts, squats, burpees, and running and focused on mountain biking (with a boot), mobility exercises, and handstand push-ups. Sometimes getting injured is a blessing in disguise, a symptom that it's time to rebalance the movement of your body to avoid injury in the future.

Here are a few tips to turn lemons into lemonade:

- Focus on correcting other nagging injuries: Maybe you were ready for a break. Was your left foot a little crooked, your IT band a bit stiff, or your back jacked up? Whip out the foam roller and get to work. Prioritize symmetry and balance and you'll come back stronger.
- Ramp up the fasting: Want to lean out quickly? Intermittent fasting can work like gangbusters. Overdo it and you might be sacrificing both energy and physical performance. But if you're not performing, you don't need as much food and risk gaining fat from inactivity. Eat less and cut some fat.
- Use your extra time to reflect and refocus: Sometimes you get in the rhythm and forget why you're doing something in the first place. What's your next goal? Have you hit a plateau? Whip out your notebook and sketch down your thoughts. You might find that you emerge with a bigger and better idea.

- Rest: We don't sleep enough. We don't always prioritize relaxation. Build in an extra meditation session. Go to the beach with friends. Take your vacation and do something crazy.
- Revisit your sense of identity: Are you putting a little too much of who you are into the fact that you're a CrossFitter, a runner, a bodybuilder, or a martial artist? This can be a good opportunity to brush up on your Spanish, learn how to play the dusty guitar that's been sitting by your desk, or hunker down and read that novel you've been meaning to read since last Christmas. Focus on another piece of who you are and you may find that you come back to your athletics refreshed and sporting a fresh new perspective.

WHAT TO DO WHEN YOU GET SICK

I know what I did wrong. Countless meetings, preparing for speaking engagements, writing books, responding to e-mails, taking care of my dog, and 19,000 other things . . . I didn't get enough sleep, and I was stressed. I just overdid it.

So, for the first time in three years, I got sick.

Even if you eat and exercise perfectly, you're still susceptible to sickness when you're run down. First, it was the headache. This one was so thick you could touch it. Right behind the eyes. Then the chills and the fever. Nothing quite like waking up in the middle of the night shivering in a pool of cold, clammy sweat. Then, of course, the incessantly stuffy nose, postnasal drip, and coughing-up of oddly colored goo. And I have to speak at a health conference in San Francisco in two days? Sweet.

The Worst Thing to Do When You're Sick

It's astonishing what we feed ourselves, our family, and our children when we're ill.

When I got the bug, here's what I didn't do. I didn't have Campbell's. Here's a list of ingredients in Campbell's Chicken Noodle Soup:

Chicken stock, enriched egg noodles (wheat flour, egg solids, niacin, ferrous sulfate, thiamine, mononitrate, riboflavin, folic acid), cooked

chicken meat, water, contains less than 2% of the following ingredients: salt, chicken fat, cooked mechanically separated chicken, monosodium glutamate, cornstarch, onion powder, modified food starch, yeast extract, spice extract, soy protein isolate, sodium phosphates, beta carotene for color, chicken flavor (contains chicken stock, chicken powder, chicken fat), flavoring, dehydrated garlic.

In the three seconds it takes to scan those ingredients, I count three probable sources of MSG, at least three GMOs, soy by-products, copious amounts of processed salt, conventional chicken parts, artificial flavors, gluten, and miscellaneous nonfood substances. This is what we feed to sick people?

Sports drinks like Gatorade and soda are another staple of sickness. First, sugar water is never good for you. Ever. But especially when you're sick.

Sports drinks and soda also contain bizarre ingredients such as brominated vegetable oil, or BVO. BVO is a chemical used as a flame retardant, but Gatorade uses it as an emulsifier.

According to "What Is That Ingredient?":

Bromine-containing sedatives resulted in emergency room visits and incorrect diagnoses of psychosis and brain damage due to side effects such as depression, memory loss, hallucinations, violent tendencies, seizures, cerebral atrophy, acute irritability, tremors, ataxia, confusion, loss of peripheral vision, slurred speech, stupor, tendon reflex changes, photophobia due to enlarged pupils, and extensor plantar responses.

Yum!

Fortunately, in response to an online petition, PepsiCo recently pulled BVO from its future drinks. Great. I'm sure whatever emulsifier they use to replace it will be clean as a whistle. . . .

So if you can't have store-bought chicken soup or Gatorade when you're sick, what should you do?

- Rest. Your body is telling you it needs some time off. And skip your workout, for Pete's sake.
- Hydrate with plenty of pure water. Have some coconut water if you like. But if you're in the camp of avoiding fake food ingredients, then there's no more important time to eat and drink clean than when you're sick.
- Eat real food as clean and fresh as possible. Bone broth is a nutrient powerhouse.
- If it feels right, try fasting. Without the burden of digestion, your body can focus its energy to fight off infection. Fasting also starves bacteria and pathogens from their main fuel source, glucose. While most infectious substances can't live without glucose, you can run on fat instead.

Alyson, bless her heart, always whips me up a bone broth when I'm under the weather. It takes less than 10 minutes to prepare, but it can cut the duration of your cold in half. It has plenty of bug-fighting goodness that will fix you right up in no time.

HOW TO MAKE BONE BROTH OR SOUP STOCK

A good broth can raise the dead.
—*South American proverb*

To heal your gut, reverse aging, or add the ultimate superfood to your diet, make like the ancients and drink a daily cup of bone broth. Broths are rich in nutrients that are difficult to source elsewhere—incredibly high in vital minerals like calcium, phosphorous, magnesium, sodium, potassium, fluoride, and sulfur. If you don't make a habit of eating cuts of meat from the whole animal "nose to tail" (and even if you do), bone broths are a must. Know in advance that the nutrients in bone broth give off a unique smell—imagine what Yoda's kitchen smells like and you'll get the right idea. Put the slow cooker in the garage if you find the smell too rich for your taste.

You can use the bones (and legs from poultry, which are rich in über-restorative collagen) from pastured chicken, grass-fed cattle, fish, crustaceans, or anything else that was RAW. Leftovers work well, too—take the picked-over carcass of a roasted fowl or the leftover bones from a roast or seafood meal. If you're in a hurry, you can even throw in a whole fish.

Directions: Place your leftovers or bones into a large slow cooker. Add a splash of vinegar to help release the minerals from the bones. Fill the slow cooker with water to cover all of the meat completely.

Set your slow cooker to low and cook for at least 6 to 8 hours, preferably longer. When we want to keep it hot, we'll often let the bones simmer for 48 hours. When the cooker is cool enough to handle, pour the broth through a sieve into a glass storage container. Season with salt and pepper to taste. Use within 5 days or freeze it for later.

Here's an easy tip to make broth into soup—a few hours before serving, add vegetables (try diced carrots, celery, parsnips, sweet potatoes, or turnips) to the simmering bones so that your resulting broth becomes an instant soup base—full of flavor and the proper nutrients (especially bone marrow) to help restore your body.

HOW TO SURVIVE THE HOLIDAYS WITHOUT GETTING A SANTA BELLY

Every year without fail, someone on TV says that you'd better stick to skinless turkey breast out of Tupperware if you don't want to pack on the pounds during the holiday season.

"Control your portions . . . avoid delicious treats . . . and eat low-fat gravy products!" they nag.

We promise ourselves to be "disciplined this year" and vow to dodge all the desserts . . . then we drink a couple of cocktails, polish off the pumpkin pie, and feel guilty and fat for the rest of the month.

Why do we overeat during the holidays? Mostly, we just eat what's around us and the get-togethers and celebrations make avoiding sweets a Herculean task. On top of that, when family is close, drama isn't far behind, and suddenly that jug of eggnog looks like a worthy friend to snuggle up with next to the fire. Emotional eating (and drinking) ensues. This is especially true when a family member or friend questions your new "diet":

"What's wrong with you? You always loved fruitcake!"

(No, you didn't.)

You'll take some flack for politely declining your aunt Nelly's fruitcake—bless her heart for making it for you—but if you don't want to eat it, you don't have to. Remember, you always have a choice—you have 100 percent free agency over every morsel that crosses your lips. If you don't enjoy the heck out of what you eat, there's no point in choking it down.

HOW TO STAY LEAN DURING THE HOLIDAYS

- Focus on satiety: During the big meals, focus on eating to get full, not stuffed. You don't need to be counting calories or analyzing the ingredients, just chill out and load your plate up with 80 to 90 percent veggies and meats—foods that will satisfy you—then leave a little room to have a treat or two. If your meal satisfies you, you'll be much less likely to overeat.
- Know your trigger foods: Acknowledge which foods might trigger a binge episode and eat something else instead.
- Plan to indulge, but not to the point of sickness: Eat your favorite foods, but dedicate yourself to enjoying the process, not fearing what might happen. Plan to eat a cookie or two, savor them, then move on. Planning ahead eliminates anxiety, reduces guilt, and allows for balanced eating and drinking.
- Separate your emotions from food: The holidays are stressful. Don't use food to cope. In your plan, figure out what you're going to do when something tweaks you

out. How about a relaxing walk? A spot o' tea? A Will Ferrell movie? Try the breathing exercise on page 332.

- Relax and enjoy yourself: Be merry. Good vibes are contagious.

Remember, if you do overeat or "accidentally" binge on sugar cookies, use that food energy to fuel a killer workout. You may even build some muscle. Play outside, get your pump on, or hit the slopes and ride your sugar high down the mountain. Be active and use the cookie calories for good, not evil.

WHAT I DO WHEN I GAIN A FEW POUNDS

Here are the first things I do when I want to drop a few pounds fast:

- Skip breakfast and work out fasted.
- Increase the intensity, frequency, or weight of my workouts.
- Cycle carbs to less than 50 grams most days, with a higher-carb re-feed day on the weekend.
- Avoid alcohol.
- Avoid sugar.
- Eat more protein-rich and fibrous produce and fewer carbs and fats.
- Sleep more until I regularly wake up without an alarm.

WHAT TO DO ABOUT ALCOHOL

Most alcohol today is nothing like the medicinal tonics, and herbal liqueurs, and other spirits served by mustachioed barmen a hundred years ago. Today's beer, liquor, mixers, and more are made with GMO corn, chemicals, and cheap alcohol that leads to fat gain, liver damage, and vicious hangovers (right?). The gut-rot you see in advertisements is closer to bathtub gin than the premium beer or liquor described on the label. Most producers of alcoholic drinks in America don't even disclose the ingredients in their products, but many are known to contain plastics, artificial colors, and chemical flavorings.

Perhaps you've read that 1 to 2 drinks a day are good for you, which may very well be true. But there's a huge difference between imbibing once a week (1 to 2 drinks a week), and every night (7 to 14 drinks a week). One or two drinks a night quickly adds up to an *extra* 2,500 calories a week or more, which could mean the difference between fat loss and fat gain.

Since it's more important to your body to be alive than sober, when you take a drink, your liver stops burning fat and starts disposing of alcohol instead. Drinking also dulls the senses and increases the appetite, which won't help with fat loss. One or two glasses of wine or a few beers here and there probably won't hurt you, but all-night bingeing will. Limit your intake to a couple of drinks a week until your reach your fat-loss goal. But if maximizing fat loss is your ultimate goal, consider abstaining or limit drinking to special occasions.

Limiting or avoiding alcohol may be the most difficult thing some of you do to reach optimal wellness. Believe me, I understand. As a musician and former frat boy, I learned how to drink from true professionals—and I was often paid in booze. I learned after one too many hangovers that it's much more rewarding to drink for taste, not buzz. When I want to drop a few pounds, alcohol is the first thing to go. But if you just can't help yourself, here's a damage control strategy.

DAMAGE CONTROL STRATEGY WHEN DRINKING

- Drink one glass of fresh, pure water for every alcoholic drink you consume. Sip, don't slug.
- Limit yourself to 1 to 2 drinks a night and favor low-sugar options like dry red wine. Drink for taste, not buzz.
- Limit your intake of calories, especially carbohydrates. You might think that you're hungry, but that's just booze hijacking your hormones, so try to fight the cravings.

- Do your best to avoid beer, but if you must, then limit yourself to just one and stay away from stouts and porters, which have high amounts of residual sugars. Dry hard cider is a decent substitute for beer.
- If you drink hard liquor, avoid sugary mixers—they add up quickly. Many margaritas have more than 400 calories a pop!
- If you drink hard liquor, avoid "well" drinks made from cheap alcohol. Tequila, whiskey, vodka, it doesn't matter: Cheap alcohols are typically made from grain alcohol with added artificial flavors and colors. Get the good stuff and skip the hangover.
- Supplement with activated charcoal before you go to sleep to help you clear the leftover booze from your system. Activated charcoal binds to toxins like alcohol, which will help eliminate it from your system before it gives you a horrible hangover.
- If you want to hold something in your hand to not look awkward at a party, here's a nice trick: Ask for sparkling water with a slice of lemon or lime—no booze but reminiscent of a refreshing vodka tonic.

ABEL'S ADVENTURE PACK

When the going gets weird, the weird turn pro.

—*Hunter S. Thompson*

I tried the "American Dream" of living in a million-dollar house, driving a Porsche, and having maids, staff, and even a concierge. But it just didn't take. After about six months, we sold off all of our belongings and decided to live lean and travel the world, living off-the-grid in the wilderness of state and national parks.

I might say that I left my fancy house, fast car, and desk job behind to live like Davy Crockett. Others might say I'm the strange fellow who lives in a trailer with his dog. Either way, this is how we choose to live, and we love it. We don't "go shopping," we brave the mountain roads into town to get *supplies*. We usually don't have running water, emulating the hardscrabble life of bygone times, when washing the dishes by hand is meaningful, carrying water is exercise, and adventure finds you every day. In a sense, we live like most people camp. We live out of a trailer that's meant to haul ATVs, but we've filled ours with guitars, adventure gear, great food, and a rambunctious yellow Lab.

Whether it's an excursion to the local coffee shop or to the top of the Rockies, I don't leave home without my pack of food, spices, herbs, supplements, and other items that support healthy habits. No matter what happens, making a good decision is as simple as reaching into my bag. If you have itchy feet and an adventurous spirit like us, I hope sharing the contents of my pack will help you in your travels.

All of the supplies on the following pages fit into the small front pocket of my carry-on backpack with my laptop, hoodie, books, recording equipment, and more. Most of these things cost a few dollars or less but can save you hundreds on the road because you won't really need to buy anything from convenience stores, restaurants, or anywhere else. Plan in advance and guarantee your success and comfort no matter where you are or what the world puts in front of you.

NONPERISHABLES	
Canned fish Nut butter / coconut butter packets Dried meat / jerky Dehydrated veggies Greens / spirulina powder Protein powder	Sometimes you get hungry and your body tells you that fasting isn't an option. Bring a few nonperishables in addition to fresh foods to make sure you never get stuck eating low-quality food just because someone put it in front of you.
SEASONING AND SPICE PACK	
Salt and pepper Chia and kelp Garlic Hot chiles Cinnamon Cocoa	Often, it's better to get fresh food from markets than to eat at a low-quality restaurant. Save money and preserve your health by seasoning fresh foods yourself. I put these in an ultra-convenient "spice missile," which cost less than 10 bucks.
Coconut oil	Salad dressing, coffee creamer, antibacterial moisturizer, hair gel, toothpaste (with baking soda and mint), deodorant, lubricant.

Activated charcoal	Detoxifying agent, antidiarrheal, hangover prevention / cure, tooth whitener.
Water bottle with charcoal pack	Five bucks for a bottle of water, you kidding me? Reduce waste and save money by carrying your own BPA-free water bottle / thermos, and drink water wherever you can find it or make teas and tonics. Charcoal pack—I use VAPUR—partially removes toxins and other nasties like chlorine, fluoride, and improves taste.
Teas, tonics, stress-reducing adaptogens	Enjoy as a tea, tonic, or in concentrated supplements. My favorites: rhodiola, gymnostemma, ginseng, kava for stress reduction, sleep, and alcohol alternative, ginger tea for upset stomach, chamomile for sleep.
Melatonin and magnesium	Carry melatonin and magnesium to reset jet lag and give your body a boost when you've been exposed to artificial light or stress at night and can't sleep. Also, it's difficult to get magnesium on the road since it's a bulky mineral, but take it at night to help your muscles recover and improve your sleep.
Ibuprofen	For aches, pains, fevers, or use as an anti-inflammatory when you overdo it or get injured.
Lacrosse ball	Use it for self-massage to roll out angry knots, keep yourself limber and healthy on the road. Use it for catch when you're bored.
Chocolate	Never get caught without chocolate. It will get you through even the roughest of days. No matter what happens, you'll feel better knowing delicious chocolate is waiting for you in your bag.

Mineral-based sunscreen	Some sun is good for you, but getting burned isn't. Keep natural, zinc-based sunscreen handy and, if you have a big nose like me, spackle it right on there and make sure you don't get fried.
Sunglasses	Nobody likes to squint. We have enough wrinkles already. Make sure to wear only glasses with UV protection, as cheap glasses without it can cause cataracts.
Blue-blocking glasses	Sometimes you have to fight fire with fire. These are great in airports or to be used at night when you're blasted with artificial light from the environment or electronics if you want to work at night or enjoy a movie.
Sea or mineral salt	Use mineral salt to flavor foods, add trace minerals, as an electrolyte on sweaty days, or as an exfoliating face scrub.
Waterproof earplugs and eye mask	You never know what's lurking in that water. Use waterproof earplugs in water that might be suspect, and use them to block excess noise with your eye mask on flights and in noisy areas to help you sleep.
Topical antibiotic	Do yourself a favor and keep a little tube in your bag. Topical agents can help treat small wounds before you're forced to take an antibiotic, which is like setting off a napalm balm in your stomach and kills off your hard-earned good gut bacteria.
Soil-based probiotic	Keep your gut bugs healthy by inviting their friends to join the party with a high-quality probiotic.
Noise-canceling headphones / noise-blocking earbuds	Wearing these on planes, trains, and buses can be the difference between feeling fried and being totally fine. Keep your stress low by blocking out the madness and rocking out with your favorite tunes, binaural beats, audiobooks, or other fun alternatives.

PEMF sleep-induction device	It sounds crazy, but for me sometimes it's the difference between tossing and turning for hours and conking out in five minutes. Try the EarthPulse on the "Sleep 4" setting.
GMO-free xylitol gum	Sometimes I just want to keep eating, but this gives me something to satisfy my oral fixation, especially after meals when I know my body is full but my mouth still wants to eat. Bonus—keeps your breath fresh.
Spork	Sporks are awesome. I'm not sure why every restaurant insists on giving us fourteen forks with every meal, but be friendly to the planet and say you don't need one. And way better than eating sardines with your hands.

PARTING WORDS

In 1958, our family farm was written up in the *Ladies' Home Journal*. "It wasn't a perfect life," my grandmother says, but one that "convinces you that you're needed."

A DAY ON THE FAMILY FARM

At 5:30 a.m. on a snowy New Hampshire morning, Horace and Marion Bascom wake to the "baby alarm" from upstairs. In the tiny 150-year-old farmhouse's one downstairs bedroom, the thermometer reads 4 degrees, "four above nothing!" Dairy farmer Horace gulps a glass of milk and spreads home-churned butter on a thick slab of Marion's baked-yesterday bread. He is off to the barn to milk 27 cows before breakfast at 9 a.m.

Marion helps stack logs on a hand-built sled carrier. At home, first-born son Donnie is in charge of brothers and sisters. If all behave well, everybody can make mint or maple candy in the evening—a special treat supervised by Marion.

Marion wanted to see the world as an Army nurse, became a farmer's wife instead, is now family barber, sewing expert, jelly maker (100+ jars a year)—"a life that convinces you that you're needed."

Marion has a cup of coffee (with "lots of milk in it" as a token to her husband's work) and braces for a descent of blue-eyed children from the attic bedrooms. After chores and hot whole-grain oatmeal with maple syrup tapped from the trees outside, the older children board the 7:45 bus to school.

Marion prepares an after-milking breakfast for Horace and readies pork and beans to cook in the oven for lunch. By 9:30 a.m., the sink is full of dishes to be washed—and washed, and washed (by hand)—her least favorite job.

Between chores and blizzards—time to feed pets, hunt torn evergreen branches to be holiday decoration. A week ahead of Christmas, Marion begins baking sugar cookies and cranberry bread "to feast all the friends who come to help us hunt a tree."

Amidst the dishes and jackets and milk pails, hair ribbons and mismatched boots and bits of kindling in the small homestead on the harsh New Hampshire hills, Horace reads his heavy black Bible before each family meal as his six children and wife bow their heads.

"We thank Thee, Lord," Horace may say, "for this good bread and the strength that comes from it." Bascoms have always worked the stubborn New Hampshire earth. "An old woman at church," Horace tells his wife, "told me last Sunday she'd sung next to five generations of Bascoms. When she was a little girl, my great-grandfather and grandfather sang bass and tenor."

In a child-filled house with flaking paint and cracked walls, her still-slim 128 pound, 5'4" frame moves energetically through the day, with hanging clothes outside and piling logs outside "recreation."

"It's a chance to get away from the children once in a while."

Marion, who couldn't cook when she married as a city girl out of Boston at 23, canned 800 jars of fruit and vegetables last year, made 100 jars of jams and jellies, including wild grape (picked in the hills), crab apple, strawberry, and orange-carrot marmalade. In the cellar, a year-long stock of preserves glints in brilliant colors in the semi dark. A food locker in town holds sides of Horace's home-grown beef. From poultry-farming neighbors, Bascoms buy fresh fowl tagged at a low 15 cents a pound, cracked eggs for 35 cents a dozen. The milk supply is plentiful 30 yards from the back door. Nine-year-old Donnie churns the butter.

"And everybody helps weed the garden, when it gets weeded." Usually everybody is too busy with other chores, and the plants shift for themselves. Organic farmer Horace, opposed to using poisonous sprays, has a special pride in their perfection. "We organic farmers are a minority," Horace says, but an enlightened one, he feels, respecting Nature's own equilibrium and refusing to chemically adulterate any food.

Tomatoes hot from the sun, crisp white and red cabbages, crunchy carrots and cucumbers go into the salads Marion serves at each meal. "And we grow our own peas, lettuce, chicory, radishes—nobody likes them, but they come up fast!—beans, corn, broccoli, squash, parsnips, rhubarb, beets, kale, almost anything you can name" in two big gardens outside the door.

For variety, too, Marion hunts delicacies for the diet. Giant mushrooms found around maple and elm trees are fried in butter. "Boiled milkweed sprouts taste like young asparagus, and sometimes we have dandelion greens with salt pork. Or lamb's-quarters—a weed that tastes just like spinach." With her chicken pies, beef stews, applesauce cakes, 7 young Bascoms have sprouted as healthily as the garden. For extra food, Bascoms have kept as many as 20 geese, broody hens to hatch the eggs.

All year long the stoves go to provide hot water in a too-small tank that can't be converted to electricity for lack of funds. The milk check, almost $1,000 a month, leaves less than $150 a month for all family expenses. The rest goes to pay debts, and Marion spends a great deal of her time budgeting.

Laundering and ironing for nine people, cleaning house, canning harvests, raising children, helping saw wood are only part of Marion's work. Meals are a big job. 7 a.m. breakfast for the 7 children, 9-o'clock breakfast for Horace, hot meal at 1 for strength until sundown, 4 p.m. after-school snacks, a hot meal at 7 p.m. for the children (who had only sandwiches at noon—school lunches cost 25 cents each), a final meal for Horace at 8:30 p.m.

For the vast majority of human existence, food was fresh and grew nearby. Until quite recently, our food came from the family garden, the village greengrocer, butcher, or fishmonger. Eggs were laid by the clucking chickens roaming around the backyard, digging up grubs and pecking at seeds. Fresh fish were sourced from the pond at the end of a line on a lazy Sunday afternoon.

Before the era of industrial food production, food was simple. Only the wealthy could afford packaged food, sweets, and baked goods made from processed white flour. Fruit was something you found in the bottom of your Christmas stocking, and ice cream took all day to churn. Food "processing" was done in the home using ancient techniques that preserve or enhance nutrients, such as sprouting, fermenting, canning, salting, or smoking. The homestead was a place of *production*, not consumption.

Those were the good old days, before corporate agribusiness nuked victory gardens with Roundup. Industrialization, processing, and the development of artificial flavorings, preservatives, dyes, and other additives brought on a new and frightening era where natural, fresh, real ingredients from the earth were replaced by waste products from the petroleum and chemical industries. Our wholesome family meals were swapped for chemically adulterated food products designed to keep us hungry for more. These days, the ingredient lists on bags and boxes in the supermarket read more like inventory from Walter White's chemistry lab than anything you'd recognize as real food.

In contrast to the idyllic farms and happy cows you see on food labels, modern agriculture was not built on the sweat, love, and toil of the farmer in his field, but on the strategic planning of Fortune 500 corporations. The sweetness of today's cookies and pies taste comes not from the skill of the cook, but the tinkering of white-coated scientists who design their products to be as addictive as possible. They know exactly what will keep us coming back for more: industrial salt, processed fat, artificial flavors, and concentrated sugar, and now these pernicious ingredients seem to be in everything. But we've had enough.

There's a movement afoot. Can you feel it? It's a monumental shift back to fresh, old-fashioned, real food. We're tired of being manipulated by Big Food's deceptive marketing and flavors designed in labs. We're sick of mistreated animals and processed foods devoid of real flavor and real nourishment. It's time to bring back the family dinner and remember that cooking is a gift and a tremendous opportunity to nourish the people you love.

As a responsible shopper, you have the power to change the way things are. So grab your recycled shopping bag. We're taking to the farmers' market in droves. Vote with your dollar and *demand* high-quality food. Your family has the right to be healthy, active, and well fed, and our collective future depends on it.

There are now more than four thousand local farmers' markets in the United States, and the number has doubled in ten years. Backyard and patio gardening is cool again, even for the hipsters. Volunteers are rejuvenating cities with community gardens. Organic sales are growing, we're working hard to get real food back into the schools, and our cooking apps are outselling Angry Birds. Some of us are even foraging in our own backyards—learning about edible plants, berries, herbs, and mushrooms, and gathering these free foods wherever they grow naturally. As Mom says, it doesn't get much cheaper than "eating the weeds." It doesn't get much healthier, either.

You can be a part of this incredible movement, too. The book you're holding in your hands right now has everything you need to make it happen. There is no perfect time to start. It might as well be now. Embrace the journey—it will last the rest of your life.

Before I sign off, I have a small request for you. If you know someone who might enjoy this book—a friend, family member, or coworker—please share it with them. And if you'd like the free recipes, cooking classes, exercise videos, and other downloadable resources we prepared to accompany this book, please visit wilddietbook.com to join in the fun.

In health and happiness,
Abel James

NOTES

PART I

. . . current research shows that a leaky gut is one of the major . . .

de Kort, Selvino, Daniel Keszthelyi, and A. A. M. Masclee. "Leaky gut and diabetes mellitus: what is the link?" *Obesity Reviews* 12, no. 6 (June 2011): 449–58.

Fasano, Alessio. "Leaky Gut and Autoimmune Diseases." *Clinical Reviews in Allergy & Immunology* 42, no. 1 (February 2012): 71–78.

The average forty-year-old man in 1960 . . .

FastStats: Body Measurements. Centers for Disease Control and Prevention. Accessed November 2, 2014. http://www.cdc.gov/nchs/fastats/body-measurements.htm.

Ogden, Cynthia L., Cheryl D. Fryar, Margaret D. Carroll, and Katherine M. Flegal. "Mean Body Weight, Height, and Body Mass Index, United States 1960–2002." *Advance Data from Vital and Health Statistics* 347 (October 2004).

One in three U.S. children born in 2000 will become diabetic . . .

"Number of Americans with Diabetes Projected to Double or Triple by 2050." Centers for Disease Control and Prevention. Press release. October 22, 2010. Accessed November 2, 2014. http://www.cdc.gov/media/pressrel/2010/r101022.html.

Olshansky, S. J., D. J. Passaro, R. C. Hershow, J. Layden, B. A. Carnes, J. Brody, L. Hayflick, R. N. Butler, D. B. Allison, and D. S. Ludwig. "A Potential Decline in Life Expectancy in the United States in the 21st Century." *New England Journal of Medicine* 352, no. 11 (March 2005): 1138–45.

Since agribusiness began genetically altering wheat in 1960, concentrations of zinc, copper, iron, and magnesium plummeted . . .

Fana, Ming-Sheng, Fang-Jie Zhaoa, Susan J. Fairweather-Taitc, Paul R. Poultona, Sarah J. Dunhama, and Steve P. McGratha. "Evidence of decreasing mineral density in wheat grain over the last 160 years." *Journal of Trace Elements in Medicine and Biology* 22 (2008): 320.

Why is the same company that manufactured Agent Orange, a highly toxic herbicide responsible . . .

Martin, Michael F. "Vietnamese Victims of Agent Orange and U.S.-Vietnam Relations." *Congressional Research Service*. August 29, 2012. 22–23.

According to the Non-GMO Project . . .

"What is GMO? Agricultural Crops That Have a Risk of Being GMO." Non-GMO Project. Accessed January 15, 2015. http://www.nongmoproject.org/learn-more/what-is-gmo/.

Since nearly all the soy produced in the United States and Canada is . . .

"Recent Trends in GE Adoption: Adoption of genetically engineered crops in the United States, 1996–2014." United States Department of Agriculture Economic Research Service. July 14, 2014. Accessed January 7, 2015. http://www.ers.usda.gov/data-products/adoption-of-genetically-engineered-crops-in-the-us/recent-trends-in-ge-adoption.aspx.

FDA loopholes allow food manufacturers to manipulate the nutrition facts . . .

Silverglade, Bruce, and Ilene Ringel Heller. *Food Labeling Chaos: The Case for Reform.* (Center for Science in the Public Interest: Washington, D.C., 2010), xiii, ix, x. http://www.cspinet.org/new/pdf/food_labeling_chaos_report.pdf.

Scientists frequently inject lab rats with MSG to literally *induce* obesity . . .

Hernández, J. A. Fernandez-Tresguerres. "[Effect of monosodium glutamate given orally on appetite control: A new theory for the obesity epidemic.] [Translated from Spanish.]" *Anales de la Real Academia Nacional de Medicina* 122, no. 2 (2005): 341–55; discussion 355–60.

And that's just the short list . . .

"Flavor Ingredients Fact Sheet." Vigon International. Accessed January 15, 2015. http://www.vigon.com/flavor-ingredients.aspx.

Today, the U.S. Department of Agriculture reports . . .

USDA. *Agriculture Fact Book 2001–2002.* USDA: Washington, D.C., March 2003: 20. http://usda.gov/factbook/2002factbook.pdf.

Aspartame (NutraSweet) was discovered in the 1980s . . .

Steginik, Lewis D., and L. J. Filer, Jr. *Aspartame: Physiology and Biochemistry.* (New York: Food Science and Technology 1984), 3.

After a twenty-one-year-old male gorilla named Brooks died of heart failure in 2005 . . .

Gabel, David A. "Captive Gorillas Succumbing to Human Disease." *Environmental News Network.* February 22, 2011. http://www.enn.com/wildlife/article/42383.

PART II

In fact, regardless of overall weight, men with waists exceeding 40 inches . . .

"Classification of Overweight and Obesity by BMI, Waist Circumference, and Associated Disease Risks." National Heart, Lung, and Blood Institute. http://www.nhlbi.nih.gov/health/educational/lose_wt/BMI/bmi_dis.htm.

A recent study found that about 49 percent . . .

Barksdale, J. *Pharmacotherapy,* 19 (May 1999): 573–581.

Another study, published in the *Journal of Urology* . . .

Burchardt, M. *Journal of Urology,* 164 (October 2000): 1188–1191.

For example, commonly prescribed drugs that treat high blood pressure . . .

Schooling, C. Mary, Shiu Lun Au Yeung, Guy Freeman, Benjamin J. Cowling. "The effect of statins on testosterone in men and women, a systematic review and meta-analysis of randomized controlled trials." *BMC Medicine* 11, no. 1 (May 2013): 3–7.

. . . wrong species of bacteria in lab mice can even make them gain fat . . .

Yin, Ya-Ni, Qiong-Fen Yu, Nian Fu, Xiao-Wei Liu, and Fang-Gen Lu. "Effects of four Bifidobacteria on obesity in high-fat diet induced rats." *World Journal of Gastroenterology* 16, no. 27 (July 2010): 3394–401.

The average American age forty-five and older . . .

Barrett, Linda. "Prescription Drug Use Among Midlife and Older Americans." *AARP Research* (April 2005): 4.

Today, more than 67 percent of us in the United States are overweight or obese . . .
"Statistical Fact Sheet 2013 Update: Overweight & Obesity." American Heart Association. http://www.heart.org/idc/groups/heart-public/@wcm/@sop/@smd/documents/downloadable/ucm_319588.pdf.

One study showed that while fasting for twenty-four hours, human growth . . .
Intermountain Medical Center. "Routine periodic fasting is good for your health, and your heart, study suggests." *ScienceDaily.* Accessed May 20, 2011. www.sciencedaily.com/releases/2011/04/110403090259.htm.

"97 percent of the most common class of cold cereals . . ."
"Children's Cereals: Sugar by the Pound: Cereals Contain Far More Sugar than Experts Recommend." Environmental Working Group. May 15, 2014. Accessed November 3, 2014. http://www.ewg.org/research/childrens-cereals-sugar-pound/cereals-contain-far-more-sugar-experts-recommend.

Some studies show that breakfast can actually boost hunger . . .
Hatori, Megumi, Christopher Vollmers, Amir Zarrinpar, Luciano DiTacchio, Eric A. Bushong, Shubhroz Gill, Mathias Leblanc, Amandine Chaix, Matthew Joens, James A. J. Fitzpatrick, Mark H. Ellisman, Satchidananda Panda. "Time-Restricted Feeding without Reducing Caloric Intake Prevents Metabolic Diseases in Mice Fed a High-Fat Diet." *Cell Metabolism* 15, no. 6 (June 2012): 848–60.

. . . eating low-carb boosts the body's response . . .
Volek, Jeff S., Matthew J. Sharman, Dawn M. Love, Neva G. Avery, Ana L. Gómez, Timothy P. Scheett, William J. Kraemer. "Body composition and hormonal responses to a carbohydrate-restricted diet." *Metabolism* 51, no. 7 (July 2002): 864–70.

PART III

Impressed by their epic feats of athleticism during the hunt, he wrote . . .
de Vaca, Álvar Núñez Cabeza. *The Account: Álvar Núñez Cabeza de Vaca's Relación.* Translated by Martin A. Favata and José B. Fernandez (Houston: Arte Público Press, 1993): 44, 56, 59.

This routine is based on science developed by the Japanese Olympic . . .
Tabata I., K. Irisawa, M. Kouzaki, K. Nishimura, F. Ogita, and M. Miyachi. "Metabolic profile of high intensity intermittent exercises." *Medicine & Science in Sports & Exercise* 29, no. 3 (March 1997): 390–95.
Pottenger, Francis M. Jr. *Pottenger's Cats.* (Lemon Grove, CA: Price-Pottenger Nutrition Foundation, Inc., 1983).

PART IV

Now, type 2 diabetes is a full-blown epidemic . . .
American Diabetes Association. "Economic Costs of Diabetes in the U.S. in 2012." *Diabetes Care* 36, no. 4 (April 2013): 1033–46.

In fact, research shows that some saturated fat can . . .
Geleijnse, Johanna M., Cees Vermeer, Diederick E. Grobbee, Leon J. Schurgers, Marjo H. J. Knapen, Irene M. van der Meer, Albert Hofman, and Jacqueline C. M. Witteman. "Dietary intake of menaquinone is associated with a reduced risk of coronary heart disease: the Rotterdam Study." *The Journal of Nutrition*, 134, no. 11 (November 2004): 3100–5.

In fact, you're just as likely to have a heart attack . . .
Bathum, Lise, René Depont Christensen, Lars Engers Pedersen, Palle Lyngsie Pedersen, John

Larsen, and Jørgen Nexøe. "Association of lipoprotein levels with mortality in subjects aged 50 + without previous diabetes or cardiovascular disease: A population-based register study." *Scandinavian Journal of Primary Health Care* 31, no. 3 (September 2013): 172–80.

And in some studies, high cholesterol is . . .

Hamazaki, T., H. Okuyama, Y. Ogushi, and R. Hama. "Cholesterol Issues in Japan—Why Are the Goals of Cholesterol Levels Set So Low?" *Annals of Nutrition and Metabolism* 62, no. 1 (January 2013): 32–36.

In the Thai language, "How are you?" translates . . .

Gomez, Kwanchai A., *"Rice, The Grain of Culture"* (The Siam Society Lecture Series, the Siam Society, Bangkok, Thailand, September 20, 2001).

While hunter-gatherers in the Australian outback . . .

Brand-Miller, J. C., and S. H. Holt. "Australian Aboriginal plant foods: A consideration of their nutritional composition and health implications." *Nutrition Research Reviews* 11, no. 1 (June 1998): 5–23.

. . . it's common for factory farms to feed their cows industrial poultry litter . . .

The Code of Federal Regulations of the United States of America. (Washington, D.C.: U.S. Government Printing Office, 1970): 98.

One Harvard study found that healthy men and women . . .

Hu, F. B., M. J. Stampfer, E. B. Rimm, et al. "A prospective study of egg consumption and risk of cardiovascular disease in men and women." *Journal of the American Medical Association* 281, no. 15 (1999): 1387–94.

But several thousand years ago, about 40 percent of us adapted the ability . . .

"Lactose Intolerance." Genetics Home Reference. May 2010. http://ghr.nlm.nih.gov/condition/lactose-intolerance.

PART VII

In a study in the 1970s in Ann Arbor, Roger S. Ulrich . . .

Ulrich, Roger. "Human responses to vegetation and landscapes." *Landscape and Urban Planning* 13 (1986): 29–44.

But willpower is weak, and that's why 92 percent of New Year's resolutions fail . . .

Norcross, J. C., M. S. Mrykalo, and M. D. Blagys. *"Auld lang Syne*: Success predictors, change processes, and self-reported outcomes of New Year's resolvers and nonresolvers." *Journal of Clinical Psychology* 58, no. 4 (April 2002): 397–405.

Bromine-containing sedatives resulted in emergency . . .

"What is brominated vegetable oil?" What Is That Ingredient? Accessed November 3, 2014. http://whatisthatingredient.com/ingredient.php?id=65.

ACKNOWLEDGMENTS

The Wild Diet is a highly collaborative work. There are many to thank—my fans, family, and friends—and all of you inspired me to write this book more than you know. I thank you all deeply for your many contributions, hard work, and damn-the-torpedoes belief that the message of health and happiness needs to get out there. This book would have been impossible to write without each and every one of you. I sincerely hope it leaves a legacy we can all be proud of.

First, I'd like to thank my lovely wife, Alyson, for the recipes, love, and back rubs that made this book possible; Mom and Dad for being guinea pigs, sharing our family recipes, and many late-night conversations (with too much wine) that made their way into the manuscript; Mark and Lindsay for helping us get dirt under our fingernails; Nan and Horace Bascom for inspiring us to live in harmony with the land; the Bridge family for incredible support and hospitality (and plenty of vitamin C); Megan, Gigi, Andrea Ho, and the publicity team for saving this silly book; Peter Hoppenfeld for playing Bad Cop; Tyler Archer for making magic happen every day; the multitalented Melinda Bryce who helped cook, write, and research this book into existence; and Peter Nesbitt for making sure nothing blows up while we live off the grid.

I'd also like to thank Denny Hemmingson for the best thank-you note I've ever received; the Tim McGraw band—Deano, Billy, Tim, Adam—for making health cool again; Tucker Max for telling me the truth about how books really get published; Tim Ferriss for standing by his beans; Dave Asprey for putting butter in my coffee; the Dartmouth Aires for inspiring me to abandon all shame; Ruth Wahl for accidentally convincing me not to become a spy; Leonard Strickman for telling me he didn't like my day job; Tobias for guiding me through a crazy world; Pedram Shojai for breaking my foot so grandmaster Carl could heal it; George Bryant for making the best pulled pork on earth; Michael Lovitch and Wallis Carter for never pulling a punch; Dr. Sara and David Gottfried for great wine and inappropriate dancing; Jonathan Bailor for his uncanny Arnold Schwarzenegger impression; Michael Fishman for inspiring thousands to kick the sugar habit; Mark Sisson for showing me the ropes; Alan Christianson for being a forty-year-old kid; Paul Jaminet for deep conversations; Ori Hofmekler for championing fasting before it was fashionable; Danny Dreyer for teaching me how to run without legs; Jamie Tardy for always finding an excuse for a get-together; Ryan Lee for reminding me to always put my family first; Jimmy Moore for humbly accepting my very first interview; Dean Dwyer for always making us smile; my friends at Dartmouth College, New Hampton, Sphinx, Sigma Phi Epsilon for showing me that real learning happens in the woods; and the Environmental Working Group for fighting the good fight.

I'm deeply indebted to the American Red Cross for helping me get back on my feet after losing everything in an apartment fire; Miss Teen Utah for convincing me to try my first green smoothie; the Bascom family for showing us a proper feast; Aunt Kate, who taught us how to bake love right into cookies; Matt Fenton for being an incredible role model without knowing it; Derek Senft for bleaching my hair; Trevor Lowell for showing me how to have a great time in the woods; Ryan Chesley for showing me how to write while furiously pacing around the room; Dave Potter for teaching me how to make pancakes from scratch; John French for keeping it warm; Tom Waits, Johnny Cash, and Greg Brown for inspiring me to use my voice; Jillian Bennett for convincing me to dance and sing; Carl Orr, who taught me humility through the ritual of tea; Scott King and David Gagne for showing me that sometimes playing music is healthier than eating lunch; Marc Elbaum for teaching me about life through music; Rick Elkin, who showed me how to be happy with fewer things; Matt Cheney, who forced me to read terrible poetry; and of course, Bailey, for reminding me every day that an unexpected tromp through the woods is just what the doctor ordered.

Thank you once again for the incredible work, guidance, and insight that made this book possible. I am in deep gratitude to you all.

358 ACKNOWLEDGMENTS

INDEX

activity. *See* exercise and activity
adventure pack, 342–46
adventures, 329
aging, 58–59, 61
Ahi Tuna, Seared, with Sesame-Ginger Asparagus, 193–95
alcohol consumption, 340–42
Alfredo, Cashew Cream, with Zucchini Noodles, 219–20
aloe vera juice, *in* Green Juice Detox, 248
Alyson's Coffee Cake, 256–57
anabolic effects, 67, 78, 101
animal nutrition
   dog food recipes, 322–25
   fasting, 320–21, 326
   feeding guideline, 322
   foods to avoid, 326
   native natural diet, 38–39
   processed pet food, 316–18
   raw food experiments, 109
   raw meat and bones, 318–20
antiaging, 58–59, 61
antibiotics, 54
Apple Cider Donuts, 255–56
apples
   Field Green Salad with Apples and Buttered Pecans, 215–17
   Old-Fashioned Apple Pie, 262–64
   Pear, Apple, and Rosemary Spa Water, 246

Artichokes, Roasted, Baked Pesto Salmon with, 197–200
artificial flavoring, 31–32
artificial sweeteners, 37
Arugula, Beef Tenderloin with Buttered Onions, Horseradish, and, 181–83
Asparagus, Sesame-Ginger, Seared Ahi Tuna with, 193–95
athletes
   carb consumption, 105, 311–12
   high-intensity exercise, 80–81, 82–83
   injuries, 333–35
avocados
   Bison Taco Salad with Avocado, 170–72
   Chipotle Steak and Veggie Fajitas with Fresh Guacamole, 167–69
   Creamy Cilantro-Lime Smoothie, 237
   Fish Tacos with Mango-Avocado Salsa, 203–4
   Parmesan Shrimp Lettuce Wraps with Avocado, 195–97
   Swordfish with Spicy Peach Salsa, 209–10

bacon
   Bacon-Wrapped Scallops and Sweet Slaw, 200–202

Hearty Pancake Breakfast, 228–30
Hot-as-the-Devil Eggs, 280–81
Ultimate Bacon Burger, 172–74
bacteria in human microbiome, 53–55, 136
Baked Pesto Salmon with Roasted Artichokes, 197–200
Balsamic Mustard Greens, Beef Brisket with, 174–77
Balsamic-Roasted Sweet Potatoes, Farmer's Omelets with, 230–32
bananas, *in* Spiced Blueberry Smoothie, 239–40
BBQ Sauce, Wild, *for* Pulled Pork Sliders, 159
beans and legumes
   proper preparation, 123
   secondary choices, 139
   to soak, 271–72
beef
   Beef Brisket with Balsamic Mustard Greens, 174–77
   Beef Supreme (for dogs), 322
   Beef Taco Salad with Avocado (swap suggestion), 172
   Beef Tenderloin with Buttered Onions, Horseradish, and Arugula, 181–83
   Chimichurri Steak and Roasted Brussels Sprouts, 183–85

beef (*cont.*)

Chipotle Steak and Veggie Fajitas with Fresh Guacamole, 167–69

Dried Beef Liver Treats (for dogs), 324

Spicy Beef Chili with Mashed Sweet Potato, 179–81

Steak and Eggs (for dogs), 325

Sun-Dried Tomato Meatballs with Zucchini Noodles, 188–90

Ultimate Bacon Burger, 172–74

beet greens, *in* Strawberry "Milk Shake," 239

beets

Ginger Lamb Chops with Roasted Vegetables, 186–88

Strawberry "Milk Shake," 239

Sweet Potato Hash, 221–22

bell peppers

Chipotle Steak and Veggie Fajitas with Fresh Guacamole, 167–69

Creamy Roasted Vegetable Soup, 217–19

Farmer's Omelets with Balsamic-Roasted Sweet Potatoes, 230–32

Roasted Red Pepper Mini Pizzas, 226–28

Spicy Beef Chili with Mashed Sweet Potato, 179–81

berries

Beef Brisket with Balsamic Mustard Greens, 174–77

Cucumber-Strawberry Spa Water, 244–45

Nan's Blueberry Salad, 264–65

Rosemary-Raspberry Smoothie, 238

Spiced Blueberry Smoothie, 239–40

Strawberry "Milk Shake," 239

beverages. *See* drinks

Big Food. *See also* processed foods

Betty Crocker character, 24

deceptive marketing statements, 27–28

distortion of nutrition facts, 28–29, 34, 59

factory farming, 111, 114–15, 118

profit motive, 14–15, 39

Birthday Cake with Whipped Chocolate Topping, 259–60

bison

Bison Taco Salad with Avocado, 170–72

Wild Shepherd's Pie, 177–79

blueberries

Nan's Blueberry Salad, 264–65

Spiced Blueberry Smoothie, 239–40

bone broth or stock, 337–38

Bone Marrow, Roasted, 278

Bones, Raw Meaty (for dogs), 323

brain growth, 78

Brazil nuts, 51

Bread, Pumpkin, 267–68

breads, packaged, 18–19

breakfast

dangers of, 59–60

green smoothies for, 112–13

Hearty Pancake Breakfast, 228–30

low-carb choices, 62

Brisket, Beef, with Balsamic Mustard Greens, 174–77

broccoli

Creamy Roasted Vegetable Soup, 217–19

Green Monster Frittata with Bruschetta, 213–15

Immune-Boosting Veggie-Full Soup, 222–24

Slow-Cooker Chicken with Roasted Broccoli and Mushrooms, 164–66

Brown Rice, 274–75

Bruschetta, Green Monster Frittata with, 213–15

Brussels Sprouts, Roasted, Chimichurri Steak and, 183–85

Burger, Ultimate Bacon, 172–74

burpees exercise, 83

Butter Pecan Ice Cream, 266

cabbage

Bacon-Wrapped Scallops and Sweet Slaw, 200–202

Creamy Chopped Slaw, *for* Pulled Pork Sliders, 159

Simple Sauerkraut, 276–77

cakes

Alyson's Coffee Cake, 256–57

Birthday Cake with Whipped Chocolate Topping, 259–60

Carrot Cake, 257–59

calories

in alcoholic drinks, 341

calorie restriction, 57–58, 125

liquid sugar calories, 36, 310

numbers on nutrition facts labels, 28–29

in nutrient-poor processed foods, 15–16

zero-calorie artificial sweeteners, 37

Caprese Salad, Lemon Kalamata Chicken Breasts with, 154–56

carbohydrates

for athletes, 311–12

in body's storage of fat, 94–95, 102–3

categories, 103

glycemic effect, 23–24, 60, 105–6, 121–22

ketogenic diet, 311

net carbs, 103, 106

slow-burning versus quick-burning, 105–6

timing of consumption, 62, 106, 122

carrots

Carrot Cake, 257–59

Cashew Cream Alfredo with Zucchini Noodles, 219–20

Creamy Roasted Vegetable Soup, 217–19

Immune-Boosting Veggie-Full Soup, 222–24

Mom's Homemade Chicken Soup, 150–52

Peaches 'n' Cream Smoothie, 242

Thai Carrot Curry Soup with Zucchini Chips, 224–26

Wild Shepherd's Pie, 177–79
cashews
    Cashew Cream Alfredo with
        Zucchini Noodles, 219–20
    Peanut Butter Chocolate
        "Cheesecake" with
        Hazelnut Crust, 250–51
    to soak and dehydrate, 269
cauliflower
    Creamy Roasted Vegetable
        Soup, 217–19
    Low-and-Slow Rubbed Ribs
        with Whipped
        Cauliflower, 162–63
    Spicy Chicken Thigh Stir-Fry
        and Cauliflower Fried
        Rice, 148–50
celery
    Creamy Cilantro-Lime
        Smoothie, 237
    Creamy Roasted Vegetable
        Soup, 217–19
    Green Juice Detox, 248
    Mom's Homemade Chicken
        Soup, 150–52
    Virgin Bloody Mary Smoothie,
        240–41
cheddar cheese, in Ultimate
        Bacon Burger, 172–74
cheese. See also dairy foods
    Chicken Parmesan with Mixed
        Greens, 143–45
    Lemon Kalamata Chicken
        Breasts with Caprese
        Salad, 154–56
    Nan's Blueberry Salad, 264–65
    Parmesan Shrimp Lettuce
        Wraps with Avocado,
        195–97
    Roasted Red Pepper Mini
        Pizzas, 226–28
    Smoked Salmon and Kale
        Salad, 211–12
    Ultimate Bacon Burger, 172–74
"Cheesecake," Peanut Butter
        Chocolate, with Hazelnut
        Crust, 250–51
Cherry-Chocolate Smoothie, 241
chicken
    Chicken Half (for dogs), 323
    Chicken Parmesan with Mixed
        Greens, 143–45

Cornish Game Hens with
        Sautéed Green Beans,
        157–58
    Curried Chicken and Onions
        with Butter-Fried
        Parsnips, 152–54
    Lemon Kalamata Chicken
        Breasts with Caprese
        Salad, 154–56
    Mom's Homemade Chicken
        Soup, 150–52
    Mustard-Roasted Chicken
        Legs with Peach Salad,
        146–47
    Slow-Cooker Chicken with
        Roasted Broccoli and
        Mushrooms, 164–66
    Spicy Chicken Thigh Stir-Fry
        and Cauliflower Fried
        Rice, 148–50
children, Wild Diet for, 314–16
Chili, Spicy Beef, with Mashed
        Sweet Potato, 179–81
Chimichurri Steak and Roasted
        Brussels Sprouts, 183–85
Chipotle Steak and Veggie
        Fajitas with Fresh
        Guacamole, 167–69
chocolate
    Birthday Cake with Whipped
        Chocolate Topping,
        259–60
    Chocolate-Cherry Smoothie,
        241
    Choco-nut Cookies, 252
    Mint Chip Ice Cream, 261–62
    Peanut Butter Chocolate
        "Cheesecake" with
        Hazelnut Crust, 250–51
    Peanut Butter Chocolate
        Chunk Cookies, 253
Choco-nut Cookies, 252
cholesterol, 97–98, 116
Cilantro-Lime Smoothie,
        Creamy, 237
circadian rhythm, 69–70
Citrus Spa Water, 245
coconut, shredded
    Carrot Cake, 257–59
    Choco-nut Cookies, 252
coconut, young, in Lime in the
        Coconut, 247–48

coconut milk
    Butter Pecan Ice Cream, 266
    Coconut Whipped Cream,
        268–69
    Hearty Pancake Breakfast,
        228–30
    Mint Chip Ice Cream, 261–62
    Peaches 'n' Cream Smoothie,
        242
    Peanut Butter Chocolate
        "Cheesecake" with
        Hazelnut Crust, 250–51
    Pumpkin Pie, 254–55
    Spicy Chicken Thigh Stir-Fry
        and Cauliflower Fried
        Rice, 148–50
    Thai Carrot Curry Soup with
        Zucchini Chips, 224–26
Coffee, French-Pressed Fatty,
        249
Coffee Cake, Alyson's, 256–57
cookies
    Choco-nut Cookies, 252
    Peanut Butter Chocolate
        Chunk Cookies, 253
corn in processed foods, 19–20
Cornish Game Hens with
        Sautéed Green Beans,
        157–58
cravings, 15, 33, 126
cream cheese, in Nan's
        Blueberry Salad, 264–65
Creamy Cilantro-Lime
        Smoothie, 237
Creamy Roasted Vegetable Soup,
        217–19
cucumbers
    Cucumber-Basil Smoothie, 236
    Cucumber-Strawberry Spa
        Water, 244–45
    Green Juice Detox, 248
    Virgin Bloody Mary Smoothie,
        240–41
Curried Chicken and Onions
        with Butter-Fried
        Parsnips, 152–54
cyclical eating. See Fasting and
        Feasting

dairy foods
    for building muscle mass, 119
    digestibility, 119–20

dairy foods (*cont.*)
    fermented options, 120
    impediment to fat loss, 119,
        120
    secondary choices, 138
    in vegetarian diet, 313
dandelion greens, *in* Chocolate-
        Cherry Smoothie, 241
dehydration of nuts and seeds,
        269–71
desserts
    Alyson's Coffee Cake, 256–57
    Apple Cider Donuts, 255–56
    Birthday Cake with Whipped
        Chocolate Topping,
        259–60
    Butter Pecan Ice Cream, 266
    Carrot Cake, 257–59
    Choco-nut Cookies, 252
    ice cream flavor variations,
        262
    Mint Chip Ice Cream, 261–62
    Nan's Blueberry Salad, 264–65
    Old-Fashioned Apple Pie,
        262–64
    Peanut Butter Chocolate
        "Cheesecake" with
        Hazelnut Crust, 250–51
    Peanut Butter Chocolate
        Chunk Cookies, 253
    Pumpkin Bread, 267–68
    Pumpkin Pie, 254–55
Detox, Green Juice, 248
Dirty Dozen and Clean Fifteen
        produce, 301–2
dog nutrition
    Beef Supreme, 322
    Dried Beef Liver Treats, 324
    Eggshell Calcium Supplement,
        325
    fasting for dogs, 320–21,
        326
    feeding guideline, 322
    foods to avoid, 326
    Half Chicken, 323
    processed dog food, 316–18
    raw meat and bones, 318–20
    Raw Meaty Bones, 323
    Steak and Eggs, 325
Donuts, Apple Cider, 255–56
Dried Beef Liver Treats (for
        dogs), 324

drinks
    alcoholic, 340–42
    brominated vegetable oil in,
        336
    Chocolate-Cherry Smoothie,
        241
    Citrus Spa Water, 245
    Creamy Cilantro-Lime
        Smoothie, 237
    Cucumber-Basil Smoothie,
        236
    Cucumber-Strawberry Spa
        Water, 244–45
    French-Pressed Fatty Coffee,
        249
    Ginger-Lemongrass Tea, 243
    Green Juice Detox, 248
    green smoothies, 112–13,
        233–34
    Lemon Water, 246
    Lime in the Coconut, 247–48
    liquid sugar calories, 36, 310
    Minted Melon Smoothie, 235
    Peaches 'n' Cream Smoothie,
        242
    Pear, Apple, and Rosemary
        Spa Water, 246
    Rosemary-Raspberry
        Smoothie, 238
    Spiced Blueberry Smoothie,
        239–40
    staple varieties, 136
    Strawberry "Milk Shake," 239
    Virgin Bloody Mary Smoothie,
        240–41
    water, 307–10, 331

eating out, 302–3
eggs
    Eggshell Calcium Supplement
        (for dogs), 325
    Farmer's Omelets with
        Balsamic-Roasted Sweet
        Potatoes, 230–32
    Green Monster Frittata with
        Bruschetta, 213–15
    Hard-Boiled Eggs, 279
    Hot-as-the-Devil Eggs, 280–81
    label terminology, 117
    nutrients in, 116
    staple varieties, 135
    Steak and Eggs (for dogs), 325

    Sweet Potato Hash, 221–22
    in vegetarian diet, 313
environmental design, 329–32
epi-genetics, 43
erectile dysfunction, 51–52
exercise and activity
    adventure pack for, 342–46
    adventures, 329
    anabolism, 67, 78, 101
    burpees, 83
    enjoyable activities, 77, 87
    environmental design for,
        331–32
    exercise machines, 76
    fasted exercise, 66
    full-body movements, 78–79,
        84–85
    guidelines, 291–92
    high-intensity interval
        training, 81–83
    hill sprints, 82–83
    hormonal response, 76–77, 78
    human capabilities, 75–76
    injuries, 333–35
    intensity versus endurance,
        80–81
    for leanness and well-being,
        77–78
    muscle growth by women,
        47–48
    overtraining, 81
    post-workout nutrition, 67,
        106
    proper form, 79–80
    standing, 328
    to start exercise program,
        86–87
    strength workouts, 84–86
    visualization for, 333
    Wild Diet for athletes, 311–12

Fajitas, Chipotle Steak and
        Veggie, with Fresh
        Guacamole, 167–69
Farmer's Omelets with
        Balsamic-Roasted Sweet
        Potatoes, 230–32
Fasting and Feasting. *See also*
        feasts
    antiaging effect, 58–59
    benefits of cyclical eating,
        55–57

to break fast, 67
calorie restriction, 57–58, 125
delay of hunger, 60–61
energizing effect, 62–63
fasted exercise, 66
fasting for athletes, 311
fasting for dogs, 320–21, 326
fasting for women, 50, 66
feast guidelines, 288–90
foods for fasting phase, 64–65
plan and menu, 68–69
recalibration of circadian
    rhythm, 69–70
recognizing true hunger,
    61–62
skipping meals, 65
snacks, 305–6
versus standard eating
    pattern, 64
weight gain from prolonged
    fasting, 125
when to avoid fasting, 66
Fat-Burning Man podcast, 6
fat gain
    from alcohol consumption,
        341–42
    body storage sites and health
        risks, 47, 50
    from grains, 23–24
    from MSG, 30
    from prolonged fasting, 125
    role of carbohydrates, 94–95,
        102–3
fat loss. *See also* Wild Diet
        challenge
    basic premise, 13
    calorie counting, 28–29
    exercise for, 66, 77, 78–79
    fad diets, 13–14
    with high-fat diet, 96–97
    with ketogenic diet, 311
    sex differences, 46–49
    tips for, 49–52, 291
    visualization exercise for,
        332–33
    water consumption for, 307–10
    with Wild foods, 93–94
fats, dietary
    benefits, 96–97
    for cooking and eating cold,
        98–99
    omega-3s, 99–100

processed fats and oils, 26–27,
    100
saturated fat and cholesterol,
    97–98
staple varieties, 136
Fatty Coffee, French-Pressed,
    249
feasting. *See* Fasting and
    Feasting; meals
feasts
    beef, bison, and lamb, 167–90
    Beef Brisket with Balsamic
        Mustard Greens, 174–77
    Beef Taco Salad with
        Avocado (swap
        suggestion), 172
    Beef Tenderloin with
        Buttered Onions,
        Horseradish, and Arugula,
        181–83
    Bison Taco Salad with
        Avocado, 170–72
    Chimichurri Steak and
        Roasted Brussels Sprouts,
        183–85
    Chipotle Steak and Veggie
        Fajitas with Fresh
        Guacamole, 167–69
    Ginger Lamb Chops with
        Roasted Vegetables,
        186–88
    Spicy Beef Chili with
        Mashed Sweet Potato,
        179–81
    Sun-Dried Tomato Meatballs
        with Zucchini Noodles,
        188–90
    Ultimate Bacon Burger,
        172–74
    Wild Shepherd's Pie, 177–79
    chicken, pork, and bacon,
        143–66
    Bacon-Wrapped Scallops
        and Sweet Slaw, 200–202
    Chicken Parmesan with
        Mixed Greens, 143–45
    Cornish Game Hens with
        Sautéed Green Beans,
        157–58
    Curried Chicken and Onions
        with Butter-Fried
        Parsnips, 152–54

Ginger Pork Chops with
    Roasted Vegetables (swap
    suggestion), 188
Hearty Pancake Breakfast,
    228–30
Hot-as-the-Devil Eggs,
    280–81
Lemon Kalamata Chicken
    Breasts with Caprese
    Salad, 154–56
Low-and-Slow Rubbed Ribs
    with Whipped
    Cauliflower, 162–63
Mom's Homemade Chicken
    Soup, 150–52
Mustard-Roasted Chicken
    Legs with Peach Salad,
    146–47
Pulled Pork Sliders, 159–61
Slow-Cooker Chicken with
    Roasted Broccoli and
    Mushrooms, 164–66
Spicy Chicken Thigh Stir-
    Fry and Cauliflower Fried
    Rice, 148–50
Ultimate Bacon Burger,
    172–74
desserts, 250–69
    Alyson's Coffee Cake,
        256–57
    Apple Cider Donuts, 255–56
    Birthday Cake with
        Whipped Chocolate
        Topping, 259–60
    Butter Pecan Ice Cream, 266
    Carrot Cake, 257–59
    Choco-nut Cookies, 252
    ice cream flavor variations,
        262
    Mint Chip Ice Cream,
        261–62
    Nan's Blueberry Salad,
        264–65
    Old-Fashioned Apple Pie,
        262–64
    Peanut Butter Chocolate
        "Cheesecake" with
        Hazelnut Crust, 250–51
    Peanut Butter Chocolate
        Chunk Cookies, 253
    Pumpkin Bread, 267–68
    Pumpkin Pie, 254–55

feasts (*cont.*)
    for dogs, 322–25
        Beef Supreme, 322
        Dried Beef Liver Treats, 324
        Eggshell Calcium
            Supplement, 325
        Half Chicken, 323
        Raw Meaty Bones, 323
        Steak and Eggs, 325
    drinks, 233–49
        Chocolate-Cherry Smoothie,
            241
        Citrus Spa Water, 245
        Creamy Cilantro-Lime
            Smoothie, 237
        Cucumber-Basil Smoothie,
            236
        Cucumber-Strawberry Spa
            Water, 244–45
        French-Pressed Fatty
            Coffee, 249
        Ginger-Lemongrass Tea, 243
        Green Juice Detox, 248
        green smoothies, 112–13,
            233–34
        Lemon Water, 246
        Lime in the Coconut, 247–48
        Minted Melon Smoothie,
            235
        Peaches 'n' Cream
            Smoothie, 242
        Pear, Apple, and Rosemary
            Spa Water, 246
        Rosemary-Raspberry
            Smoothie, 238
        Spiced Blueberry Smoothie,
            239–40
        Strawberry "Milk Shake,"
            239
        Virgin Bloody Mary
            Smoothie, 240–41
    grains
        Brown Rice, 274–75
        Grandma's Oatmeal, 273–74
    seafood, 191–212
        Bacon-Wrapped Scallops
            and Sweet Slaw, 200–202
        Baked Pesto Salmon with
            Roasted Artichokes,
            197–200
        Fish Tacos with Mango-
            Avocado Salsa, 203–4

        King Prawns and Seared
            Garlic Zucchini Spears,
            204–6
        Lemon-Garlic Snapper,
            207–8
        Macadamia-Crusted Cod
            with Tender Greens,
            191–93
        Parmesan Shrimp Lettuce
            Wraps with Avocado,
            195–97
        Seared Ahi Tuna with
            Sesame-Ginger
            Asparagus, 193–95
        Smoked Salmon and Kale
            Salad, 211–12
        Swordfish with Spicy Peach
            Salsa, 209–10
    snacks and bites
        Hard-Boiled Eggs, 279
        Hot-as-the-Devil Eggs,
            280–81
        protein options, 305–6
        Roasted Bone Marrow, 278
        Simple Sauerkraut, 276–77
    vegetable dishes, 213–32
        Cashew Cream Alfredo with
            Zucchini Noodles, 219–20
        Creamy Roasted Vegetable
            Soup, 217–19
        Farmer's Omelets with
            Balsamic-Roasted Sweet
            Potatoes, 230–32
        Field Green Salad with
            Apples and Buttered
            Pecans, 215–17
        Green Monster Frittata with
            Bruschetta, 213–15
        Immune-Boosting Veggie-
            Full Soup, 222–24
        Roasted Red Pepper Mini
            Pizzas, 226–28
        Sweet Potato Hash, 221–22
        Thai Carrot Curry Soup with
            Zucchini Chips, 224–26
    vegetarian substitutions, 313
fermented foods
    dairy options, 120
    for healthy gut environment,
        53, 55
    Simple Sauerkraut, 276–77
    staple varieties, 136

Field Green Salad with Apples
    and Buttered Pecans,
    215–17
fish. *See* seafood
Fish Tacos with Mango-Avocado
    Salsa, 203–4
flavors, "natural," 31–32
flour from modern wheat, 16–17
flour secondary choices, 139
food as medicine, 91–92
food intolerances and
    sensitivities, 55
food labels
    deceptive marketing
        statements, 18, 27–28
    egg label terminology, 117
    on high-quality packaged
        foods, 287–88
    ingredients containing GMOs,
        22–23
    ingredients containing MSG,
        30–31
    manipulation of nutrition
        facts, 28–29, 34, 59
    pet food ingredients, 317–18
food manufacturers. *See* Big
    Food
food shopping. *See* shopping
food staples and secondary
    choices, 132–40
"free" meals, 124–27
French-Pressed Fatty Coffee,
    249
Frittata, Green Monster, with
    Bruschetta, 213–15
fruit. *See also specific types*
    daily limit for fat loss, 121
    Dirty Dozen and Clean
        Fifteen, 301–2
    to pick, 122–23
    secondary choices, 137
    sugar in, 121
fruit juice, 36

genetic factors, 43–44
Ginger Lamb Chops with
    Roasted Vegetables,
    186–88
Ginger-Lemongrass Tea, 243
Ginger-Mint Tea, 244
glycemic effect of carbohydrates,
    23–24, 60, 105–6, 121–22

GMOs (genetically modified organisms)
  Bt corn, 19–20
  commercial products containing, 21–22
  common GMO ingredients, 22–23
  highest-risk crops, 23
goat cheese, *for* Roasted Red Pepper Mini Pizzas, 226–28
grains
  Brown Rice, 274–75
  fat gain from, 23–24
  Grandma's Oatmeal, 273–74
  modern wheat and flour, 16–18
  secondary grain and flour choices, 139
  to sprout, 272–73
  sprouted and fermented, 17
grapefruit
  Citrus Spa Water, 245
  Hearty Pancake Breakfast, 228–30
Green Beans, Sautéed, Cornish Game Hens with, 157–58
Green Juice Detox, 248
greens. *See also specific types*
  Chicken Parmesan with Mixed Greens, 143–45
  Macadamia-Crusted Cod with Tender Greens, 191–93
  prioritizing in daily diet, 112
green smoothies, 112–13, 233–34
growth hormones
  age-related decline, 50, 58
  boosting through fasting and exercise, 52, 58–59, 66, 67, 68
  synthetic, in conventionally raised animals, 23, 100, 110, 114
Guacamole, Fresh, Chipotle Steak and Veggie Fajitas with, 167–69
gut bacteria, 53–55, 136

Hard-Boiled Eggs, 279
hazelnuts
  Peanut Butter Chocolate "Cheesecake" with Hazelnut Crust, 250–51

to soak and dehydrate, 269
heart disease, 97–98
Hearty Pancake Breakfast, 228–30
heirloom produce and livestock, 110–11
high blood pressure, 51–52
hill sprints, 82–83
holiday overeating, 338–40
honeydew, *in* Minted Melon Smoothie, 235
hormones. *See also* growth hormones; insulin
  cholesterol component of, 97
  effects of fasting, 57, 125
  exercise and, 76–77, 78, 81, 84–85
  fat-friendly diet and, 96
  gender differences, 47, 48, 50
  morning meals and, 60
  testosterone, 47, 50–52
Hot-as-the-Devil Eggs, 280–81
hunger
  appetite distortion from processed foods, 15–16, 33
  foods and snacks to curb, 65, 99, 306
  induced by MSG, 30–31
  from insulin spike, 60, 62, 95, 105
  to manage false hunger, 61–62
  training body to expect food, 60, 68
hydration, 307–10

ice cream
  Butter Pecan Ice Cream, 266
  flavor variations, 262
  Mint Chip Ice Cream, 261–62
illness
  antibiotic treatments, 54
  bone broth for, 337–38
  Mom's Homemade Chicken Soup for, 150–52
  pervasiveness in developed world, 11–12
  to survive, 335–37
Immune-Boosting Veggie-Full Soup, 222–24
industrial food. *See* Big Food; processed foods
injuries, to survive, 333–35

insulin
  elevation from dairy foods, 119, 120
  insulin resistance, 95–96
  spike following carbohydrate consumption, 60, 62, 105
  stabilization of, 92–93, 106
  in storage of body fat, 94–95
interval training, 77, 81–83

juice, packaged, 36
Juice Detox, Green, 248

kale
  Beef Brisket with Balsamic Kale (swap suggestion), 177
  Immune-Boosting Veggie-Full Soup, 222–24
  Macadamia-Crusted Cod with Tender Greens, 191–93
  Minted Melon Smoothie, 235
  Peaches 'n' Cream Smoothie, 242
  Rosemary-Raspberry Smoothie, 238
  Smoked Salmon and Kale Salad, 211–12
ketogenic diet, 311
King Prawns and Seared Garlic Zucchini Spears, 204–6

lactose intolerance, 119
lamb
  Ginger Lamb Chops with Roasted Vegetables, 186–88
  Wild Shepherd's Pie, 177–79
Lemon-Garlic Snapper, 207–8
Lemon Kalamata Chicken Breasts with Caprese Salad, 154–56
Lemon Water, 246
lettuce wraps
  Fish Tacos with Mango-Avocado Salsa, 203–4
  Parmesan Shrimp Lettuce Wraps with Avocado, 195–97
lifestyle. *See* Wild lifestyle
Lime in the Coconut, 247–48

Liver Treats, Dried Beef (for dogs), 324
Low-and-Slow Rubbed Ribs with Whipped Cauliflower, 162–63

macadamia nuts
  Macadamia-Crusted Cod with Tender Greens, 191–93
  Mint Chip Ice Cream, 261–62
mahimahi, *in* Fish Tacos with Mango-Avocado Salsa, 203–4
Maltz, Maxwell, 332
Mango-Avocado Salsa, Fish Tacos with, 203–4
Marrow, Roasted, 278
meals. *See also* feasts
  cyclical timing, 55–56
  Fasting and Feasting versus standard eating pattern, 64
  feast guidelines, 288–90
  "free" meals, 124–27
  holiday overeating, 338–40
  home cooking, 131–32
  at restaurants, 302–3
  sample meal plan, 294–95
  to savor, 303–5
  skipping, 65
Meatballs, Sun-Dried Tomato, with Zucchini Noodles, 188–90
meats. *See also specific types*
  from heirloom livestock, 110–11
  organs and offcuts, 115–16
  secondary choices, 137
  staple varieties, 134
  from wild or pastured versus factory-farmed animals, 113–15
Melon Smoothie, Minted, 235
men, fat loss in, 46–49, 50–52
microbiome, human, 53–54
minerals and trace elements, 107
Mint Chip Ice Cream, 261–62
Minted Melon Smoothie, 235
Mom's Homemade Chicken Soup, 150–52

mozzarella cheese
  Chicken Parmesan with Mixed Greens, 143–45
  Lemon Kalamata Chicken Breasts with Caprese Salad, 154–56
  Roasted Red Pepper Mini Pizzas, 226–28
MSG (monosodium glutamate), 30–31
muscle mass
  anabolism following workout, 67
  dairy and egg consumption for, 119
  fasting and interval workouts, 58–59
  recovery and growth during sleep, 71
  strength workouts, 77, 84–86
  visualization exercise, 332–33
  in women, 47–48
mushrooms
  Chipotle Steak and Veggie Fajitas with Fresh Guacamole, 167–69
  Farmer's Omelets with Balsamic-Roasted Sweet Potatoes, 230–32
  Immune-Boosting Veggie-Full Soup, 222–24
  Roasted Red Pepper Mini Pizzas, 226–28
  Slow-Cooker Chicken with Roasted Broccoli and Mushrooms, 164–66
Mustard Greens, Balsamic, Beef Brisket with, 174–77
Mustard-Roasted Chicken Legs with Peach Salad, 146–47

Nan's Blueberry Salad, 264–65
"natural" flavors, 31–32
90/10 rule in Wild Diet, 124
Non-GMO Project, 21, 23
noodles
  Cashew Cream Alfredo with Zucchini Noodles, 219–20
  secondary choices, 140
  Sun-Dried Tomato Meatballs with Zucchini Noodles, 188–90

nori, *in* Immune-Boosting Veggie-Full Soup, 222–24
nuts
  Baked Pesto Salmon with Roasted Artichokes, 197–200
  Brazil nuts, reproductive health and, 51
  Butter Pecan Ice Cream, 266
  Carrot Cake, 257–59
  Cashew Cream Alfredo with Zucchini Noodles, 219–20
  Choco-nut Cookies, 252
  Field Green Salad with Apples and Buttered Pecans, 215–17
  Macadamia-Crusted Cod with Tender Greens, 191–93
  Mint Chip Ice Cream, 261–62
  Nan's Blueberry Salad, 264–65
  Peanut Butter Chocolate "Cheesecake" with Hazelnut Crust, 250–51
  as snack, 120–21
  to soak and dehydrate, 269–71
  staple varieties, 135

Oatmeal, Grandma's, 273–74
oils. *See* fats, dietary
Old-Fashioned Apple Pie, 262–64
olives
  Lemon-Garlic Snapper, 207–8
  Lemon Kalamata Chicken Breasts with Caprese Salad, 154–56
  Mustard-Roasted Chicken Legs with Peach Salad, 146–47
omega-3 fats, 99–100
organically raised foods
  to avoid GMOs, 20, 21
  heritage livestock, 111
  produce choices, 301–2
  standard of quality, 110
organ meats, 115–16
overeating during holidays, 338–40

Pancake Breakfast, Hearty, 228–30

Parmesan Shrimp Lettuce
    Wraps with Avocado,
    195–97
Parsnips, Butter-Fried, Curried
    Chicken and Onions with,
    152–54
pathogenic bacteria, 53, 54
peaches
    Mustard-Roasted Chicken
        Legs with Peach Salad,
        146–47
    Peaches 'n' Cream Smoothie,
        242
    Swordfish with Spicy Peach
        Salsa, 209–10
peanuts
    allergic reaction to, 121
    Peanut Butter Chocolate
        "Cheesecake" with
        Hazelnut Crust, 250–51
    Peanut Butter Chocolate
        Chunk Cookies, 253
    to soak and dehydrate, 270
Pear, Apple, and Rosemary Spa
    Water, 246
pecans
    Butter Pecan Ice Cream, 266
    Carrot Cake, 257–59
    Field Green Salad with Apples
        and Buttered Pecans,
        215–17
    Nan's Blueberry Salad, 264–65
    to soak and dehydrate, 270
pets. *See* dog nutrition
pies
    Old-Fashioned Apple Pie,
        262–64
    Pumpkin Pie, 254–55
pineapple
    Carrot Cake, 257–59
    Creamy Cilantro-Lime
        Smoothie, 237
    Cucumber-Basil Smoothie,
        236
    Nan's Blueberry Salad, 264–65
pine nuts
    Baked Pesto Salmon with
        Roasted Artichokes,
        197–200
    to soak and dehydrate, 270
Pizzas, Roasted Red Pepper
    Mini, 226–28

pork. *See also* bacon
    Ginger Pork Chops with
        Roasted Vegetables (swap
        suggestion), 188
    Low-and-Slow Rubbed Ribs
        with Whipped
        Cauliflower, 162–63
    Pulled Pork Sliders, 159–61
Pottenger, Francis, Jr., 109
Prawns, King, and Seared Garlic
    Zucchini Spears, 204–6
probiotic bacteria, 53, 54, 55,
    103, 120
processed foods. *See also* Big
    Food
    appetite distortion from,
        15–16, 33
    beverages, 36, 336
    breads, 18–19
    corn in, 19–20
    fats and oils, 26–27, 100
    GMO ingredients, 21–23
    gut damage from, 55
    imitation meats, 313
    MSG in, 30–31
    "natural" flavors in, 31–32
    pet food, 316–18
    shelf life of, 29
    soups, 335–36
    soy products in, 25–26
    sugars in, 33–35
    wheat processing, 16–17
produce. *See* fruit; vegetables
protein
    consumption guideline, 101–2,
        290
    importance of, 48, 101
    for post-exercise nutrition, 67
    secondary supplement choices,
        138
    snacks, 305–6
    for vegetarians, 48
Pulled Pork Sliders, 159–61
Pumpkin Bread, 267–68
Pumpkin Pie, 254–55

Raspberry-Rosemary Smoothie,
    238
Raw Meaty Bones (for dogs),
    323
recipes. *See* feasts
restaurant meals, 302–3

Ribs, Low-and-Slow Rubbed,
    with Whipped
    Cauliflower, 162–63
Rice, Brown, 274–75
rice, faux, *in* Spicy Chicken
    Thigh Stir-Fry and
    Cauliflower Fried Rice,
    148–50
rice types and quality, 104
Roasted Bone Marrow, 278
Roasted Red Pepper Mini Pizzas,
    226–28
Rosemary-Raspberry Smoothie,
    238
Rosemary Spa Water, Pear,
    Apple, and, 246

salads
    Bacon-Wrapped Scallops and
        Sweet Slaw, 200–202
    Beef Tenderloin with Buttered
        Onions, Horseradish, and
        Arugula, 181–83
    Bison Taco Salad with
        Avocado, 170–72
    Creamy Chopped Slaw, *for*
        Pulled Pork Sliders, 159
    Field Green Salad with Apples
        and Buttered Pecans,
        215–17
    Lemon Kalamata Chicken
        Breasts with Caprese
        Salad, 154–56
    Mustard-Roasted Chicken
        Legs with Peach Salad,
        146–47
    Nan's Blueberry Salad,
        264–65
    Smoked Salmon and Kale
        Salad, 211–12
salmon
    Baked Pesto Salmon with
        Roasted Artichokes,
        197–200
    Smoked Salmon and Kale
        Salad, 211–12
Sauerkraut, Simple, 276–77
Scallops, Bacon-Wrapped, and
    Sweet Slaw, 200–202
seafood
    Bacon-Wrapped Scallops and
        Sweet Slaw, 200–202

seafood (*cont.*)
  Baked Pesto Salmon with
    Roasted Artichokes,
    197–200
  Fish Tacos with Mango-
    Avocado Salsa, 203–4
  King Prawns and Seared
    Garlic Zucchini Spears,
    204–6
  Lemon-Garlic Snapper, 207–8
  Macadamia-Crusted Cod with
    Tender Greens, 191–93
  Parmesan Shrimp Lettuce
    Wraps with Avocado,
    195–97
  Seared Ahi Tuna with Sesame-
    Ginger Asparagus, 193–95
  secondary choices, 137
  Smoked Salmon and Kale
    Salad, 211–12
  staple varieties, 134
  Swordfish with Spicy Peach
    Salsa, 209–10
  in vegetarian diet, 313
  whole fish, 118
  wild-caught versus farmed,
    118
seeds
  Creamy Cilantro-Lime
    Smoothie, 237
  Minted Melon Smoothie, 235
  Rosemary-Raspberry
    Smoothie, 238
  as snack, 120
  to soak and dehydrate, 270
  Spiced Blueberry Smoothie,
    239–40
  staple varieties, 135
Sesame-Ginger Asparagus,
    Seared Ahi Tuna with,
    193–95
7-minute Wild Interval Workout,
    81–83
sex differences in fat loss, 46–49
Shepherd's Pie, Wild, 177–79
shopping
  cost of high-quality foods,
    299–302
  deceptive label statements, 18,
    27–28
  Dirty Dozen and Clean Fifteen
    produce varieties, 301–2

egg label terminology, 117
ingredients containing GMOs,
    22–23
ingredients containing MSG,
    30–31
labels on high-quality
    packaged foods, 287–88
manipulated data on nutrition
    facts labels, 28–29, 34, 59
to pick produce, 122–23
real food, 287–88
secondary choices, 137–40
staple foods, 132–36
shrimp
  King Prawns and Seared
    Garlic Zucchini Spears,
    204–6
  Parmesan Shrimp Lettuce
    Wraps with Avocado,
    195–97
Simple Sauerkraut, 276–77
sleep, 69–71
Sliders, Pulled Pork, 159–61
Slow-Cooker Chicken with
    Roasted Broccoli and
    Mushrooms, 164–66
Smoked Salmon and Kale Salad,
    211–12
smoothies
  Chocolate-Cherry Smoothie,
    241
  Creamy Cilantro-Lime
    Smoothie, 237
  Cucumber-Basil Smoothie,
    236
  green smoothies, 112–13,
    233–34
  Minted Melon Smoothie, 235
  Peaches 'n' Cream Smoothie,
    242
  Rosemary-Raspberry
    Smoothie, 238
  Spiced Blueberry Smoothie,
    239–40
  Strawberry "Milk Shake,"
    239
  Virgin Bloody Mary Smoothie,
    240–41
snacks, 305–6, 314–15
Snapper, Lemon-Garlic, 207–8
soaking and dehydrating nuts
    and seeds, 269–71

soups
  bone broth or stock, 337–38
  canned soup ingredients,
    335–36
  Creamy Roasted Vegetable
    Soup, 217–19
  Immune-Boosting Veggie-Full
    Soup, 222–24
  Mom's Homemade Chicken
    Soup, 150–52
  Thai Carrot Curry Soup with
    Zucchini Chips, 224–26
soy processing, 25–26
spa waters
  Citrus Spa Water, 245
  Cucumber-Strawberry Spa
    Water, 244–45
  Lemon Water, 246
  Pear, Apple, and Rosemary
    Spa Water, 246
Spiced Blueberry Smoothie,
    239–40
Spicy Beef Chili with Mashed
    Sweet Potato, 179–81
Spicy Chicken Thigh Stir-Fry
    and Cauliflower Fried
    Rice, 148–50
Spicy Peach Salsa, Swordfish
    with, 209–10
spinach
  Beef Brisket with Balsamic
    Spinach (swap
    suggestion), 177
  Cucumber-Basil Smoothie,
    236
  Green Juice Detox, 248
  Green Monster Frittata with
    Bruschetta, 213–15
  Macadamia-Crusted Cod with
    Tender Greens, 191–93
  Wild Shepherd's Pie, 177–79
sprouted and fermented grains,
    17
starchy vegetables
  for athletes, 311
  glycemic effect, 121–22
  secondary choices, 138
Steak, Chipotle, and Veggie
    Fajitas with Fresh
    Guacamole, 167–69
Steak and Eggs (for dogs),
    325

strawberries
Beef Brisket with Balsamic
Mustard Greens, 174–77
Cucumber-Strawberry Spa
Water, 244–45
Strawberry "Milk Shake," 239
strength training, 77, 84–86
sugar
avoidance of, for fat loss, 13
in breakfast foods, 59
in food processing, 33–35
in fruit, 121
nutrient-dense and minimally
processed alternatives,
37–38, 140
support of pathogenic
bacteria, 53
transformation into body fat,
93–94
Sun-Dried Tomato Meatballs with
Zucchini Noodles, 188–90
Sun-Dried Tomato Pesto, for
Baked Pesto Salmon with
Roasted Artichokes, 198
sweeteners. See also sugar
artificial sweeteners, 37
nutrient-dense and minimally
processed options, 37–38
secondary choices, 140
sweet potatoes
Creamy Roasted Vegetable
Soup, 217–19
Farmer's Omelets with
Balsamic-Roasted Sweet
Potatoes, 230–32
Ginger Lamb Chops with
Roasted Vegetables,
186–88
Spicy Beef Chili with Mashed
Sweet Potato, 179–81
Sweet Potato "Buns," for
Pulled Pork Sliders, 159
Sweet Potato Hash, 221–22
Wild Shepherd's Pie, 177–79
Swiss Chard Salad, Smoked
Salmon and (swap
suggestion), 212
Swordfish with Spicy Peach
Salsa, 209–10

Tacos, Fish, with Mango-
Avocado Salsa, 203–4

Taco Salad, Bison, with Avocado,
170–72
tea
Ginger-Lemongrass Tea, 243
Ginger-Mint Tea, 244
testosterone, 47, 50–52
Thai Carrot Curry Soup with
Zucchini Chips, 224–26
tomatoes
Bison Taco Salad with
Avocado, 170–72
Green Monster Frittata with
Bruschetta, 213–15
Lemon-Garlic Snapper, 207–8
Lemon Kalamata Chicken
Breasts with Caprese
Salad, 154–56
Spicy Beef Chili with Mashed
Sweet Potato, 179–81
tomato sauce, for Chicken
Parmesan with Mixed
Greens, 143
Virgin Bloody Mary Smoothie,
240–41
tomatoes, sun-dried
Sun-Dried Tomato Meatballs
with Zucchini Noodles,
188–90
sun-dried tomato pesto, for
Baked Pesto Salmon with
Roasted Artichokes,
198
Tuna, Seared Ahi, with Sesame-
Ginger Asparagus, 193–95
Turkey Taco Salad with Avocado
(swap suggestion), 172

Ultimate Bacon Burger, 172–74

vegetable dishes
Cashew Cream Alfredo with
Zucchini Noodles, 219–20
Creamy Roasted Vegetable
Soup, 217–19
Farmer's Omelets with
Balsamic-Roasted Sweet
Potatoes, 230–32
Field Green Salad with Apples
and Buttered Pecans,
215–17
Green Monster Frittata with
Bruschetta, 213–15

Immune-Boosting Veggie-Full
Soup, 222–24
Roasted Red Pepper Mini
Pizzas, 226–28
Sweet Potato Hash, 221–22
Thai Carrot Curry Soup with
Zucchini Chips, 224–26
vegetables. See also specific
types
Dirty Dozen and Clean
Fifteen, 301–2
glycemic effect of starchy
vegetables, 121–22
green and non-starchy staple
varieties, 133
to pick, 122–23
secondary starchy choices, 138
starchy vegetables for athletes,
311
vegetarian and vegan diets, 48,
312–13
Virgin Bloody Mary Smoothie,
240–41
visualization exercise, 332–33
vitamins
common deficiencies, 108
in maintenance of health,
106–7
synthetic enrichment of
bleached flour, 18, 30

walnuts
Choco-nut Cookies, 252
to soak and dehydrate, 271
watercress, in Creamy Cilantro-
Lime Smoothie, 237
waters
Citrus Spa Water, 245
Cucumber-Strawberry Spa
Water, 244–45
Lemon Water, 246
Pear, Apple, and Rosemary
Spa Water, 246
pure water for hydration,
307–10, 331
wheat processing, 16–17
Whipped Cream, Coconut,
268–69
Wild Diet. See also Fasting and
Feasting
basic philosophy and
principles, 14, 44, 92–93

Wild Diet (*cont.*)
  beans and legumes,
    123
  body fat burning and storage,
    93–96
  carbohydrates, 102–6
  dairy foods, 119–20
  dietary fats, 96–100
  eggs, 116–17
  fish and seafood, 118
  "free" meals, 124–27
  fruit, 121
  greens, 112–13
  lapses, 127
  meats, 113–16
  90/10 rule, 124
  nuts and seeds, 120–21
  organic, fresh, and seasonal
    foods, 110–12
  for pets, 316–21
  protein, 101–2
  secondary food choices,
    137–40
  staple foods, 132–36
  starchy vegetables, 121–22
  variety, 107–8

vitamins, minerals, and trace
    elements, 106–7
Wild Diet challenge
  adoption of new way of eating,
    285–86
  exercise, 291–92
  feast guidelines, 288–90
  foods to avoid, 290–91
  maintenance of desired
    weight, 296
  purging pantry of low-quality
    foods, 287
  results to expect, 292–93
  sample meal plan, 294–95
  shopping, 287–88
  tips to maximize fat loss, 291
  to track progress, 286–87
Wild lifestyle
  adventure pack for support of
    healthy habits, 342–46
  connection with nature,
    327–29
  of James family, 342–43,
    347–49
  simple versus industrialized
    food, 349–50

website for resources on, 351
  in world of modern
    technology, 45
Wild Shepherd's Pie, 177–79
women
  fasting, 50, 66
  fat loss, 46–50
workouts. *See* exercise and
    activity

young coconut, *in* Lime in the
    Coconut, 247–48

zucchini
  Cashew Cream Alfredo with
    Zucchini Noodles, 219–20
  King Prawns and Seared
    Garlic Zucchini Spears,
    204–6
  Spicy Beef Chili with Mashed
    Sweet Potato, 179–81
  Sun-Dried Tomato Meatballs
    with Zucchini Noodles,
    188–90
  Thai Carrot Curry Soup with
    Zucchini Chips, 224–26